Clinical Studies
in
Culture Conflict

Edited by

Georgene Seward, Ph.D.

ASSOCIATE PROFESSOR OF PSYCHOLOGY
UNIVERSITY OF SOUTHERN CALIFORNIA

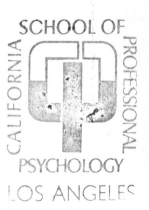

THE RONALD PRESS COMPANY • NEW YORK

Library of Congress Catalog Card Number: 58-9806
PRINTED IN THE UNITED STATES OF AMERICA

For BARBARA

"To put the whole problem on a broader base"

Foreword

Within the last two decades the description and the understanding of human behavior have been facilitated by the progressively explicit development of the theory, methods, and experiments of the sciences studying the social interaction and organization of men. In our society, the transition from the reliance upon a common sense knowledge about social man to the increasing use of the contemporary fund of information and thought developed by social scientists is in active occurrence. Moreover, as social science comes of age the task of achieving a general integrating theory about human action, embracing at least the scientific disciplines dealing with body, personality, society, and culture, must now be pursued with urgent scholarship and research.

The studies detailed in this book afford concrete and practical illustrations of how this comprehensive consideration of behavior broadens the general understanding of human conflict. Particularly for those who are engaged actively in the transactions of the many formal helping processes existing in our society, these descriptions of the social class and cultural determinants of human distress and unease provide another dimension to the ordinary ways of considering health and disease.

What is needed for most professional workers engaged in the various applications of behavioral science knowledge is not less emphasis upon psychodynamic description of individual behavior or a chronic engagement in ideological warfare in defense of a personalized and ego-involved theory. A comprehensive theoretical stance from which to view any specific behavioral event; an understanding of how society and culture get into not only the person but his body as well, and of how the body gets into person and culture; a recognition that the individual's internal reality, no matter how distorted idiosyncratically by the uniquely physiological and psychological determinants of the learning experience, is nevertheless an internalization of social and cultural reality —these are some of the basic needs of all students of human behavior for which these writings provide a palpable satisfaction.

EDWARD STAINBROOK, Ph.D, M.D.

HEAD, DEPARTMENT OF PSYCHIATRY,
UNIVERSITY OF SOUTHERN CALIFORNIA
SCHOOL OF MEDICINE, LOS ANGELES

Preface

Since the war, the closer collaboration among the various social sciences has led the clinical team of psychologist, psychiatrist, and social worker to recognize the need for a better understanding of their patients' backgrounds in the interest of more adequate diagnosis and treatment. In some progressive institutions, anthropologists have been added to the teams. In my own work with students in the clinical psychology training program at the University and the Veterans Administration, the importance of taking cultural factors into account in handling members of minority groups has been repeatedly demonstrated. An attempt to delineate some of the problems encountered was the purpose of my *Psychotherapy and Culture Conflict* (The Ronald Press, 1956), which is a textual presentation of the main psychological differentials among certain ethnic groups. But the practitioner also needs case material to bring home to him the specific ways in which culture may affect personality, thereby distorting the diagnostic picture and confounding treatment.

Diagnostic difficulties arise from a number of cultural sources. A "symptom" may not be pathological at all, but rather a benign adaptation to a malignant cultural situation, as dramatically portrayed in the "psychotic" ego splitting which made survival possible for many inmates of German concentration camps. Another example is the Negro's suspicion of Caucasians in the deep South, which in that setting more often represents realistic vigilance than paranoid delusion. At the opposite extreme, pathology may be mistaken for health. Examples of such "malignant adjustment" may be found in certain Negroes' accommodation to the subservient role forced upon them.

Diagnosis is not only a matter of behavioral meaning; it also depends on the correct interpretation of test performance. In transcultural application of psychological techniques, necessary allowances must be made for basic differences in *Weltanschauung*. An obvious illustration is the caution we have learned to use in interpreting a low IQ, which may signify either lack of ability or of opportunity according to such background differentials as bilingualism and schooling. Less familiar are the subtler subcultural shadings of responses on projective techniques.

In an effort to make socioclinical problems more concrete, I have collected in the present volume a series of case studies from professional colleagues in psychology, psychiatry, and anthropology who have had a rich experience with patients of diversified cultural origin. The present material has been restricted to conflicts associated with ethnic minority status. Such special subcultures as the homosexual, the gifted, the élite, the rustic, the aged, and innumerable others lie beyond the scope of this book. Those selected fall in essentially the same categories as in the previous volume, including the Negro, the displaced European Jew and Gentile, the American Indian, the Japanese, and, in addition, a Spanish-speaking group.

Because culture conflict problems are neither defined nor restricted by ethnic grouping, an introductory chapter with illustrations from the case studies has been included to provide a frame of reference for them. Moreover, a brief preview is presented at the beginning of each major section of the book, and an integrative "postscript" at the end.

Originally a special section dealing with that ubiquitous American phenomenon, social mobility, was planned. It was found, however, to be so intrinsic a part of all culture conflict problems that it had to be treated as a covariant with other aspects of the cases. Thus, upward mobility oriented toward better jobs and higher status was part and parcel of the struggle of the typical minority group member to find an identity within the dominant cultural stream. Downward mobility was analogously tied in with failure to achieve the desired status, or with loss of a stable frame of reference.

Since the first impact of the culture comes through the home, the earliest signs and most serious forms of conflict with it are reflected in children's problems which often become exacerbated at adolescence. To highlight the primary sources of culture conflict, cases from early developmental periods have been included. Both sexes are also represented because of the different stresses to which men and women are subjected in the various subcultures.

A wide range of psychopathology is covered by the cases making up the present volume so that cultural complications in diagnosing and treating a variety of conditions may be demonstrated. In preparing his report, each contributor was asked to follow a prescribed set of points, and to keep the length of his chapter within rather flexible limits, with the exception of one fairly complete psychoanalytic study which was given more space than the others.

With respect to diagnostic techniques, the selection was left to the discretion of each contributor, according to the demands of the particular problem under consideration. In some instances, heavy reliance is placed on informal interviewing; in those at the other extreme, extensive batteries of standard tests are used. Since this volume was designed as a manual, sample records are appended at the end of each diagnostic study. In some, the results of repeated testing are given to show changes correlated with therapy or acculturation.

Originally intended as a diagnostic manual, the chief emphasis of the book has remained diagnostic. In the majority of cases, the *result* of psychotherapy has been assessed by diagnostic instruments. In a few, the emphasis has been *procedural*, with hour-by-hour analysis of patient–therapist interaction. While the theoretical frame of reference of the therapy in most cases is psychoanalytical, broadly interpreted, the particular application varies from the briefest supportive measures to intensive depth analysis, depending on the needs of the case.

Documentation of the case studies has been uniformly omitted on the assumption that the most relevant literature has been covered in the preceding textual volume, *Psychotherapy and culture conflict.* Some further sources are referred to in the two introductory chapters.

The contributors are for the most part actively engaged in clinical practice. The majority are also identified with the field of socioclinical research through their publications. The case reports represent a multidisciplinary approach in which psychiatrist, psychologist, social worker, and, in many cases, anthropologist, have given the benefit of their specialties.

As for the patients themselves, they have been so carefully disguised with respect to names, places, dates, and other identifying marks that any resemblance to themselves aside from the nuclear features of their problems is purely coincidental. The privilege granted us of using this invaluable human material by the institutions that "cleared" it for us, is most gratefully acknowledged. The authors would also like to express their personal thanks to their assistants in preparing the individual studies. In the interest of maintaining the patients' anonymity, however, those immediately concerned with the case material must also remain anonymous.

The present volume is designed to fill the need for a case book of clinical studies in culture conflict which will serve as a diagnostic aid during training and in practice to the clinical psychologist, psychiatrist, and social worker in the handling of problems involving culture conflict.

GEORGENE SEWARD

Los Angeles, California
May, 1958

Contributors

Charlotte G. Babcock, M.D.
PROFESSOR OF PSYCHIATRY
UNIVERSITY OF PITTSBURGH SCHOOL OF MEDICINE

Gertrude Baker, Ph.D.
CLINICAL PSYCHOLOGIST
V.A. NEUROPSYCHIATRIC HOSPITAL, LOS ANGELES

Lauretta Bender, M.D.
PRINCIPAL RESEARCH SCIENTIST IN CHILD PSYCHIATRY
NEW YORK DEPARTMENT OF MENTAL HYGIENE
PROFESSOR OF CLINICAL PSYCHIATRY
NEW YORK UNIVERSITY COLLEGE OF MEDICINE

Isaac Berman, A.B.
TRAINEE, CLINICAL PSYCHOLOGY PROGRAM
UNIVERSITY OF SOUTHERN CALIFORNIA

Trent E. Bessent, Ph.D.
CHIEF PSYCHOLOGIST
METROPOLITAN STATE HOSPITAL, NORWALK, CALIFORNIA

Charlotte Buhler, Ph.D.
ASSISTANT CLINICAL PROFESSOR OF PSYCHIATRY
UNIVERSITY OF SOUTHERN CALIFORNIA SCHOOL OF MEDICINE

Aaron H. Canter, Ph.D.
CHIEF CLINICAL PSYCHOLOGIST
PHOENIX V.A. HOSPITAL AND MENTAL HYGIENE CLINIC
PSYCHOLOGICAL CONSULTANT
GOOD SHEPHERD SCHOOL FOR GIRLS, PHOENIX, ARIZONA

William A. Caudill, Ph.D.
LECTURER ON SOCIAL ANTHROPOLOGY
DEPARTMENT OF SOCIAL RELATIONS, HARVARD UNIVERSITY
RESEARCH ASSOCIATE, DEPARTMENT OF PSYCHIATRY
HARVARD MEDICAL SCHOOL

Norman L. Farberow, Ph.D.
CLINICAL PSYCHOLOGIST
V.A. MENTAL HYGIENE CLINIC, LOS ANGELES

Alan J. Glasser, Ph.D.
CHIEF PSYCHOLOGIST
REISS-DAVIS CLINIC FOR CHILD GUIDANCE, LOS ANGELES

A. William Hire, Ed.D.
CONSULTANT IN CLINICAL PSYCHOLOGY
MASSACHUSETTS MEMORIAL HOSPITAL, BOSTON
ASSOCIATE PROFESSOR OF CLINICAL PSYCHOLOGY
BOSTON UNIVERSITY GRADUATE SCHOOL AND SCHOOL OF MEDICINE

George W. Hohmann, Ph.D.
CLINICAL PSYCHOLOGIST
LONG BEACH V.A. HOSPITAL, LONG BEACH, CALIFORNIA
ASSISTANT CLINICAL PROFESSOR OF PSYCHOLOGY
UNIVERSITY OF CALIFORNIA AT LOS ANGELES

H. Elston Hooper, Ph.D.
CLINICAL PSYCHOLOGIST
LONG BEACH V.A. HOSPITAL, LONG BEACH, CALIFORNIA
DIRECTOR, PSYCHOLOGICAL SERVICE CENTER OF THE SOUTH BAY
REDONDO BEACH, CALIFORNIA

Franklin R. McDonald, Ph.D.
ASSOCIATE CLINICAL PSYCHOLOGIST IN PSYCHIATRY
PSYCHIATRIC UNIT, LOS ANGELES COUNTY GENERAL HOSPITAL

Howard E. Mitchell, Ph.D.
CHIEF PSYCHOLOGIST, CHILD GUIDANCE CLINIC
LANKENAU HOSPITAL, PHILADELPHIA
ASSOCIATE IN RESEARCH, DEPARTMENT OF PSYCHIATRY
UNIVERSITY OF PENNSYLVANIA SCHOOL OF MEDICINE

Sol Nichtern, M.D.
DEPARTMENT OF PSYCHIATRY
NEW YORK UNIVERSITY COLLEGE OF MEDICINE
PSYCHIATRIST IN CHARGE OF CHILDREN'S WARD
BELLEVUE PSYCHIATRIC HOSPITAL, NEW YORK

Leonard B. Olinger, Ph.D.
LECTURER, UNIVERSITY OF SOUTHERN CALIFORNIA
CONSULTANT, UNITED CEREBRAL PALSY FOUNDATION, LOS ANGELES

Marvin K. Opler, Ph.D.
VISITING PROFESSOR OF ANTHROPOLOGY (SOCIAL PSYCHIATRY) IN THE
DEPARTMENT OF PSYCHIATRY, CORNELL UNIVERSITY MEDICAL COL-
LEGE AND THE PAYNE WHITNEY PSYCHIATRY CLINIC, NEW YORK
HOSPITAL

Channing Orbach, A.B.
TRAINEE, V.A. CLINICAL PSYCHOLOGY PROGRAM
UNIVERSITY OF SOUTHERN CALIFORNIA

Horace M. Peak, Ph.D.
SENIOR CLINICAL PSYCHOLOGIST
PATTON STATE HOSPITAL, PATTON, CALIFORNIA

Carl H. Saxe, Ed.D.
CLINICAL PSYCHOLOGIST
V.A. NEUROPSYCHIATRIC HOSPITAL, LOS ANGELES

Georgene Seward, Ph.D.
ASSOCIATE PROFESSOR OF PSYCHOLOGY
UNIVERSITY OF SOUTHERN CALIFORNIA
PSYCHOLOGICAL CONSULTANT
U. S. VETERANS ADMINISTRATION

Edwin S. Shneidman, Ph.D.
CHIEF FOR RESEARCH, PSYCHOLOGY SERVICE
V.A. NEUROPSYCHIATRIC HOSPITAL, LOS ANGELES
RESEARCH ASSOCIATE
UNIVERSITY OF SOUTHERN CALIFORNIA

Jerome L. Singer, Ph.D.
WILLIAM ALANSON WHITE INSTITUTE OF PSYCHIATRY,
PSYCHOANALYSIS, AND PSYCHOLOGY
LECTURER AND ASSOCIATE, GUIDANCE LABORATORY
TEACHERS COLLEGE, COLUMBIA UNIVERSITY

Vita S. Sommers, Ph.D.
CLINICAL PSYCHOLOGIST
V.A. MENTAL HYGIENE CLINIC, LOS ANGELES

Contents

Part VI. New World Symphony and Discord

PART I

CULTURE AND CLINICAL PRACTICE

1

Culture-Personality Dynamics: Orientation

Georgene Seward

CULTURAL DIFFERENCES IN PSYCHODYNAMICS

CULTURE IN PERSONALITY THEORY.   Recognition of the importance of including cultural factors in personality theory-making was the great advance over earlier thinking of such pioneers as Sapir and Benedict. The next step is to go beyond description in order to show the specific ways that "culture invades physiology" and affects the developing person. The status level of the family in the social hierarchy determines the particular mode of child rearing conventionally followed (Sears, *et al.*, 1957). The scope of this early socialization also includes the more informal but probably more effective training by the age peers. From such diverse learning experiences with the specific patterns of identification they produce, there gradually emerge differences in expressive styles, ego defense systems, and moral controls (Miller and Swanson, 1956).

In *Psychotherapy and culture conflict* (Seward, 1956), an attempt was made to demonstrate in general terms some of these relationships with selected subcultures in contemporary United States. The present volume gets "down to cases," indicating specifically how this process works through the person-to-person interaction among individuals within

3

the small groups that make up their immediate environment.

The cases reported below are grouped, as the Preface indicates, according to ethnic minority, but it should be emphasized that membership in a minority per se does not constitute or define a problem. In the last analysis each problem is inevitably personal and unique.

We might have organized our cases according to the personality schema which follows and in terms of which we shall try to analyze the cases. Since, however, certain of these problems occur more commonly under certain subcultural pressures than others, it seemed useful to group them according to the more familiar ethnic categories.

IDENTIFICATION. The innermost core of personality is a feeling of identity. This may be positive, negative, or ambivalent, and each could be rated along an intensity continuum. On the identification pattern depends the individual's self concept as well as his attitude toward others. This will become increasingly evident from the variability in identification among the cases to be presented.

EXPRESSIVE STYLES. Wide cultural variability is found in the expressive styles permitted. Marked differences between Irish and Italians, for example, are even reflected in a different configuration of their respective schizophrenic symptomatology (Opler & Singer, 1956). Among our cases, we also note striking contrasts in style of impulse expression. There is the direct acting out of the Puerto Rican boys (Chapter 11), which has its counterpart at the adult level in the lower-class Puerto Rican man (Chapter 10). Such behavior is too crude, however, to be tolerated by the middle-class "companion piece" described in the same chapter. The second young man had to pay for his higher status by holding his impulses under such rigid control that their only outlet was in bizarre symbolism.

EGO DEFENSE SYSTEMS. Another way in which the social milieu affects personality is in terms of certain predilections it fosters for type of ego defense, and correlatively, for type of psychopathology on failure of the defenses to hold. We are reminded in this connection of the high incidence of certain psychophysiological reactions reported by Ruesch (1951) among lower-middle-class patients for whom status striving is especially intense. A case in point is the Filipino (Chapter 12) whose desperate struggle to "make good" against all odds was interrupted only by recurrent attacks of tuberculosis from which he was unaccountably slow to recover, despite his impatience. Somatization is more clearly a defense in the Nisei, Ichiro (Chapter 16).

Although a comprehensive, systematic survey is out of the question at this time, a few more examples from our clinical studies should at least give some inkling of the variation in styles of ego defense in relation to cultural emphases. Another of our cases, a young Jewish man (Chapter 19), experienced so much pressure from his subculture to be "an intellectual" that intellectuality became a defense, concealing and rendering ineffectual his underlying warmth and skill in interpersonal relationships.

We should also call attention to the Hopi girl (Chapter 7) who, when threatened by her own unacceptable hostilities, resorted to a culturally supported trancelike dissociative reaction. Or again, the Navajo veteran (Chapter 8) who faced the stress of paraplegia according to his stoic upbringing by denying his grief, thereby adding the paralysis of his emotions to the paralysis of his limbs.

In the cases of the Kibei young man and the Issei old man (chapters 13 and 14), a parallel may be drawn since they both leaned heavily in characteristic cultural style on suppressive defenses until their weakened egos could no longer support the crescendo of frustration to which they had been subjected and they collapsed into psychosis.

MORAL CONTROLS. Cultural differences in moral values and controls are also generously supplied in our case studies. In the Nisei who attempted suicide (Chapter 15), we see an angry woman reared in the Oriental mores requiring feminine passivity and subordination to men. Since open hostility toward her husband would have been "wrong," her only recourse was passive aggression which she expressed by a suicidal "attack" on her husband.

Differences in moral code are again conspicuous in the six-year-old Jewish boy (Chapter 18) who was thrown into serious conflict over differences in the interpretation of orthodoxy *within* his own ethnic group.

ARTICULATION PATTERNS BETWEEN SUBCULTURE AND MAIN CULTURE

When subcultural differences in personality structure are complicated by the double identities involved in minority adaptation to majority standards, we have to take account of the resulting interaction. We may distinguish several separable patterns of identification of the individuals involved, with their inner subculture and outer main culture. In general, we may start with the paradoxically sounding assumption that the more firmly an individual is embedded in his primary ingroup, the better integration he may be expected to make with the dominant culture. On the other hand, in cases where the individual has negative or ambivalent identifications, he is likely to find himself without an identity in the larger community. Basic differences in orientation may be variously combined. While certain subcultures are more susceptible to some of the identification patterns to be described, this is not a categorical *given,* but must be analyzed clinically in the individual case. The particular kind of identification so determined will serve as an important clue to diagnosis and guide to treatment. At least three patterns of sub–main cultural interaction may be distinguished.

CONGRUENCE. The first type represents a form of positive interaction characterized by a high level of resilience and based on strong identifications with the original group which are temporarily threatened from the outside by the necessity of regrouping in a new environment. In such cases the individual usually possesses sufficient ego strength and flexibility to enable him to adapt to the new culture and find secondary identities there. In certain instances, the adaptation may go to the extreme of overidentification with the new models. Sometimes the centripetal force is accelerated by an ejective push from the homeland as in the displaced European woman (Chapter 20) who was not satisfied until she had acquired the protective coloration of her adopted culture.

Among certain minorities, the adjustment to the dominant group may be on the level of certain social values and adaptive mechanisms. The individual may fit comfortably and acceptably into the pattern of life around him while basic differences in character structure, religion, and certain customs shared with others from the same subculture remain untouched. Such was the situation in which many Nisei found themselves after relocation (Caudill and De Vos, 1956). In the Nisei teacher of *English* (Chapter 16), we have a variation on this theme where acceptance and apparent adjustment were attained at great inner cost.

RESISTANCE. Where the subculture is so disfavored that the main culture constitutes a continuous threat, we may expect a healthy resistance, provided that the basic identification is firm. In minorities such as those of Mexican origin who take pride in their cultural heritage, the members have a core identity that serves as a bulwark against their difficulties in coping with the dominant group. A poignant example of ability to resist cultural attack was the little Negro boy who had been reared as white (Chapter 3). His strong white identification ironically served as a defense against the ambivalence and confusion involved in changing to the far less desirable Negro identity. In fact, he achieved a better adjustment in this extraordinarily difficult situation than many a Negro whose ego is torn from the beginning by doubt, ambivalence, and self-rejection.

AMBIVALENCE. In cases of submerged subcultures which fail to give their members a rationale for positive identification, there will be few inner resources with which to combat the unmitigated threat from without. Individuals reared in such subcultures can hardly escape ambivalence in their self concepts. This is still unfortunately true of the Negro American who, through his inevitable internalization of the prevailing negative attitudes, incorporates self-hatred into the very core of his ego. This ego split is a "fault" on which is built the precarious structure of his personality. As we have just pointed out, the Negro boy reared as white acquired this type of attitude toward himself only after he found out that he was a Negro with all its undesirable social connotations, but fortunately this had been superseded by the development of a basically strong ego.

Confusion is often added to ambivalence, as in the woman of Negro-Indian background (Chapter 6), where the differing role models introduced an added dimension to the culture conflict. At the extreme of confusion we find the person who has lost whatever identification he once had. These are people of low initial ego strength who have fought a losing battle to establish and maintain an identity. An example here would be the English war bride who lost her moorings among her Armenian in-laws.

Further complications of the kinds of culture conflict we have been discussing come from age and sex differences, each of which may be thought of as a separate subculture. In other words, the impact of a culture will be different for men and women, young and old. In the present volume, no systematic comparisons along these lines will be attempted although we have made passing reference to differences between children and adult Puerto Ricans, Negroes, and Jews, younger and older men of Japanese background, and men and women of several subcultures.

PSEUDOCULTURAL EFFECTS

The person working professionally with members of submerged groups must be sensitive not only to real effects of the surrounding culture, but he must be equally alert to certain pseudocultural influences. In other words, he needs to avoid committing what we may call the "cultural error," by which we mean attributing a phenomenon to a cultural factor when it can be better explained without recourse to culture. Culture may thus be made to "explain" too much, in flagrant violation of parsimony as well as truth.

CULTURE CONFLICT AS A DEFENSE. One way in which this danger may arise is through the patient's defensive use of cultural material. For example, he may hide behind his minority group membership in order to rationalize his failures. It is easier to accept defeat if it can be projected onto an external situation rather than to accept personal responsibility for it. The analysis of the case in which color conflict was used as a defense (Chapter 5) is a case in point. Throughout the study the patient defended himself against all failure by saying in effect, "It isn't my fault; it's because I'm a Negro." Since, as every psychologist knows, the best rationalizations have reality support, color conflict makes a good excuse especially in the case of the Negro who constantly meets serious obstacles in his effort to rise in his world. The clinician's problem is to determine when to attribute a given failure to external versus internal barriers. Unfortunately, he must still depend on his "third ear" to pick up overtones of rationalization and overdetermination. Of the greatest value is familiarity with the problems of culture conflict.

Culture conflict has sometimes been used more offensively than defensively. Devereux (1953) cites instances in which culture was consciously made a "red herring" by the patient to distract the therapist from the central problem by taking advantage of his known anthropological interest. Certain of his Indian patients overproduced cultural material in the hope of camouflaging their underlying problems, thus, in a circuitous but effective way, resisting the therapist.

DENIAL OF CULTURE CONFLICT AS A DEFENSE. At the opposite extreme are the patients—or their therapists—who defensively deny the Negro, Mexican, or other "problem," refusing to face the consequences of ethnic discrimination. Such patients symbolically identify with the dominant group, and set up for themselves aspiration levels that are unattainable under existing conditions. Although there are no clear-cut examples of this mechanism in the present volume, it is widespread among minority group members and requires careful handling on the clinician's part to bring it to light and deal with it adequately. Where there seems to be some likelihood that opportunities previously closed to a given group may soon become available, it is worth while to train qualified individuals to be ready to pioneer in the new territory (Seward, 1956).

CULTURE CONFLICT BY CHANCE. Sometimes it is not the patient who fools the therapist but the therapist who unwittingly fools himself. This may happen when he mistakenly attributes some bit of deviant behavior to cultural rather than to idiosyncratic factors. The patient may be in a situation of stress involving certain cultural features which, however, are neither necessary nor sufficient to explain his personal dilemma. In such cases, one must dig beneath the cultural façade to get at the more personal basis of the problem. The "culture conflict" in such a case may be quite accidental. To avoid the trap of this false front, the therapist must ask himself, "Would Mr. X have behaved in this way if he were *not* Japanese, Jewish, or whatever?" To determine the delicate balance between the cultural and noncultural demands continual vigilance on the part of the therapist, as in the differentiation of cultural from individual factors in the young Nisei presented in Chapter 17.

Sometimes, although the cultural factors have clearly precipitated a major conflict, as in the English war bride (Chapter 21), they are fortuitous in the sense that something else might just as well have served as a triggering mechanism under different circumstances.

CULTURE CONFLICT BETWEEN PATIENT AND CLINICIAN

ETHNIC DIFFERENCES. Culture–personality dynamics are not confined to the patient as viewed against his own background; they also involve the patient as viewed against the clinician's background. The clinician's interaction with his patient is necessarily colored by his own frame of reference in terms of which he is bound to evaluate others. As pointed out in the previous volume, ethnic factors may lead to a variety of distortions through a failure to break through the "culture barrier" to real communication in cases of differences. Even where clinician and patient share the same broad ethnic grouping, misunderstandings may develop as between a reformed Jewish therapist and his orthodox patient (Pollak, 1952). In other cases we may find paralyzing negative counter-transference arising from hostile overidentification of therapist with the patient whom he sees as liable to reinforce the unfavorable social stereotypes of his people.

SOCIAL CLASS DIFFERENCES. More subtle cultural blocks may result from social class differences between clinician and patient because of different orientations. Since therapists are mainly drawn from the middle class, they are apt to be heavily saturated with middle-class values. An example is the concept of self-help which the middle-class therapist shares with patients of similar background but which makes the working man with his "prescription set" uncomfortable in relating to the new kind of "medicine man." Patients more like himself will impress the therapist as more suitable candidates for psychotherapy and will be selected in preference to those from different backgrounds. Recent work [1] reviewed by Seward (1956) has revealed a hierarchical stratification of patient–therapist matchings, with the patients from the higher social echelons picked for the higher status therapists while those from the lower ranks were apt to be relegated to medical students. Blue-collar workers were perceived as lacking in proper motiva-

---

[1] A full account of the Yale studies appeared too late for inclusion in our discussion: A. B. Hollingshead and F. C. Redlich, *Social class and mental illness* (New York: John Wiley & Sons, Inc., 1958).

tion and insight while those from the top strata, whose backgrounds had presumably given them better information as to what to expect from the therapeutic situation, were considered better "risks."

PROFESSIONAL VERSUS LAY "CULTURES." Within the social class cleavage between clinician and patient may be distinguished what Pollak (1956) has called a "professional subculture" which differs from the lay culture surrounding it. Every profession develops its own traditions, "lingoes," and shibboleths. The psychotherapeutic professions are no exception. Until recently they have concentrated on intrapsychic conflict to the neglect of the culture that induced it. They have tended to regard events going on inside and those going on outside the patient's skin as separate and distinct entities, instead of recognizing their functional unity. They have failed to realize that a person carries his "field properties" within him and in a sense *is* his culture. Too often they have regarded as irrelevant cultural material presented by the patient which may actually be significantly self-revealing and therapeutically of greatest usefulness. Henry (1949; 1951) has demonstrated that ordinary case records are actually ethnological accounts of American life as interpreted by *our* "natives." He points out "the significance of the common-place" and indicates that the clinician's ability to understand his patient's remarks depends on his own understanding of the cultural setting in which they inhere. By ignoring the medium in which the patient lives the culturally unsophisticated therapist is likely to set up treatment goals that are irrelevant from the patient's standpoint. People asked to give up long-honored customs in the name of a new and incomprehensible treatment will not be in a position to benefit from that treatment. Such was the situation of the Mexican patients described by Saunders (1954) who could not understand the necessity for the precious privacy demanded by their Anglo doctors. To them the natural thing was for the entire family and even the wider community to participate in a member's cure.

THE THERAPEUTIC COMMUNITY. Nowhere is the dichotomy between professional and lay culture more marked than in the traditional hospital. Here we find what amounts to a caste system separating personnel from patient populations, with class stratification on either side of the caste line. Communication across the various status barriers is very difficult and seriously interferes with treatment. One investigator (Caudill, 1952) who spent two months in a mental hospital in the role of a patient observed the patient–staff split. The patients formed cliques which increased their social interactions and served an ego-sustaining, mutually supporting function, but at the same time tended to insulate them from the hospital culture as a whole. The staff, on the other hand, often made poor contact with the patients because of their ignorance of patient life.

The therapeutic community has recently won much acclaim (Jones, 1953; Stanton and Schwartz, 1954) as the solution to the communication problem in the modern hospital. Reorganization has been suggested in order to provide informal means of transmitting and receiving information between staff and patients. Ideally the patient would have the opportunity of participating in ward management and consequently of participating in his own treatment. He would be encouraged to play the active role of a responsible group member rather than those of "old chronic," "crazy," and other regressed roles. Since psychotic behavior would no longer be reinforced, it would in time become extinguished, at least on the level of immediate social interaction.

References

CAUDILL, W. A., and DE VOS, G. 1956. Achievement, culture and personality: the case of Japanese Americans. *Amer. Anthropologist*, 58, 1102-26.

CAUDILL, W., *et al.* 1952. Social structure and interaction processes on a psychiatric ward. *Amer. J. Orthopsychiat.*, 22, 314-34.

DEVEREUX, G. 1953. Cultural factors in psychoanalytic therapy. *J. Amer. Psychoanalyt. Ass.*, 1, 629-55.

HENRY, J. 1949. Cultural objectivity of the case history. *Amer. J. Ortho-psychiat.*, 19, 655-73.

——. 1951. The inner experience of culture. *Psychiat.* 14, 87-103.

JONES, M. 1953. *The therapeutic community.* New York: Basic Books, Inc.

MILLER, D., and SWANSON, G. E. 1956. The study of conflict. In M. JONES (ed.), *Nebraska symposium on motivation.* Pp. 137-79.

OPLER, M. K., and SINGER, J. L. 1956. Ethnic differences in behavior and psychopathology. *Int. J. soc. Psychiat.*, 2, 11-23.

POLLAK, O. 1952. *Social science and psychotherapy for children.* New York: Russell Sage Foundation.

——. 1956. *Integrating sociological and psychoanalytic concepts; an exploration in child psychotherapy.* New York: Russell Sage Foundation.

RUESCH, J., *et al.* 1946. Chronic disease and psychological invalidism. *Psychosom. Med. Monogr.*, p. 191.

SAUNDERS, L. 1954. *Cultural difference and medical care.* New York: Russell Sage Foundation.

SEARS, R. R., MACCOBY, ELEANOR E., and LEVIN, H. 1957. *Patterns of child rearing.* Evanston, Ill.: Row, Peterson & Co.

SEWARD, GEORGENE. 1956. *Psychotherapy and culture conflict.* New York: The Ronald Press Co.

STANTON, A. H., and SCHWARTZ, M. S. 1954. *The mental hospital.* New York: Library of Behavioral Science.

2

Psychodiagnosis Across the Culture Barrier

Gertrude Baker

RELATION OF TESTS TO BACKGROUND

THE CASE HISTORY AS A METHOD OF SCIENCE. Only very limited data on the relationship of cultural background to psychodiagnosis are available to the clinician. In diagnosing the culturally distant patient probably the most common procedure is to rely heavily on intensive study of the individual case, combining inferences from tests with whatever knowledge is available about the particular background. While this is often an uncertain procedure, it is nevertheless a necessary approach to the development of a broad understanding of personality and psychopathology.

Individual case study has as important a place in scientific investigation as any other approach, a position which has been taken by Henry A. Murray (1947; 1955), who said,

. . . as the science of man becomes more truly scientific, more psychologists will devote more time . . . to the careful analysis of critical events in the lives of the objects whose behavior it is their function to interpret and predict. (1955, p. 11)

In no case study is there more opportunity to observe variability and uniqueness than in that of individuals subjected to cross-cultural stress. From close perusal of such histories, knowledge and deeper insight into all cultures is not only enhanced, but also a better separation of those factors in personality that are culturally rather than biologically determined becomes possible.

THE FOCUS FOR CLINICAL STUDY. The ways in which an individual resembles or differs from members of his culture are, of course, of clinical significance because of their implications concerning his social adaptation. In the clinical study of members of different cultures it is wise to keep in mind that the main focus is on the individual and not on his culture, although the cultural context in which the individual is found needs to be understood in order to assess whether the adjustment is adaptive or otherwise (Seward, 1956).

The individual's history alone often leads to valid diagnostic conclusions, particularly if the history is complete enough and extended sufficiently in time. Psychodiagnostic tests also, without the supplementary facts from the case history, can lead to valid diagnostic conclusions. However, the superiority of the integration of case history material with diagnostic test data over the use of either alone is something that few clinical psychologists would dispute. In the area of culture conflict, to attempt analysis of diagnostic test findings without a knowledge not only of the history but of the cultural setting from which the individual comes and in which he finds himself at the time of testing is to invite serious error. In no field is the exercise of "blind" test interpretation more inappropriate (Hallowell, 1956; Klopfer, 1954).

COMPLEXITY OF VARIABLES. Many interdependent factors influence the data of the test protocols. Among these, to name the more obvious ones, are the culture or subculture itself, the social stratification within the particular culture, the dynamics of the individual's relationship with his family and his present environment. Separating the various effects of these influences from one another is very difficult, if not impossible, because of the complicated interaction among the variables. The case history may be of considerable help in assessing the interaction, although it may itself be distorted by a succession of biases inasmuch as it must be obtained by someone from someone about someone.

The factors of constantly changing cultural, social, and economic relationships such as are found in complex, heterogeneous societies like our own complicate the task of the clinician and add to the necessity for close attention to individual events. A striking illustration is afforded by the Negro, whose pathology often is determined by his reaction to social issues (Odum, 1954).

THEORETICAL LIMITATIONS

GAPS IN PERSONALITY THEORY.   It is seldom easier to state what we do not know than what we do know, but it is sometimes more profitable to try, especially when little in the way of factual data is available. It might be well to begin with the problem of personality in our culture. Psychological scientists stress the need for personality theory in terms of which to construct studies of personality. In the field of projective techniques they ask for perceptual theory. Anthropologists have repeatedly warned psychologists and psychiatrists that theories of personality, and notably psychoanalytic theory as developed by Freud, may not prove adequate when applied cross-culturally. Thus, what we "know" about one culture may be true only for that culture, and it may be true only for a given time span during which that culture did not change. And if any sampling biases occurred in the collecting of the data that contributed to the development of the theory, caution would have to be exercised in applying the theory to other samples from the same culture.

INADEQUACY OF NORMATIVE DATA.   We do not have any large-scale, stratified, systematic studies of normal subjects of the American population using projective techniques. In spite of this fact, projective techniques are among the most widely used instruments in clinical studies, and they are also the most frequently approved instruments for personality studies of normal individuals in other cultures. In a recent book, Hallowell (1956) gives his argument for the use of the Rorschach as the most culture-free of the techniques now available for personality study. Presented with close attention to existing personality and perceptual theory, it is integrated with his own and others' experience in the cross-cultural application of the method. Most of the existing Rorschach samples of individuals from cultures other than our own are relatively small, and the incidence of abnormal individuals within the samples is even smaller. So far we have learned very little about the clinical or abnormal case in those cultures differing most significantly from our own—the preliterate societies (Demerath, 1955).

Another significant gap in our test knowledge concerns the effect of social class affiliation upon responses to tests other than the projective techniques. Although it has frequently been demonstrated that such affiliation affects test responses (Auld, 1952), it is still not customary to provide separate norms based on large samples of each of the social classes for the personality and intelligence tests in common use. Perhaps this omission is due to a need to adhere wishfully to the fictional ideal that America is a land without social inequalities. It would be more truly idealistic—as well as realistic—to determine exactly where, how, and why the American ideal breaks down, in order to correct the existing deficiencies. That deficiencies exist can hardly be concealed at the clinical level, and perhaps it is the obligation of the clinical psychologist in particular to demand the sort of test norms that are clinically and socially meaningful.

THE CLINICIAN'S DILEMMA

If the above analysis of the situation is correct, the clinician's position begins to look pretty uncomfortable. He is frequently called upon to evaluate the degree and nature of psychological disturbance in individuals of his own culture, and in so doing he relies much more upon his knowledge of pathology than upon any systematic knowledge of how the "well" person looks on psychological tests. He is much more rarely called upon to evaluate the degree of disturbance in an individual from a culture widely different from his own. When such occasion arises, he has available only scattered information about the test findings on small samples of that individual's culture, and he probably has no clinical studies on either a group or individual basis for that culture. For the subcultures within his own culture, information is sporadic at best, and because of differences in populations and methodology it often seems to be contradictory.

How then should the psychodiagnostician proceed when confronted with a patient from a divergent culture? In the literature many warnings can be found regarding the possibilities for making errors, but the solutions appear to lie in the future. Obeying the exhortation that theory precedes any systematic study, the clinician would do well to consider Hallowell's carefully thought-out personality theory which emphasizes the long-neglected cultural differences. To state this theory briefly, Hallowell (1956) contends that personality organization will vary with the requirements of the particular culture because what the subject experiences and learns in his own environmental setting is what shapes the structure of his personality. From this it follows that members of a stable group exposed to the same influences should resemble each other more closely than members of another group having different social institutions and value systems.

PRACTICAL APPLICATIONS

Now how does Hallowell's personality theory assist the clinician when he is confronted with a subject from a particular cultural group differing from the one or ones the clinician has worked with in developing his personal "norms" for abnormal behavior? Should he first look up the group norms for the subject's culture, if any are available? Certainly it will be of some help to determine just how much the subject resembles or deviates from the "average" for his culture. If he deviates, does this mean he is clinically abnormal—psychotic, for instance? Not necessarily, for deviation from the average does not always imply illness; it could imply superiority in adjustment, or perhaps a special creative nonconformity.

As stated earlier, the accepted clinical approach focuses on the individual, with due consideration for the various nuances of his environment. Although Hallowell designed his theory to account for personality differences between *cultures,* there is no reason why it is not just as applicable to the clinical case study approach, nor why clinical test data should not be as useful in the verification of the theory as any other data.

Looking back a few paragraphs at the somewhat incomplete treatment of the subject of gaps in the clinician's knowledge, it can now be seen that if, in the years since psychological tests have been available, psychologists had proceeded somewhat more systematically in the acquisition of test data, using a broad cultural theory like Hallowell's as a guide, those gaps might have been filled.

SELECTION OF TESTS

Somewhere in this discussion must come the difficult question of what techniques can be used to enrich the immediate understanding of the patient who belongs to some unfamiliar culture or subculture. Should the clinician proceed under the assumption that test signs for any really serious pathology will appear the same from one culture to the next? As indicated above, this question has not yet been answered satisfactorily by any large-scale studies, and those who have considered this problem point up some of the dangers of drawing too ready conclusions.

However, since the goal is to understand the individual subject, usually in the absence of adequate criteria by which to evaluate degree of sickness and health for one of his culture, perhaps the safest approach for the clinician is to proceed with the diagnostic instruments he best understands.

RORSCHACH TECHNIQUE

TRANSCULTURAL. Hallowell (1956) would be strongly in favor of the use of the Rorschach in testing the patient with an unusual cultural problem because he believes it is the technique most free from culturally determined stimuli. It is perhaps well that the recommendation for the use of the Rorschach in the study of culture comes from an anthropologist, for a clinical psychologist might be accused of bias! Recently reported work which, though not concerned with pathology, is pertinent here is that of Kaplan (1955) and of Kaplan *et al.* (1956). These investigators found evidence to support the Hallowell personality hypothesis, while at the same time noting wide individual variability within relatively "pure" cultural groups (Indian and Mormon). This variability appeared to increase in those members most exposed to cross-cultural influences (veterans). These findings suggest that the clinician cannot expect close conformity to a modal cultural pattern when dealing with the single case. Nevertheless, it does not follow that he is justified in ignoring the patient's culture. The prediction of behavior in the form of observable acts is a more difficult process than making statements simply about personality organization. Behavior is always a consequence of the interaction of the individual with some aspect of his environment, and it is necessary to be able to anticipate what the environment will be like before attempting predictions about how an individual with a given personality organization will act.

Klopfer [1] points out that when established patterns of behavior for the individual's culture are known and the modal personality organization for the culture is also known, it is much easier to anticipate what kind of behavior to expect from an individual. When information in a given case includes a knowledge of the modal personality organization for the culture, of the sort of behavioral expression sanc-

---

[1] B. Klopfer. Personal communication to the author.

tioned by the culture, and of clinical data revealing how the subject differs from or conforms to the mode, it is often possible to anticipate areas in which difficulties will occur or other areas in which the individual will be able to function successfully. It should be kept in mind, however, that in the individual case environment will not necessarily conform to the mode for the culture. Furthermore, as a society becomes more complicated, environment also becomes more variable, making the kinds of situations to which the individual will be exposed less predictable and rendering behavior also less predictable.

An understanding of the individual's cultural background is essential for a valid use of the Rorschach inasmuch as the indefiniteness of the blots invites the projection of a wide variety of objects and symbols. The need for an extensive knowledge of the practical and symbolic significance of the majority of animate and inanimate objects for each particular culture has been emphasized by many writers, and in the case of the Rorschach this is particularly true for animals because of the very high incidence of animal responses (Klopfer and Kelley, 1942; Hallowell, 1955, 1956; Henry, 1941; Goldfarb, 1945). The habits of animals unknown to the clinician and the culturally stereotyped attitudes toward particular animals need to be known.

SUBCULTURAL. Applied to American culture, nothing more academic is required for the interpretation of animal responses, to continue our example, than a memory of nursery rhymes, visits to the zoo or farm, and an occasional trip to the movies or viewing of TV to keep up with the latest role in which Mickey Mouse and his fellows are being cast. It is just as well to keep in mind, however, that the stereotypes change with the times and that one needs to keep up with the "new look" in nursery tales.

Once the stereotype is learned, however, it is unsafe to cease exploration of meaning, for the meaning that is private for the individual needs to be determined, and its importance increases as the individual deviates from the norm. Some items will be far more affect-laden for either the individual or for the culture or subculture, and such items have great projective value. An example is that well-known domestic animal, the pig, which symbolizes a great variety of private and cultural values. To name only a few: he can be a sign of plenty to the southern share-cropper—an emblem of the only time meat is found on the table—whereas to an educated New England city dweller the appearance of a pig in his protocol may represent conflict over what he regards as his "baser instincts." To the Jew the pig could be a symbol of his guilt over failure to live up to the religious dietary prohibitions of his fathers. An occasional psychologist might even project the pig as a symbol of intelligence, knowing that this is one of the more "brainy" of laboratory animals, whereas to the row-crop farmer the pig may be a psychopath who respects neither fences nor ditches. Thus, many are the variations from the narrow stereotype of the pig as a derogatory symbol.

The fairly common practice of having the subject free-associate to the response is of value in getting at individual meanings. Unsophisticated subjects, however, especially those with subcultural backgrounds, may find this awkward or difficult, and it is often better to determine the subject's experience with the animal or object by more or less indirect inquiry. For example, when a young man gave the response to Card VI, "This is the skin off a lamb that did not have the displeasure of being deprived of his tail," the examiner observed, "I see you are aware that lambs are born with long tails." The patient replied, "Oh yes, I used to cut the little fellows' tails off." This informal conversation led to some very significant reminiscences about his early life.

SUPRACULTURAL.   Aside from the objects and symbols of specific cultural significance which appear as manifest Rorschach content, there are certain supracultural indices of health or pathology which hold in any culture. Ego organization, reality contact, affective disturbances, and conflict, indicate how well the individual is adjusting to whatever demands his culture is making upon him. The capacity to cope with the environment in order to survive is a human requirement that is not bounded by any culture. But, of course, the environment has to be understood in order to assess the individual's adjustment to it. If the subject lives in a simple homogeneous culture, he may not need to show signs of a strong ego in order to exist there in a relatively healthy state, but such an individual is surely headed for trouble if he migrates to a more complicated and demanding environment, for migration of this sort frequently places a severe strain on even a good ego.

Klopfer (1954) regards "form-level" and certain indications of ego defense as the best signs of ego strength, and Beck (1946) employs the score, "F+," as his corresponding index. Thus, attention to reasonable accuracy of fit of the concept to the chosen blot area seems to be a sign of an ego that pays attention to reality considerations that should be applicable to all individuals irrespective of cultural affiliation. This does seem to be the case in the studies that have been reported for adults. For the clinic patient, this means that extreme fluctuations in form-level or poor form perception indicate difficulties in ego mastery regardless of the cultural group to which the patient belongs.

Examination of the literature reviewed by Hallowell (1955; 1956) leads to the suggestion that perhaps the areas that create the most perplexity in transcultural application of the Rorschach are those of affect and interpersonal relations. The problem here seems to lie in determining what levels and kinds of affect and what sorts of interpersonal relations conform to cultural expectation. It is of the utmost importance to know the whole context in which the patient is found before evaluating his test responses in terms of pathology.

With respect to conflict, its amount and nature depend on the kinds of pressures exerted by a particular culture on its members. Signs of conflict appear most persistently in the protocols of individuals constantly exposed to cross-cultural stresses as Goldfarb (1951) has pointed out in relation to the Negro American. The Negro-Indian half-breed presented in the present volume (Chapter 6) is an excellent example of the same thing. This poor woman revealed in her Rorschach the severe conflict that was clinically observable in her behavior. It was manifested in the "splitting" and "tearing" attributed to the blots, in crude color responses, in anxiety reactions to shading, and the generally depressive content throughout, as in her perception on Card VIII of "two drops of water leaking through the earth into somebody's casket."

A more thorough understanding of the problems related to affect, interpersonal relations, and conflict depends on the development of more precise approaches to the evaluation of Rorschach responses, as exemplified by De Vos' (1952) system for quantifying affective responses, based on his recent study of the Japanese.

THEMATIC TESTS

TAT. Hallowell (1955; 1956) feels that picture-thematic tests can be applied to many cultural groups, although when used in preliterate societies, they may present more difficulties than the Rorschach. A discussion of the many modifications of the Thematic Apperception Test (TAT) (Murray, 1943) is beyond the scope of this chapter. As with the Rorschach, interpretation of thematic tests needs to be made with greater caution and with more attention to value systems of the particular culture as cultural distance gets greater.

Interpersonal conflicts and feelings about social status often come out clearly. An example from this volume is the psychoneurotic young adult Nisei (Chapter 16), the eldest son of Japanese parents, whose conflict over his cultural mixture led to his disidentification with Japanese culture. In his story to TAT Card 7BM, which he entitled "Youth and Age," there is no need to resort to "clinical intuition" to discover this conflict:

. . . There is a chasm between them because of their different backgrounds and education. There have not been violent outbursts, but rather a series of disagreements extending over many years. However, as the son grows up he learns that underlying their many disagreements is love. His reactions to his father have been magnified and distorted. . . .

MAPS. Deprived individuals who come from lower social classes frequently are so concrete that they have a difficult time applying imagination to pictures. The result is a description of the scene rather than a story. Even mere description, however, frequently reveals clearly how the subject views his environment. For the concrete individual, the Make A Picture Story Test (MAPS) (Shneidman, 1951) is particularly desirable, since he is presented with materials he can manipulate, and the emphasis is directed toward the somewhat more concrete problem of setting up a situation rather than toward the perhaps more threatening suggestion that he use his imagination to make up a story.

Regardless of the concreteness of the individual, the manner in which he undertakes the responsibility for organizing his own social scene can be extremely revealing from the standpoint of determining the nature of his interpersonal relations and his identifications. This is well exemplified below in the psychotic Mexican-American youth (Chapter 9). This patient's figure selections are indicative of a dichotomous attempt at identification, with failure to identify realistically with his own social class. All his ego-ideal identifications were with Americans of a higher status than himself; that is, the heroes of his stories were middle-class non-Mexican Americans. Individuals belonging to minority groups were chosen for the role of villain and placed well below himself in social status. For example, in the *Street Scene* a colored female figure is "a B-girl going into the tavern"; a colored male figure is "a wino"; another minority group figure is "a jitterbug," and a Mexican figure is "a pachuco."

THEMATIC VARIATIONS. The thematic technique has been adapted for use with different cultural groups, e.g., for Negroes (Thompson, 1949) and Indians (Henry, 1947). For children, the chief forms are the Michigan Picture Test

(Hartwell *et al.*, 1953) and the Children's Apperception Test (CAT) based on animal pictures (Bellak, 1954). The CAT proved very helpful in revealing the manifest content of an orthodox Jewish boy's conflicts reported in the present volume (Chapter 18).

In general, the great value of all the thematic techniques is obtaining in the subject's own words his reactions to social situations and environmental settings. The greater the cultural distance between subject and examiner, the more necessary it is to obtain the subject's own statement regarding these factors.

COMPLETION TECHNIQUES

SENTENCES.   While sentence completion techniques might be of limited applicability in the testing of preliterate subjects in their native environments, such instruments can be applied orally regardless of whether the subject reads or writes. Like thematic tests, they give the subject's own verbalizations about a great variety of relationships, such as cultural differences in attitude towards sex, obligations of males and females in their cultural roles, sources of anxiety, needs, and so on. For example, in our case of color conflict in an ambitious, psychoneurotic young Negro (Chapter 5), areas of difficulty come out readily: *Charlie was happiest when:* he was busy; *My greatest fear is:* poverty; *When told to keep his place, Henry:* moved; *John thought his future:* looked black.

FABLES.   A number of variations of the completion technique are available for different age groups. For younger children the Despert-Fine Fables (Fine, 1948) is very effective in eliciting projections.

DRAWING TESTS

FIGURE DRAWINGS.   While it might be expected that freehand drawings would be a culture-free medium and consequently very useful as a clinical technique, in the writer's experience, data of this kind are often confusing and become more confusing as cultural distance increases. We know that art forms vary greatly from culture to culture, and who is to judge what is bizarre? [2] Despite these difficulties, the clinician may often "spot" signs of culture conflict in such tests as the Draw-A-Person (DAP) (Machover, 1948). The little boy referred to above in connection with the CAT drew a person rich in the symbolism of the religion which was causing him so much conflict. Variations of the free-drawing technique such as the House-Tree-Person (HTP) (Buck, 1948) also offer possibilities of cross-cultural application.

BENDER GESTALT. Drawings that are copied, such as the Bender Gestalt (Pascal & Suttell, 1951), may be somewhat more useful clinically, but preliterate adults and children sometimes take liberties, such as rotating figures if it seems easier to reproduce the drawing at a different angle. Unless visual-motor difficulties are extreme, the productions are very difficult to evaluate. Allowance often needs to be made for inexperience in using a pencil. In the case of sophisticated subjects belonging to slightly different cultural backgrounds, evaluation appears to conform to usual clinical practice. An example of the usefulness of the Bender Gestalt drawings to rule out organic visual-motor impairment occurs in the aging schizophrenic Issei (Chapter 14). Since the *Gestalten* were well reproduced, the disturbance in body image revealed by the Draw-A-Person probably can be safely attributed to his schizophrenia.

NEWER PROJECTIVE DEVICES

The need to learn about the individual's point of view—how he sees the world and regards its objects and what his feelings are—has been stressed here. A method intended for this purpose and designed for cross-cultural use is Hanfmann and Getzels' (1955) Episodes Test, which they adapted from Sargent's (1953) Test of Psychological Insight. The subject is offered a description of an interpersonal situ-

---

[2] See Linton (1955) for drawings.

ation and asked to predict the developments and outcome. One advantage of the method is that the subject is not asked about his own actions but about what someone else might do. By directing attention away from the self, defensiveness is reduced.

Another intriguing method is the Make Believe Questions adapted by Farberow and Shneidman from Sarbin's (1955) role theory, and demonstrated below in their Nisei suicidal woman (Chapter 15). Although in this technique, the response is given in the first person, the "make believe" character of the task presumably reduces the guardedness of the subject, and yields revealing dynamic data.

Other techniques that appear promising from the standpoint of personality study and afford considerable freedom for expression of cultural differences are the Horn-Hellersberg Test (1950), Buhler's World Test (1951), and Lowenfeld's Mosaic Test (1954).

WECHSLER INTELLIGENCE SCALES

Even intelligence tests, particularly those administered individually, can be employed quite profitably in many cases, provided that qualitative as well as quantitative analyses are included. For example, tests like the Wechsler Scales (1944, 1949, 1955) that are quite culture-bound and therefore of very limited value in determining an alien subject's potential ability can reveal better than almost any other instruments what the subject is faced with in adapting to like situations in the new culture.

SUBCULTURAL INTERPRETATIONS.   In the case of the transplanted subject, the intelligence test that is well standardized for the new environment is often very useful in pointing out which deficits are significantly related to external reality factors, as opposed to internal conflicts. For example, when the cause of a very low arithmetic score is explored, it might be discovered that an apparently "neurotic" anxiety and insecurity about accepting a particular job had been due to the subject's realistic concern over some expected arithmetical requirements for the position, since his schooling had been so limited that he did not learn the rules for working arithmetic problems. In such a case, a course in basic arithmetic might turn out to be the best "therapeutic" recommendation arising from diagnostic testing. Many times such subjects are unaware of the availability of the opportunity and the ease of overcoming such deficits, which they frequently have more or less internalized as part of a negative self concept.

Verbal abstraction tests in which the subject is asked how two things are alike give information about the quality of his thinking, whether or not he is able to reach an abstract level, provided, of course, that he is familiar with the objects for which the likeness is to be stated. To evaluate the response, however, it would not be enough to know that the subject is familiar with the object. Both the significance of the object in the culture or subculture and to the subject as an individual should be known. To the average American who has never known real want, an orange and a banana may be alike because they are both fruit. But the fact that both are edible may seem the more important likeness to the man who spent his childhood during the depression in the "dust bowl" area of the Southwest or to the deprived Negro whose dreams of a better life include "a roof that doesn't leak" and "something to eat every day" (Sutherland, 1942).

Giving a concrete reply in cases of this kind does not necessarily imply a real defect in the ability to assume an abstract attitude, such as might be due to low intelligence or brain damage. But a knowledge of the subject's background is part of the additional information needed to evaluate whether the reply constitutes a serious defect in capacity to perceive abstract relationships or whether it constitutes a concrete initial approach to any new situation that comes from having faced the hard realities of a deprived existence. Sometimes both factors are present, and such cases are, of course, the ones that give the most trouble diagnostically.

APPLICATIONS. An example of the practical application of Wechsler-Bellevue (Wechsler, 1944) test findings is perhaps in place here. While working in the New York area, the writer noted that Negroes from the rural South, who had had very poor schooling, gave on two forms of the Wechsler test a high frequency of scores on the Comprehension and Picture Completion subtests that were well above the mean for the remainder of their subtest scores. Southern rural poor whites with limited schooling also tended to do exceptionally well on Picture Completion, but scored more nearly around their mean on Comprehension. In contrast to these, native Puerto Ricans tested in a similar setting frequently scored below their mean on Comprehension and functioned erratically on Picture Completion. No statistics are available for these impressions, but discussion with other clinicians indicated that they had made similar observations.

The differences noted can imply certain cultural differences: In the case of the uneducated but alert farmer, whether white or colored, the high Picture Completion could denote reliance upon keen observation in order to cope with his particular environment. Weather and crop conditions are often unpredictable, and he has to be alert to signs of change and to meet emergencies.

The Negro farmer or sharecropper, unlike the white, has the additional need to watch his step socially very closely, to be aware of regulations, and to pay keen attention to the values of others in order to conform and keep out of trouble. Hence, perhaps, the elevated Comprehension score.

The Puerto Ricans who gave the most erratic performances and the significantly low Comprehension scores were mostly from poverty-ridden districts comparable to slums, where as children they grew up with little supervision. Their test results reflected not only their deprived backgrounds and bilingual handicaps, but also a lack of motivation to achieve on the tests that is a rare finding in the more competitive American culture. A nonpsychotic Puerto Rican might appear "impaired" in his intellectual functioning on the tests in somewhat the same way as a regressed but not bizarre psychotic from the American culture would appear. For this reason, the psychiatric status of these individuals was often very difficult to evaluate. The unpredictable performance of José, a ten-year-old schizophrenic Puerto Rican boy, reported below (Chapter 11), is a good illustration of the difficulty encountered in making a clinical evaluation of one of his culture. In schizophrenia, an erratic, unpredictable test performance is common; however, the authors note, "His poorest performances occurred on tests which were weighted with everyday meaning appropriate to American culture." It is difficult to determine how much of the deficit might be attributable to schizophrenia and how much to the inappropriateness of the test for one of his culture.

IMPLICATIONS. These intelligence test findings probably are not without their implications for adjustment. For example, in the case of the Puerto Ricans, the lack of motivation that often resulted in failure to make a good showing on the tests, while perhaps representing a good adaptation to an environment that would yield little in return even if one were ambitious, could lead to serious difficulties in competing in the United States labor market. The subject might become very disturbed and baffled by rejections for behavior that to him seemed perfectly normal. His relatively poor understanding of social comprehension items peculiar to the northern culture could create an unfavorable impression about his character and lead to unfavorable reactions from members of the new culture, thus increasing his stress.

On the other hand, the southern Negro farm boy who moves to the city and shows alertness and awareness of the social requirements of his society might be expected to compete rather well in spite of poor education and thus to adapt with less emotional upheaval.

Another example of how the problem of cultural affiliation complicates the problem of test interpretation is afforded in this volume by the delinquent, adolescent Hopi girl (Chapter 7). Her Wechsler Performance I.Q. is 21 points higher than her Verbal I.Q. Better performance ratings are common in cases of acting-out sociopathic personalities, in whom the motor development often exceeds the development in verbal comprehension. Here, however, where the girl's cultural and educational background would be likely to lead to a deficit in the kind of information required on the verbal scale, it would not be valid to attach the same significance to her poor verbal rating as if she belonged to a group comparable to that on which the test was standardized.

CULTURE-FREE TESTS OF INTELLIGENCE

Space does not permit a thorough treatment of the use of intelligence tests for cross-cultural problems; [2] however, the applicability of an easily administered nonverbal technique like the Porteus Maze Test should be noted (Porteus, 1950). Porteus claims that this test is a good measure of both intelligence and planning ability, and it does not require literacy. He reports its successful application to American Indians and Australian Bushmen. In his opinion, the test was fair to these subjects, since some of them did better than American whites. Among the nonverbal tests of general intelligence that are well adapted for cross-cultural use, the Raven Progressive Matrices (PM) (Raven, 1947) is becoming increasingly popular for all ages.

In an attempt to get away from the middle-class loadings of the other verbal tests, Davis and Eells (Eells *et al.*, 1951) have constructed a new scale, the Davis-Eells Games, presumably free from social class bias. It is still too early to evaluate its usefulness.

CONCLUSION

The aim of this chapter has not been to supply an exhaustive inventory of tests suitable for use in assessing ethnic differences and conflict, but merely to describe certain types of techniques available, and to note some of the indications for their applicability.

---

[2] Work on the Negro has been recently summarized in Audrey Shuey, *The testing of Negro intelligence* (Lynchburg, Va.: J. P. Bell & Co., 1958).

As psychologists become more conscious of the need for culture-free techniques in ideal clinical practice, and more cognizant of the limitations of culture-bound methods no matter how rigorously standardized on middle-class citizens, undoubtedly progress will be made through the development of tests such as those discussed above. The use of local norms, particularly in the case of achievement tests, has become an approved practice. In the field of personality study those techniques that afford the broadest possible expression of individual differences will yield the most accurate and complete picture of the individual subject. Once this picture is obtained, it should be possible to compare it with norms established for the particular technique not only on the well but also on the sick of the subject's own cultural group. According to Opler and Singer (1956), the clinician needs to be alerted to "distinctive cultural patternings in illness processes."

References

AULD, F. 1952. Influence of social class on personality test responses. *Psychol. Bull.*, 49, 318-32.

BECK, S. J. 1946. *Rorschach's test.* New York: Grune & Stratton, Inc.

BELLAK, L. 1954. *The TAT and CAT in clinical use.* New York: Grune & Stratton, Inc.

BUCK, J. N. 1948. The H-T-P test. *J. clin. Psychol.*, 4, 151-59.

BUHLER, CHARLOTTE, KELLY, GAIL, and CARROL, HELEN. 1951. World Test standardization studies. *J. child Psychiat.*, 2 (Sect. 1).

DEMERATH, N. J. 1955. Schizophrenia among primitives. In A. M. ROSE (ed.), *Mental health and mental disorder: a sociological approach.* New York: W. W. Norton & Co., Inc. Pp. 215-22.

DE VOS, G. 1952. A qualitative approach to affective symbolism in Rorschach responses. *J. proj. Tech.*, 16, 133-50.

EELLS, K., DAVIS, A., HAVIGHURST, R. J., HERRICK, V. E., and TYLER, R. W. 1951. *Intelligence and cultural differences: a study of cultural learning and problem solving.* Chicago: University of Chicago Press.

FINE, R. 1948. Use of the Despert Fables (revised form) in diagnostic work with children. *Rorschach res. Exch.*, 12, 106-18.

GOLDFARB, W. 1945. The animal symbol in the Rorschach test and an animal association test. *Rorschach res. Exch.*, 9, 8-22.

―――. 1951. The Rorschach experiment. In A. KARDINER and L. OVESEY (eds.), *The mark of oppression.* New York: W. W. Norton & Co., Inc. Pp. 318-30.

HALLOWELL, A. I. 1955. *Culture and experience.* Philadelphia: University of Pennsylvania Press.

HALLOWELL, A. I. 1956. The Rorschach technique in personality and culture studies. In B. KLOPFER, et al., Developments in the Rorschach technique. Vol. II. New York: World Book Co. Pp. 458-544.

HANFMANN, EUGENIA, and GETZELS, J. W. 1955. Interpersonal attitudes of former Soviet citizens, as studied by a semi-projective technique. Psychol. Monogr., 69, No. 4 (Serial No. 389).

HARTWELL, S. W., HUTT, M., ANDREWS, GWEN and WALTON, R. E. 1953. The Michigan Picture Test. Chicago: Scientific Research Associates.

HELLERSBERG, ELIZABETH F. 1950. The individual's relation to reality in our culture (an experimental approach by means of the Horn-Hellersberg Test). Springfield, Ill.: Charles C. Thomas.

HENRY, J. 1941. The Rorschach technique in primitive culture. Amer. J. Orthopsychiat., 11, 233.

HENRY, W. E. 1947. The thematic apperception technique in the study of culture-personality relations. Genet. Psychol. Monogr., 35, 3-135.

KAPLAN, B. 1955. Reflections of the acculturation process in the Rorschach test. J. proj. Tech., 19, 30-35.

KAPLAN, B., RICKERS-OVSIANKINA, MARIA A., and JOSEPH, ALICE. 1956. An attempt to sort Rorschach records from four cultures. J. proj. Tech., 20, 172-80.

KLOPFER, B. 1954. Rorschach hypotheses and ego psychology. In B. KLOPFER, et al., Developments in the Rorschach technique. Vol. I. New York: World Book Co. Pp. 561-98.

KLOPFER, B., and KELLEY, D. M. 1942. The Rorschach technique. New York: World Book Co.

LINTON, R. 1955. The tree of culture. New York: Alfred A. Knopf, Inc.

LOWENFELD, MARGARET. 1954. The Lowenfeld Mosaic Test. London: Newman Neame, Ltd. New York: The Psychological Corp., Inc.

MACHOVER, KAREN. 1948. Personality projection in the drawing of the human figure. Springfield, Ill.: Charles C. Thomas.

MURRAY, H. A. 1943. Thematic Apperception Test manual. Cambridge: Harvard University Press.

————. 1947, 1955. Introduction. In A. BURTON, and R. E. HARRIS (eds.), Clinical studies of personality. Vols. I and II. New York: Harper & Bros.

ODUM, H. W. 1954. On diagnosis and direction in certain national and southern issues in the United States. J. soc. Issues, 10, 4-12.

OPLER, M. K., and SINGER, J. L. 1956. Ethnic differences in behavior and psychopathology: Italian and Irish. Int. J. soc. Psychiat., 2, 11-22.

PASCAL, G., and SUTTELL, BARBARA J. 1951. The Bender-Gestalt test. New York: Grune & Stratton, Inc.

PORTEUS, S. D. 1950. The Porteus Maze test and intelligence. Palo Alto, Calif.: Pacific Books.

RAVEN, J. C. 1947. Progressive Matrices (1947). London: H. K. Lewis & Co., Ltd.

SARBIN, T. 1954. Role theory. In G. LINDZEY (ed.), Handbook of social psychology. Cambridge, Mass.: Addison-Wesley Publishing Co., Inc. Pp. 223-58.

SARGENT, HELEN D. 1953. The Insight test. New York: Grune & Stratton, Inc.

SEWARD, GEORGENE. 1956. *Psychotherapy and culture conflict.* New York: The Ronald Press Co.

SHNEIDMAN, E. S. 1951. A manual for the MAPS test. *Proj. tech. Monogr,.* 1, No. 2.

SUTHERLAND, R. L. 1942. *Color, class and personality.* Washington D.C.: American Council on Education.

THOMPSON, C. E. 1949. The Thompson modification of the TAT test. *Rorschach res. Exch.,* 13, 469-78.

WECHSLER, D. 1944. *The measurement of adult intelligence.* (3d ed.) Baltimore: The Williams & Wilkins Co.

———. 1949. *Wechsler Intelligence Scale for Children.* New York: The Psychological Corp., Inc.

———. 1955. *Manual for the Wechsler Adult Intelligence Scale.* New York: The Psychological Corp., Inc.

PART II

COLOR AND CONFLICT

Preview

We selected the Negro minority as the starting point for our analysis of cultural influences on personality development because in this group the impact of the dominating culture has made its deepest and most devastating penetration. With no specific culture of its own, beyond the forgotten echoes of African drums, around which to ingroup, the Negro sub-"culture" has had to pull itself up by its own bootstraps. As a consequence, Negro Americans present in extreme form the ambivalent problems outlined in Chapter 1, and need special understanding for their treatment.[1]

In this part three cases will be presented whose problems are all related to their ethnic grouping, but in different ways.

---

[1] For a more extensive general discussion of the Negro patient in terms of his social background and of his clinical problems, the reader is referred to Georgene Seward, *Psychotherapy and culture conflict* (New York: The Ronald Press Co., 1956).

3

A Negro Child Reared As White

Alan J. Glasser

A SUCCESSION OF PARENTS

PRESENT PROBLEM. Wendell is an eight-year-old boy troubled and confused by problems of racial identification. Though his skin is a very light chocolate hue he has tight, curly, dark brown hair and obvious Negroid facial characteristics. Adopted by a middle-class white couple two days after birth, he was relinquished by them at five years of age and adopted by a Negro couple one year later. Early in 1956 his school referred these parents to the clinic. The mother stated in her application that Wendell's "overactivity, and inability to complete school assignments, his refusal to obey and his tendency to lie" were problem areas for which she was requesting help. One month after application she called and with great agitation stated that Wendell had "stolen" a bicycle, so the intake study was commenced at this point.

NATURAL PARENTS. Wendell, born May, 1948, was independently adopted out of state at two days of age. His natural mother, aged twenty-one and unmarried, was a salesgirl in a ten-cent store. Her own mother had died when she was two and she had lived with a father, stepmother, and five half-brothers and sisters until she left home at the age of seventeen. She was said to be pleasant, intelligent, and well liked. Her ethnic background, as described to the adoptive parents, was Danish, German, and Spanish. She had light brown hair, hazel eyes, and a light olive skin and looked completely Caucasian. The natural father was described by her as having blond hair and blue eyes, but for reasons that became ever more apparent this statement is quite certainly false.

WHITE FOSTER FAMILY. Adoption was arranged by the natural mother's physician, who noted in Wendell at birth what appeared to be Negro characteristics and, it is believed, communicated this to the adoptive parents, Mr. and Mrs. Brown. They, however, refused to pay any attention to it, stating that they loved dark-skinned babies, that they had a distant kinship with someone of Cherokee Indian blood, and that anyway many people on both sides of their family were dark-complexioned.

The adoptive mother at that time was thirty-two. She was native born of German stock, and a nominal Protestant. Her education included one year of college and she was employed as a secretary in a manufacturing firm. The father, also thirty-two, was California born, and of Irish background. He had completed high school and worked for a farm equipment firm. He was a non-practicing Catholic. Wendell was welcomed by the members of the Browns' families, the maternal grandparents in particular becoming extremely fond of and interested in him.

EARLY DEVELOPMENT. Wendell's developmental history was normal, with the exception of one month spent in a body cast sometime between eight and twelve months of age. It was supposed that his hip joint was not in the socket properly, although this was not confirmed by X-rays. He weighed six pounds at birth; his mother's pregnancy and labor were uncomplicated. He took food well on the whole, although suffering from occasional colic. He walked at ten months and talked without baby talk at the same age. Although Wendell rebelled against bowel training, he was trained at about age two. Even now he is said to retain a stubborn streak toward this function. Nocturnal wetting, except for rare instances, was apparently controlled early; however, he wet his pants during the day until age five—

"just forgot to go to the bathroom." No early sleep problems were remarked by the parents.

Wendell was noticed masturbating at the age of four, but this apparently only lasted for a short period. At five he occasionally lifted little girls' dresses, but no issue was made of this. There is no information about any verbal interchange between Wendell and the parents in the early years with respect to sex.

The patient was an extremely active child from the beginning—running, jumping, and climbing all over everything. He began playing with other children, all of whom were white, at an early age and was well liked by them. Apparently these children made no mention of his physical dissimilarity. Wendell was always a very affectionate child who enjoyed being read to and cuddled. The maternal grandparents showered much love and attention upon him which he seemed to reciprocate.

SUSPICIONS OF ORIGIN. At the time when Wendell first came to them, and for a considerable period thereafter the Browns were extremely enthusiastic about him, projecting such attitudes as their wish for a college education upon the child. At the age of six months, however, Wendell's skin began to get noticeably darker, and the parents at this time first really suspected that he might be partly Negro. However, nothing at all was done about this suspicion, nor was anything said to anyone. The parents apparently preferred to ignore this possible problem than to attempt a solution. Further doubts about the boy's race were raised from time to time, but the parents could not face these, and "did not pay much attention" to the matter until Wendell reached the age of three. It was then that the slowly crystallizing suspicions, or at least, their conscious recognition, began to lead to some action on the part of the Browns. They contacted various people in the community in an effort to resolve the problem. They first talked to a judge who suggested they relinquish Wendell for readoption. Next a Negro doctor was contacted, who advised that the child be placed where he would have better opportunities when he grew up. However, a second Negro physician recommended their keeping him. A "college crowd" they knew said the Browns should keep Wendell because he was intelligent and got along well. Upon consulting a Catholic priest, they were told "God will take care of it."

GIVING UP THE BOY. This series of experiences represents almost a caricature of the dangers of directive advice giving! Thoroughly confused, the parents did nothing for several months, finally making an abortive contact with a Family Service Agency. No further contact was made with a public agency until approximately one year later when Mrs. Brown called the particular agency to which they eventually relinquished the child. Five months later, the mother called again and arrangements were made for a series of interviews which culminated in Wendell's leaving the Brown home in the summer of 1953, when he was five years old.

Although there undoubtedly had been tension between Mrs. Brown and her parents over Wendell prior to the eight-month period of intermittent agency contact, matters became increasingly strained between them during the last interval prior to giving up Wendell. It was reported by the Browns that the grandparents' affection for the child was abnormal, even replacing their love for their own children and other grandchildren. Several times they had talked Wendell's parents out of relinquishing the boy. Then, when they found they could not dissuade the Browns from the final proceedings, they suggested that the child be given to them and that they would legally adopt him. At the time of separation Mrs. Brown's mother was furious and refused to speak to her daughter for three months. In addition to these family pressures, various members of the community also suggested to the Browns that they should not give up the boy.

When the Browns first presented themselves to the agency, they appeared to be an attractive couple with many positive elements in their relationship and personalities. However, as time went on, they were unable to conceal the fact that they were profoundly unhappy, disturbed emotionally, and conspicuously lacking in stability and maturity. They appeared on the verge of divorce and they revealed that Wendell was originally taken to save their marriage. It was brought out that there had been considerable disagreement and difficulty over bringing up the child.

Some notes on the final interview before Wendell was given up may help to clarify and accentuate this picture. The mother cried throughout most of the interview, and at the same time little or no affection was shown between herself and her husband. It appeared that the couple had had endless troubles with respect to health, work, home, and family relationships. There seemed to be nothing for them to look forward to. The father slumped in his chair, apparently dissociating himself from the proceedings. He showed no emotion in the discussion over boarding care placement, nor did he respond to his wife in any way. Parenthetically, the parents readily agreed to pay all boarding home costs. Extreme ambivalence characterized Mrs. Brown's attitude even at this late date—"I don't want to let him go, but it's best for him. I'll never get over my real feelings."

By Christmas of 1953, six months after Wendell's departure, the parents had not yet resolved their feelings about the boy and were still feeling hurt and upset. There was some talk of selling their home and moving to a new city for a fresh start. They and the maternal grandparents sent expensive Christmas presents to Wendell in his boarding home. Mrs. Brown's feelings several months later were unchanged. She could not forget the boy—"is he really Negro?" This ambivalent state of mind persisted up to her final relinquishing him to a Negro couple. It was reported that later on Mr. Brown thought he saw him in a group of "poor children" and "nearly went to pieces." Mrs. Brown subsequently went to an astrologist who told her that Wendell would be great some day and that she would know him.

SELF-DOUBTS REGARDING IDENTITY. Although Wendell felt completely a part of the Brown family in their all-white neighborhood and was accepted without question by his playmates, there had been incidents in stores and markets from time to time when he had heard slurring remarks about himself and/or his mother. During the period prior to his removal from this home he was obviously becoming increasingly aware that something was wrong. In May, 1953, he asked his mother whether he was colored. She could not bear to answer him and said nothing to him. At no time was any mention made of his racial characteristics or skin pigmentation.

Mrs. Brown couldn't face telling Wendell about leaving, and apparently kept putting it off until a month or so prior to the act. All she was able to say to him was, "We can't keep you—you'll be in a home where you'll be happy." She was amazed that though he appeared not to understand why he had to leave, he took it so well, showing no outward emotion about it at all. However, it was at this time that he first started to suffer from nightmares.

TRANSITIONAL HOMES. Because the agency felt that Wendell was very much confused about his rejection by his parents it was decided to place him in a white boarding home. Upon removal to this home no outward signs of conflict could be discerned, although he had appeared anxious about becoming acquainted on a previous visit. He kissed his mother goodbye only on request, and during the placement talked about going back home, though he refused to talk to his parents. Wendell remained in this boarding home for only a month—not being well accepted because he was "too bright." He was transferred, again without outward emotional signs, to another white boarding home in August, 1953.

RESPONSE TO NEW WHITE FOSTER PARENTS. Wendell, although hyperactive and tense, apparently made a fairly good adjustment in this home, forming a close attachment to the foster mother. During this period his dependency needs were expressed in an extraordinary fondness for milk. He wanted it at school when the other children received it, even though he got an ample supply at home. He even stole money from a little girl on the school bus in order to get the additional milk. However, he was able to curb this behavior when it was explained that the foster mother couldn't afford to give him the milk money. He demanded a great deal of love and affection and put anything and everything into his mouth. His adjustment in kindergarten that year was said to be good on the whole, despite his exorbitant demands for attention. He was very curious about sex at this time and was hard to discipline. The outstanding feature of his behavior during this period was his need for almost ceaseless physical activity.

THE QUESTION OF COLOR AGAIN. When Wendell asked the new foster mother about his appearance, in response to being called "black boy" and "Negro" by other children, she told him that he was a little darker than they and that this could be a good thing. The social worker on the case also talked to the child about this problem, telling him that they were looking for a mother and father who were dark like him. The word "Negro" was not used, since it was felt that Wendell wouldn't understand it and, further, the agency was not sure of his ultimate placement. It was felt that he was gradually understanding and accepting his situation, and the impression was that he was not worried about it. He appeared, it was said, to be identifying himself with Mexican and Spanish children. Nevertheless, Wendell still wondered from time to time why he was not living with his former foster parents, and a year after leaving them he wanted them to be informed that he was all right. He also mentioned the maternal grandparents once in a while.

The child found it very hard also to accept the fact that some day he'd be leaving the new foster home. For a long time the foster mother let him think he could remain, but some time before the separation she was able to prepare him for it in answer to his query, "Will I be placed before you die?" He seemed to accept the explanation that he would be placed where he would "match" with satisfaction, expressing the hope that his new parents would be brown since "the other ones weren't."

NEGRO FOSTER PARENTS. By the middle of 1954 the agency had settled on a new pair of adoptive parents, this time Negro. The timing was fortunate since the foster family was moving out of town. This new adoptive couple, the Smiths, had come to the agency the previous fall, and after an extended period of contact it was felt they were ready to accept Wendell as a son. The Smiths were an attractive couple who appeared to present few obstacles to a successful placement. Mrs. Smith, a well-dressed, very light-skinned woman of forty, had a clerical position in city offices. She was a high school graduate and reported a warm, happy family life in childhood. The father, thirty-eight and dark-skinned, was a college graduate employed in a civil service position.

Mrs. Smith said she had taken care of children and felt she knew enough about them to do a good job. She was much more cautious about the adoption, however, than her husband who wanted to rush in immediately, talked of taking two children, and so on. The Smiths took great pride in their two-bedroom home, liked to have the lawn and interior immaculate at all times, though later denied the importance of this. Like many middle-class Negroes, this couple was excessively conforming, particularly in "keeping up with the Jones's," but this was not regarded as an important obstacle. Religion, as for the original parents, was only nominal.

Wendell was told in June, 1954, that the social worker had found parents for him. He was given an opportunity to ventilate his feelings about his original parents and to explain that his future parents would look like him. He saw a colored man and said, "He's a nice, good man; mother and father will be like that." Wendell was taken to meet the Smiths in the town where they resided, and his reaction seemed positive. He bragged and was happy after this visit, but on the way back to the foster home he ate a large amount of candy, seemed confused, and did not ask any questions about his parents-to-be. The confusion persisted after his return to the foster home. Although he was very anxious to be settled in his new home the old one was in his thoughts and he said, "Tell them (the Browns) that I'm all right."

RIGHT ABOUT FACE. On placement Wendell seemed frightened and nervous. Sleep patterns were disturbed—he cried, jumped, and had muscle spasms. He was afraid of closed doors and dreamed about dragons attacking him. He tore up toys and scratched the furniture. Gradually this behavior was said to have diminished. The Smiths live in a mixed neighborhood and Wendell was quickly accepted by white, Oriental, and Negro children.

School adjustment was only minimal. While teachers reported that Wendell was bright and imaginative, his attention span was said to be very limited and he had a tendency to become easily fatigued. He would go to extremes to get attention. At home he confused the parents by his "lies" and stories. When not allowed to take a bicycle to school, he "stole" a bike and rode it home. He never cried when whipped and appeared happy as a lark afterwards, giving his parents a feeling of hopelessness about controlling him. The parents' attitude toward all of Wendell's naughtiness was overmoralistic; the mother asked, for example, "If he steals now, what will he do later?" Her attitude was that God had sent her this problem and that she must endure it.

Wendell's sexual activity included masturbating in his parents' presence, but he soon stopped this when admonished. He was curious to see his mother naked, and enjoyed taking showers with his father. When he asked about birth, he was told that God plants a seed under the mother's heart and that the doctor takes it out.

In adjusting to this new setting Wendell became quite attached to an aunt of Mr. Smith's, possibly with some transference from his former "grandmother." This new grandmother figure died in January, 1956. His parents told him nothing about it and he inadvertently learned the truth at school. The parents then confirmed the fact, telling Wendell that Aunt B was now an angel. Subsequently he developed pains similar to those she had been suffering.

When the agency worker tried to contact the parents a few months after Wendell's placement, she found them uncooperative and far less eager than previously to communicate. They seemed increasingly anxious concerning Wendell's acting out and aggressive behavior and their inability to handle it. It was the worker's impression that they wished they could relinquish him.

Approximately a year after Wendell's placement the Smiths applied for help at a school guidance center. Subsequently they placed him in a parochial school which made them ineligible for school guidance. He seemed to get along fairly well in parochial school but was expelled when he rang the church bell. Replaced in public school, his hyperactivity became completely unacceptable; he was excluded from class, and the school doctor suggested a tranquilizing drug.

In the summer of 1955, despite their troubles with Wendell, the Smiths were given the final adoption papers. Wendell was present at the court proceedings and listened very intently to everything that was said. Since his formal adoption his behavior has shown no noticeable change. At the time of placement Mrs. Smith had said that she would give up working for a year in order to stay home with Wendell, but she returned to work within a few months, and since then no arrangements for supervising him at home during the day have proved satisfactory. At present he is unsupervised from 11:30 A.M. to 5:00 P.M., and has to make his own lunch.

Now, two years after leaving them, Wendell still speaks of his first foster parents and grandparents. Mrs. Smith feels that he still thinks of himself as white rather than Negro. Once when she said to him, "We're both the same color—brown," he replied, "No, we're both white."

The overconforming, status conscious, moralistic atmosphere of the Smith household, in contrast to the warm, relaxed milieu at the previous foster homes, has not been conducive to identification with the new parents and the ethnic group they represent. In fact, their stern and rock-bound respectability is a common form of social defense erected by middle-class Negroes against identification with the Caucasian stereotype of Negro. The inevitable communication of their own ethnic ambivalence could hardly fail further to confuse Wendell. With neither a strong identity based on a feeling of ingroup belongingness, nor a consistent pattern of values to internalize, the child's confusion, restlessness, and acting out behavior are not difficult to understand.

PSYCHODIAGNOSIS

DIAGNOSTIC CONTACTS. Wendell was seen for two diagnostic play interviews at the clinic in addition to undergoing extensive psychological testing. Mr. Smith brought him to the appointments. Wendell was very active during the waiting periods, though not destructive, and Mr. Smith exclaimed repeatedly in Wendell's hearing about his naughtiness: "He's impossible . . . isn't he awful? . . . ," etc. The contrast between Mr. Smith's endless verbal complaints and Wendell's innocuous behavior was so great that it even led to comments of surprise on the part of the office staff.

At the first interview Wendell, who was expensively dressed, appeared self-possessed and adequate, greeting the interviewer by name and spontaneously admiring the toys. He did not play very long with any of them, and several times ran into other offices to collect more. He also ran to the waiting room and playfully threatened his father with two guns. When asked why he felt he was coming to the clinic he said things were pretty good but he gets into mischief sometimes. His parents had told him to mind the interviewer and do what he was told. When it was suggested that the clinic could help Wendell, he said he thought that was right, but that he had been frightened about coming, thinking "it was a spooky old house where they scare you." At this point he rushed forward with hands lifted menacingly in the manner of a spook.

PLAY INTERVIEW. In Wendell's second interview his behavior was very similar to that seen before. He reacted negatively to broken dolls and toys, particularly to a Negro doll which had arms missing, though this doll had excited him before he saw it was damaged. He put scotch tape over the baby doll's genitals to "keep the blood and water from coming out." Finding another baby he taped it down because it was too jumpy and nervous, then threw it in the wastebasket. When it was stated that parents really don't do that to their children, Wendell answered, "That's what they feel like doing sometimes." When asked about school, he said he was excluded because he was too jumpy. In both interviews Wendell was quite demanding and intolerant of limits and begged to take toys home with him.

PSYCHOLOGICAL TESTING. Behavioral data from the psychological testing sessions give a somewhat different picture from that of the play interviews. The hyperactivity and mischievousness complained of by his teachers and parents were present in these sessions, but they decreased considerably after the first interview. It is noteworthy that Wendell reacted quite satisfactorily to the setting of limits in the test situation, and it was the impression of the examiner, who was a woman, that he could relate very well to adult women.

During the testing he was quite restless, and he showed little frustration tolerance on tasks demanding patience and thought. It was observed, however, that he was able to relax and stay quiet during periods of no pressure. On several occasions, after completing tests Wendell asked to have a children's book read to him. He sat as close as possible, leaning against the examiner's arm, and was completely quiet for twenty minutes at one of these times. When in the course of testing Wendell was permitted to handle the dolls, he did so in a very aggressive manner, pulling limbs off, jamming metal clips into their joints, etc., although during other play periods he happily and quietly modeled clay or played with little dolls. To call his attention back to the tests was easy, but to keep it there for more than five minutes was almost impossible. At one point Wendell asked why the mother doll was pink when the papa and boy dolls were a different color, remarking, "Her color is pale. She's too pale."

The psychological tests administered to Wendell included the Wechsler Intelligence Scale for Children, the Rorschach, Thematic Apperception, House-Tree-Person, Draw-A-Person, and Make-A-Picture-Story tests.

Intellectually he functioned within the normal range, attaining a full-scale I.Q. score on the WISC of 93 (see Test Summary A). While his performance throughout the test was fairly consistent and even, there were two factors in the test situation that might have tended to depress the results slightly. First, his unusually low frustration tolerance resulted in his giving up almost immediately on challenging items. Second, his restlessness made for extreme distractibility, preventing him from giving sufficiently sustained attention to the tasks in hand. On the whole, however, it was felt that the test gave a fairly reliable appraisal of Wendell's intellectual functioning.

The projective findings confirmed and emphasized the problem areas so apparent in Wendell's history. Primarily he has an overwhelming sense of rejection by parental figures. In addition, he feels very keenly his exclusion from school, which has intensified his sense of not being an acceptable person. His response to TAT Card 6BM illustrates his feelings of maternal rejection. A death wish toward the mother and need for the grandmother found their way into his story for Card 18GF. Here the unacceptable idea of the mother's death is transformed into sleep.

It is significant that on both the TAT and the Rorschach (Test Summaries A and B) the stimuli usually associated with the father, Cards 7BM and IV, respectively, were completely rejected. Card 8BM elicited a story which the patient entitled "Operation before Death," that seemed to deal ambivalently with rather transparent but unacceptable death wishes. Again, as in the fantasy to Card 18GF, the hero is saved from death by a tour de force at the end.

A positive attitude toward school suggesting a wish for acceptance is revealed in the story produced in response to Card 1.

Illustrating his profound sense of emotional deprivation were responses to the HTP Test. In answer to the question of what the person he drew needed most, he replied, "tender care." One leaf on his tree was dead from "not watering it." On the TAT, a feeling of loneliness pervades his story for Card 13B. His emotional deprivation is further reflected in his Rorschach where, instead of good human figures, he sees monkeys, angels, mummies, and headless men. The only woman (Card I) is "holding two eagles without any head," and the only man (Card X) is "a big fat man. With a skinny head (and skinny legs)."

It is also noteworthy that on the WISC, the only object assembly that he was unable to achieve was the *face*.

These factors are, of course, inseparably a part of Wendell's relationship with past and present parents and other authority figures. While originally he seems to have had a perception of the mother figure as warm and loving, this picture is changing. He now sees Mother as critical, domineering, and moralistic. He wants desperately to feel free and relaxed, but his mother never stops pushing him toward the "straight and narrow." His resentment of this is overlaid by strong feelings of guilt for being a bad boy.

Wendell exhibits no feeling of closeness to a father. He feels he does not know one—both in the literal sense of not knowing his present father well, and in the deeper sense of not knowing what a real father is. In general he finds male adults threatening. The Rorschach and TAT clearly show his "castration anxiety," as in the headless figures already noted, as well as in "two little pincher bugs," with pinchers "to grab ahold," and "sting rays." His feeling of being overpowered comes out even more strikingly in his TAT fantasy to Card 11. As with his feelings for his mother, he suffers from guilt for hostile and aggressive thoughts toward his father, and generally attempts to deny them. This may account for his rejection of the "father" cards already noted.

It is evident that the rigid and demanding attitude of these present parents has deeply impressed Wendell with the importance of their cultural standards as a criterion of acceptability. Throughout the testing he consistently equated being "good" (i.e., wanted) with orderliness. In the HTP Test his house is nice because it's "neat"; when shown a background of a shack in the Make-A-Picture-Story Test he refused to populate the scene, actually becoming upset and exclaiming that everyone was too neat "for that greasy old shack."

The basic conflict of his own identity is totally unresolved for Wendell. In response to the Rorschach Card IX, he described a "colored butterfly." He stopped suddenly, asking, "Did you write 'colored'?", after which he denied his butterfly response, changing it to an ant, which significantly is black. The word "colored" was apparently completely charged for him, and it may be hypothesized that he was forced to reject the "colored" response very much as he had been rejected for being colored. In another test he identified a Negro figure as "a hobo and a kidnapper." Thus it is possible that he feels his present parents were responsible for his removal from his original home. Nevertheless, in drawing a tree, Wendell stated that the tree was sick because "it's pale," and there were indications in the doll play mentioned above that he strongly associates acceptability with having color. The whole area of self-perception is unquestionably problematic for him.

In spite of Wendell's obvious and severe problems, it was felt on the basis of the testing that his good reality contact and intelligence make him a good therapeutic risk. Immediate psychotherapy was recommended, with concomitant counseling of the parents.

SUMMARY OF DIAGNOSTIC IMPRESSIONS: PROGNOSIS AND RECOMMENDATIONS. The problems for which Wendell was referred to the clinic, namely, overactivity and inability to complete school assignments, refusal to obey, and tendencies to lie, are behavior patterns which commonly go together. In Wendell's case this constellation appears to have multiple, complex determinants, some of which have their genesis in the present situation while others seem to stem from earlier experiences.

In the first place, Wendell's provocative behavior is an obvious effort to gain attention and thus the warmth and love he craves. The strict, moralistic approach of the Smiths, which contrasts with the more lenient attitudes of his original parents, goads Wendell on to "test the limits" of their love for him and unconditional acceptance. He has to change or modify behavior patterns which were learned and ingrained at a tender age in the face of rigidly conformist adults who do not appreciate his predicament. It is interesting in this connection that in the testing situation, when not under pressure, he was able to relax and conform warmly and lovingly.

Underlying Wendell's overt behavior lies an intense anxiety concerning his personal worth. His experiences of repeated rejection have resulted in his perceiving himself as one who can be discarded or thrown away without explanation. Seen in this light, Wendell's motor excesses are an attempt to deny through ceaseless activity the annihilative power of such thinking. His feeling of being a robot manipulated by others also can be denied through such self-assertive activity.

Why Wendell has chosen hyperactivity as his manner of symptomatic expression is not clear, although there are several clues in the history. Wendell was an extremely active baby from the beginning of life, and the frustration of being placed in a body cast at about the age of ten months for a whole month may have reinforced his tendency to motor activity upon release. Finally, he was said to have been rebellious during bowel training, a budding character trait which could later express itself in oppositional hyperactivity.

The culture conflict which is inextricably woven into Wendell's present personality maladjustment must have had its origin in the early months of his life. Consciously his first parents showered him with love and affection, while unconsciously they commenced, in spite of themselves, a subtle rejection which reached the community level by the time the boy was three years old, and culminated in his final relinquishment at five. Concurrent with this was an uncritical, adoring acceptance by the maternal grandparents, which strengthened his sense of family and identification with the Caucasian race.

Placement for a year in white foster homes did nothing to alter his fundamental conception of himself as white. Further, one must not neglect the inadequate explanation offered him at the time he was adopted by the Smiths, in addition to the fact that at no time has Wendell been given a real feeling for the implications of the role and status of the Negro in the United States. At all junctures in the proceedings the true reason for his dislocation was side-stepped or played down. That he has been and remains in a state of dilemma concerning the implications of the terms "Negro," "white," and "colored" is confirmed beyond doubt by the results of the diagnostic interviews and testing.

His reaction to his own use of the word "colored" on the Rorschach test, and his identification of a Negro figure as "a hobo and kidnapper" indicate that to some degree he has formed a negative attitude toward the idea of being Negro —an attitude perhaps most clearly expressed in his defensive color denial when he contradicted his mother's statement, "We're both the same color—brown," with, "No, we're both white." To what extent this attitude has resulted from earlier occurrences in his life, from interpersonal contacts outside his home, or to his unfavorable experiences in the Smith home cannot be determined, but the importance of warm and positive identification with his Negro parents as a foundation for ultimate acceptance of his racial status can hardly be overemphasized. At present he does have some feeling of "belonging" in regard to color, as evidenced by his doll play and his statements about objects being "too pale." This may prove a favorable factor in the resolution of the traumatic identification conflict in which he presently finds himself. That he has thus far reacted to this conflict by a characteristic personality pattern—namely, hyperactivity—in an effort to suppress his intense unhappiness and feeling of abandonment appears perfectly consistent with the picture we have of Wendell's development.

Unless he is able to gain some insight into his predicament through psychotherapy, the prognosis for this bright, cheerful, and affectionate little boy appears poor. The pattern of inconsistency in discipline from home to home, especially the change from the easy-going Browns to the much stricter Smiths, has been conducive to his minor acting out. Continued exclusion from school can only make matters worse, possibly leading to major acting out and the beginning of a delinquent career.

An integral part of the treatment plan for this young patient must include counseling of the parents who at present see only a bad boy. If they can be helped to understand Wendell's basic identification problems and to see the destructive impact of the extreme disciplinary change on the child's behavior, half the battle of correcting his present difficulty will have been won.

Granted the parents' cooperation, Wendell's chances of reorienting himself are good. Since his reality testing is unimpaired, and he has not yet developed paralyzing defenses, he should be easily accessible to psychotherapy. Moreover his desperate longing for a warm relationship with an adult will greatly facilitate the process. In his case, a Negro therapist is indicated to reinforce his recently acquired Negro identity. For most members of ethnic subcultures, the core identification is with the minority, while that with the dominant group is secondary. In Wendell's case, the process was reversed: his basic identification was white, while his self concept as a Negro has been a late and reluctant development. Since, however, his primary white identification was appropriate in terms of his situation in contrast to the many Negro cases where a black identity is unrealistically repudiated, there is an intact ego foundation on which to built for the future. For Wendell, therapy with an adult Negro might be profitably supported by satisfying relationships with a Negro peer group.

Test Summary

A. WISC RESULTS

Verbal Scale	Wtd. Score	Performance Scale	Wtd. Score
Information	8	Picture Completion . . .	7
Comprehension	9	Picture Arrangement . . .	9
Arithmetic	10	Block Design	9
Similarities	6	Object Assembly	11
Vocabulary	10	Coding	9
(Digit Span)	12	(Mazes)	–
Sum	55(46)*	Sum	45

Verbal Scale IQ . . . 95   Performance Scale IQ . . 93

Full Scale IQ 93

* Prorated.

Test Summary

B. THEMATIC APPERCEPTION TEST

CARD 1. Well—boy's practicing violin—just like I did—and doesn't know which string it is and when teacher comes he'll correct him and it will be all right. (Couldn't think of title.)

CARD 3 BM. 3″ I don't know this story.
            8″ I don't know. (Encouraged—any kind of story want.) I don't know—really.

CARD 4. Oh that's a love scene—the girl wants to do something and man won't let him—lady won't let man do something. (Q—what?) Don't know what man told him to do. (Q—Is there another man?) Yah, other man told him to come but wife won't let him. "The Love Scene." (Q—Married?) Uh huh.

CARD 6BM. Oh—it's Perry Como's Mother—and there's Perry Como. (Wendell sings *Hot Ziggety*.) This before he became a show star— he's asking his Mother can he do it—she says no—you're terrible—she tells him he sings songs wrong—he wanted singing lessons—wanted to sing in the band. It should be (sings *Hot Ziggety* again—indicating this is correct way to sing it). "Perry Como Sings *Hot Ziggety*."

CARD 7BM. I don't know—(encourage). No, I can't—I've never seen those two men before. (Can make up story anyway.) No— funny thing—if I never saw them I can't—I've seen Perry Como.

CARD 8BM. You tell me that story now—I can't tell you—cause he killed somebody—they're gonna kill somebody. I can tell you story now that I don't have it out (he put the card down). They're operating on the man. (Q—Who is the boy?) Same man—this is a picture of operating on him and after they're finished operating on him. (Q) A gun. (Q—Why there?) Don't know—somebody just put it there for decoration. "Operation Before Death." (Q—Who dies?) That man was very sick—had cancer (Q—Boy after?) Well, operated just in time. (Q—Die?) No—got all cancer out of him.

CARD 11. Is that upside down? I don't figure out what that is. Oh, it's a big mountain top with a big avalanche. (Q—That all?) I see two buffaloes. (Q—Creatures on path?) (Pointed to serpent.) That's the avalanche. Don't know title. (Wendell got a doll—pulled leg off—tried to put it back.)

CARD 13MF. That's a man in the dark and his wife—he has a wife who's asleep. (Q) He's sleepy too. "Sleeping Beauty."

CARD 3B. That is a boy sitting on a log cabin—barefooted Pete. (Q) He's just a barefooted Pete—that's all I know about it. "Log Cabin Pete."

CARD 15. That's a cemetery in there and that's a man rising from the dead. (Q—Why?) Goin' to Heaven—remember all good souls go to Heaven. Don't know title.

CARD 16. Make a picture of the Cross. (Q—Anything else?) No (here patient spoke softly and dramatically).

CARD 18GF. The grandmother found the woman dead—grandmother found woman asleep. (Q—What doing?) Oh—just trying to wake her up. "Sleeping Beauty."

Test Summary

C. RORSCHACH PROTOCOL

Response	Inquiry
CARD I. 5″	
Looks like a woman holding two eagles without any head.	I can see woman and two eagles—wings.
CARD II. 5″	
(Makes face)	
Two hats with a man with no head—two men with no head. Man with magic head, I think.	Hats—no head—feet together, hands. (Hats?) Way shaped that's only thing makes me think so.

Response	*Inquiry*
CARD III. 4″	
(laughs)	(He pointed out the popular figures —but each with 2 hands instead of legs)
1. 2 monkeys	1. They're grabbing hold of the bone of some dead thing. (Q) Looks like bone.
2. and a bow	2. Two little things like a bow.
CARD IV. 4″	
I don't know what that looks like.	1. I couldn't tell you what that was. (looks like now?) I don't know.
CARD V. 3″	
1. Looks like a butterfly.	1. Butterfly—2 feet, wings, head, and feelers.
CARD VI. 4″	
1. Looks like a wolf.	1. (Rejects wolf) Looks like a dinosaur with body open. (Body open?) Has to be closed body. Like you, if your body was open, you wouldn't be alive, it has to be closed.
CARD VII. 3″	
1. Looks like 2 little angels.	1. I mean 2 little Indian girls—Head —feather—feet—Big feet—Big feet Indian girls. (Alive?) No, mummies.
CARD VIII. 3″	
1. Looks like a little sweet buggy.	1. Here's head—see feet and body. (What about blot?) Don't know.
CARD IX. 3″	
1. Looks like a sweet, little pretty-colored butterfly. (Wendell asked, "Did you write "colored?")	1. Butterfly, no. I said this was an ant—see head and big eyes? Ants have pop eyes and there's the feet.
CARD X. 4″	
1. Two little pincher bugs and	1. Crab. See crabs have lot of legs and there's pinchers to grab ahold. That's their protection—sting rays here.
2. A big fat man. With a skinny head.	2. Here—and skinny legs (asked about inside details and what about blot?) Just things.

4

Psychological Flight from "Black Identity"

Franklin R. McDonald

THE SETTING

This young Negro woman was selected for presentation because her experiences exemplified the effects of sociocultural pressures from an unwholesome family situation and a negatively reinforcing social matrix. These deleterious effects on her personality development were reflected in her particular dilemma and the difficult, ambiguous, many-sided problem for all authority figures concerned with her welfare. Considered in the frame of reference of her past and present background from which she was striving to free herself, her problem seemed to take on a clearer perspective. This new perspective and understanding helped to pave the way for smoother management and more effective rehabilitation for this seriously troubled woman.

In the sequence of their contact with Mrs. W. were the social welfare workers, firemen, policemen, judge, psychiatrist, clinical psychologist, and probation officers. The social welfare workers had the problem of her promiscuity; the firemen, her attempted arson; the arresting officers, her too-ready verbal acceptance of "wrongdoing"; and the probation officers, her management over a five-year period. To psychiatrist and psychologist fell the delicate and difficult task of unravelling those aspects of her psychodynamics that were idiosyncratic from those that were attributable to her ethnic status. They shared the further responsibility of modifying conventional psychotherapeutic techniques to meet the problems growing out of her social milieu and strivings.

THE ARREST

On the day of her arrest for attempted arson, Mrs. W. noticed a slight headache developing and sought relief by taking four Anacin tablets. Some friends stopped by to encourage her to join them in a drinking party. After she had refused the invitation and had related her financial difficulties to them, all but one man left. Thereafter, Mrs. W. sat staring at the wall not thinking of anything in particular when suddenly she remarked to the man, "I ought to set the sofa on fire." She began to cry and felt she wanted to die, as her children would be better off without her. The man left and another arrived to find her crying. When asked about her difficulty she cried more intently. Thereupon he struck her across the face in an effort to stop her crying and left her by herself.

Mrs. W. recalls nothing following his departure other than walking around the immediate vicinity of her apartment. Some friends stopped her at the doorway advising her to stay out of the house as both policemen and firemen were in there. She could not recall definitely whether or not she had gone back into the apartment after being struck across the face as her "mind was a blank." She did recall definitely that the baby had been taken to a neighbor earlier in the day, the two oldest children were downstairs at the time of the fire, and the other two were over at another neighbor's home. Homicide was denied but suicide was admitted as a motive since this ". . . would probably make my mother realize how badly off I was in the need of help."

Two weeks prior to the alleged offense she was quite upset over the family situation, noticing that she "was in a family

way." Little or no money was available with which to buy
food for the children. Her youngest child was ill with pneumonia and she with influenza. The gas was turned off because of her inability to pay the bill. Her boy-friend "who
had put me in a family way" walked out with what small
savings she had, and her relief funds had been stopped temporarily. Her mother had "lost money to the bookies on the
horses" and was unable to help her financially. Unable to
pay her rent, she contacted her husband in the northern
part of the state who agreed to help her by taking four of
the children. One day prior to her offense he informed her
he would not accept the children. During her period of
retention in jail she underwent psychiatric and psychological
examinations.

BROKEN FAMILY

Typical of her lower-class Negro background, Mrs. W.
came from an "extended" family consisting of mother,
father, two aunts, a grandmother, and an older brother.
Conspicuous by his absence was the father.

THE "BAD" MOTHER. Mrs. W.'s mother is alive and forty-
five years of age. She was sixteen years old when her first
child, a boy, was born and eighteen years of age when the
patient was born. After completing the tenth grade her
first occupation was as a maid in a house of prostitution.
Mrs. W. states that her mother was quite proud that she
had worked up to become a prostitute for "white men."
She has persisted up to the present time in supporting herself by "playing the horses, and cards," donations from her
various boy-friends, and occasional maid's work.

During the few times Mrs. W. was with her mother she
and her brother were introduced to many of her mother's
boy-friends and were told to call them "Daddy." There
were many occasions on which she observed her mother engaged in sexual relations with these men. She felt badly
about "seeing my mother in bed with different men" as she

knew it was wrong, but when she tried to talk with her mother about such activities, she was told to mind her own business.

Mrs. W. was an unwanted dark-skinned daughter of a light-brown-skinned mother who called her a "millstone" and showed marked preference for her lighter-skinned son. Her mother is described as irritable, indifferent, selfish, and "always wanting to run around with men." The only time she showed the girl any affection was when the child, at the age of four, experienced a serious burn on her leg.

THE "FATHER?" The man who claimed to be her father was twenty-eight years old at the time of her birth. Mrs. W. is not certain that he is her father: "People tell me he's my father and people tell me he's not." He had finished the eighth grade and worked irregularly as a domestic laborer. He is remembered as an "irresponsible alcoholic who is still living, drinking, and working two jobs." The patient feels that he never encouraged her but made her feel inferior instead. At first she hated him, but as she became more and more aware of his weaknesses and maladjustment, she began to pity him. Few memories are retained of him except for his encouraging her to be nice to male admirers.

THE "GOOD" MOTHER. Mrs. W. was left with her maternal aunt who lived in the same city. This aunt was a Church of God in Christ minister's wife with three children in their early adolescence. She had asked her sister for permission to raise her two children as she felt that a better family life could be provided for them. From the very first Mrs. W. ". . . felt loved by her and that I was somebody because I was wanted." Her aunt is remembered as cheerful and ". . . everything that is good."

When her aunt died in the autumn of 1954 Mrs. W. threatened to break probation and suffer the punishment if she were not permitted to attend the funeral. During the burial rites she had to be forcibly restrained from jumping into the grave as her aunt was being lowered. To date she has persistently refused to accept the fact that her aunt is dead. She thinks of her and recalls her "good advice" whenever she does something that she believes or her aunt believed to be wrong.

GRANDMOTHER. Another mother figure in Mrs. W.'s early life was her grandmother, with whom she lived for some time. This woman was a staunch African Methodist-Episcopalian and is still living. She loved the patient and stood by her until she discovered that "I was a big liar. Then she began telling me right from wrong." The grandmother tried to tell the girl the facts of life and warned her against sexual play with boys. The last straw was the patient's theft from her benefactor of $300 with which she bought the sweaters and skirts she needed for acceptance in her peer group. On discovery, the girl was sent back to her mother, who was at that time in a Western gambling town.

THE SIBLING RIVAL. Her only sibling is a brother who is one and one-half years older than Mrs. W. Early memories of her brother all involve him as fighting her—behavior which has persisted up to the present time. She first became aware of her jealousy of him when she was four, on discovering her mother's preference for him. She states that they have never been close to each other but he is now attempting to effect a reconciliation by occasionally visiting her with a peace offering: "He brings over a half-a-pint whenever his wife kicks him out."

THE SOCIAL MOLD

Mrs. W. was born in 1929 in a small Midwestern agricultural and mining town. Her birthplace was near a large military fort and college. The Negro section of the small town was poor and run-down. It possessed three small churches, one Negro elementary school, and one integrated high school. There were no professional Negroes in the community and the townspeople occupied themselves by attending church, theaters, and, most frequently, "gin mills." The segment of the Negro population of which her mother and father were members catered to the soldiers' desires. There was little or no discrimination, but most of the Negroes "tried to do like what the white people were doing." This consisted of relieving themselves of working-week tensions by week-end drinking sprees and visits to houses of prostitution.

The town in which the patient's grandmother lived also was small and run-down. It was in a milling belt where most of the Negroes were employed as unskilled laborers in the various flour mills. A poor and a middle class could be distinguished within the Negro segment of this community as in the previous one. The monotony of existence was relieved only by the nightly fighting and drinking bouts which became more violent on week ends and holidays.

In the aunt's town, the Negro area was again the same sort of place—dirty, barren, and dilapidated. Community life was at a minimum. Instead were found gambling, drinking, "hell-raising," and houses of ill repute. There was one substandard elementary school and one church with a very small congregation led by Mrs. W.'s uncle.

DEVELOPMENT

GROWTH AND TRAUMA. The patient presented no difficulty at the time of birth and sustained no birth injuries. Both she and her cousin were breast fed by her mother for six months, at which time her teeth appeared. She walked at one year and was toilet trained by her maternal grandmother by one and one-half years. No bad habits were present other than biting her mother during nursing. A tonsillectomy was performed when she was ten years old and the usual childhood diseases were experienced with no sequelae.

In the course of growing up, this unfortunate girl sustained two serious injuries when she was four years old. One was a concussion with persistent, intermittent headaches, caused by a blow on the head when her brother threw a horseshoe at her. The other occurred at about the same time when she fell into an ash pit while playing with her cousins during one of her mother's sprees. She suffered a third-degree burn which nearly cost her her leg. For the following two years she could not use the disabled limb at all, and even at the present time, it swells whenever she stands for several hours. It has been badly disfigured ever since.

SCHOOL. Mrs. W. ". . . loved to go to school and never received any low grades." Her grades consisted wholly of A's and B's for subject matter, and S's for conduct. All subjects were easy for her but she was singularly outstanding in music, spelling, and physical education. She claimed that both teachers and pupils relied on her to lead in these subjects. She regards her school life as a satisfactory balance of social, athletic, and scholastic attainments.

For her various teachers distinct preferences and aversions were expressed. A male Negro home-room teacher was liked above all others ". . . because he was paralyzed from the waist down yet was so good looking, and besides he was so understanding toward me, more than to the other children." At the other extreme was a female Caucasian gym teacher whom she abhorred. This abhorrence was based on one incident of her forcing Mrs. W. to take gym against her physician's orders during the time she was convalescing from complications of her third-degree burns. Her vehemence is best exemplified by her own unique terminology: "I bit the shit out of her." Those teachers who exerted a marked or permanent influence upon her personality development were a Caucasian female art teacher and a middle-aged male history teacher. The former encouraged her to do embroidery work which she has continued up to the present time. The latter ". . . made me his pet. . . . he liked me."

Her classmates ". . . thought I was the best thing in the world. . . ." They never teased her. However, she felt embarrassed around them as "I never dressed like they did. . . . I always wanted good pretty clothes like my girlfriends and felt bad about my hand-me-downs."

She was an excellent student in school and skipped two grades. Her school adjustment and deportment were unblemished until the age of twelve years. At this time her introduction to sexual experiences far outweighed the gains from school. A high school diploma always has been her goal but was never attained, as school was terminated in the tenth grade, when she was thirteen, due to her first pregnancy.

SEXUAL SAGA. Actually an early sensitization to sexual experiences began between the ages of four and five when she witnessed intercourse between her mother and boy-friends. Active participation in sexual relations began at the age of five years with an eight-year-old cousin. All the children slept together in the same bed and the cousin's sexual play frightened her so that she told her grandmother who warned her "Never to let nobody stick nothing in me." Thereafter, Mrs. W. was always eager to play "Mommy and Daddy" with herself as the "baby." On one occasion while engaged in this pleasurable game Mrs. W. had a curiosity to play the mother role. She was ". . . caught in the act" by a neighbor who ". . . scared me to death," and was later also punished by her grandmother.

Discouraged from this activity, Mrs. W. practiced clitoral masturbation to the point of unconsciousness. This habit continued up to the age of seven years at which time her grandmother put red pepper on her fingers to stop her. Once this practice was terminated her interests turned to observing the sexual act between grown-ups and between her teen-age cousins and their girl-friends.

From the ages of ten and eleven, sexual information was sought from a twelve-year-old girl regarding two subjects of interest to her: menstruation and intercourse. When her menses appeared, however, she was not prepared and be-came frightened.

During her twelfth year her cousin, who had attempted sexual relations with her when she was five, took her to her mother's forty-year-old boy-friend who had expressed a sexual interest in her. She still recalls the incident of his taking her behind a highway signboard because ". . . it hurt when he broke my cherry." This act resulted in vaginal repair requiring seven stitches and two weeks of daily medical treatment. The bill was paid by her accoster who later married her mother.

After she had healed, regular intercourse was practiced with a fourteen-year-old boy every time she could slip away from her grandmother's watchful vigilance. This experience is described as a very pleasurable one to her since she always wanted to be with him because "I loved him." The relationship continued regularly three or four times a week until she was twelve and one-half years old when she became pregnant. She pleaded with her mother to allow the boy to marry her as they both desired marriage. However, her mother refused and sent her to her ex-husband on the ground that she ". . . was a whore." Mrs. W. has never forgiven her mother for this act. She gives this experience as her reason for engaging in sexual relations with older men and getting pregnant by them whenever an argument ensues between her and her mother.

No guilt has ever been experienced over her active sexual escapades except "Now, I'm more selective and careful in protecting myself." Since she has been in psychotherapy, sexual urgency is experienced only occasionally. Recently she has acquired an older boy-friend with whom she engages in sexual relationships once weekly with contraceptives. Her present attitude toward sexual activity is that it should be reserved for married life. She feels that her "sexual problem" has been resolved. She intends her children to receive progressive sexual education and information from the age of nine years on through puberty whenever they express any curiosity about it.

SOCIAL LIFE. Up to the age of fourteen, Mrs. W. described herself as a friendly, outgoing, intelligent, and flexible girl who enjoyed "the simple things of life."

Subsequent to this age a marked change occurred as she became increasingly burdened with feelings of depression, inferiority, and guilt. She summarizes this condition with a phrase she has repeated frequently during the initial and middle phases of psychotherapy, i.e., "I'm shy—I just don't like nobody to be looking at me . . . (long contemplative pause) . . . I guess I feel guilty." With older people she feels at ease but with authority figures she is stricken with panic, "I'm scared of all of them: police, doctors, preachers, etc. . . ."

PSYCHIATRIST'S REPORT

It was the psychiatrist's opinion that Mrs. W. was suffering from a reactive depression. Although a diagnosis of schizophrenic reaction could not be conclusively ruled out, he felt that the circumstances of the patient's life were sufficiently disturbing to have precipitated her depressed attitude and to have accounted for her emotional disturbance.

PSYCHOLOGICAL EXAMINATION

The psychological examination, conducted by the writer, consisted of a psychodiagnostic interview, a Draw-A-Person Test (with inquiry), a Sentence Completion Test,[1] and a Rorschach analysis.

BEHAVIOR AND MANNER. A mild-mannered, dark-brown-skinned Negro mother of five children, Mrs. W. was examined in a room at the county jail. Short in stature, unattractive but youthful looking, and clad in loose-drape inmate garments, her unattractiveness was accentuated by parched protruding lips, straightened but ungroomed hair, and silly mannerisms. During the examination her mood was gay, jovial, and unperturbed. With this mood the test tasks were entered into as enjoyable games although she worked at them with conscientious cooperation.

Spontaneous remarks concerned her children's welfare during her present incarceration and a plea for out-patient psychiatric treatment rather than hospitalization. On this latter point she was persistently questioning and querulous.

---

[1] The form used was developed by Dr. Bertram Forer, of The V.A. Mental Hygiene Clinic, Los Angeles, California.

If hospitalized, she pledged no cooperation as she would feel deprived of her children and ". . . forced into something that ain't right." As regards out-patient treatment, irrespective of personal inconveniences to her, wholehearted cooperation was assured ". . . as I know I'm sick in mind and need someone to get a load off my chest to."

Various traumatic episodes in her life, including the pregnancies, were discussed in a frank unashamed manner as if they were of little consequence or else were mere thoughtless actions on her part. As she states ". . . these were just part of life but I don't know why." Of her recent arson attempt, concern, responsibility, and acceptance of punishment were expressed: ". . . I must have been out of my mind. . . . I don't remember doing it yet I know I must have and I am willing to pay for my crime."

DRAW-A-PERSON TEST. The patient's guarded approach to life is reflected in her use of a stick figure to represent a person in her first drawing (see Fig. 4–1). The female figure that follows (Fig. 4–2), while indicating an appropriate sex identification, displays a damaged body image in the crooked legs. Her preoccupation with her disfigurement comes out in her reply to the inquiry (Test Summary A) concerning the "worst part." This negative self feeling contrasts with her ego ideal represented in her description of the "woman": "Well, through all her childhood up to 24 years old, she tried to be a lady. She has never been a bad girl, and doesn't run around."

SENTENCE COMPLETION TEST. On this test (see Test Summary B) the patient expressed her disillusioned views of love and sex in her negative replies to the appropriate questions, such as:

7. *A person who falls in love* never have a happy life.
29. *Most marriages* are not successful.

Her concern over her children came out in many responses, including:

24. *I used to feel down in the dumps when* I had to let my kids go.

25. *Most of all I want* is for my five children to come home
to me.

27. *At times she worried about* her children.

Her resentment of her mother was especially frank in:

4. *I used to feel I was being held back by* my mother.

Throughout this test runs a pervasive feeling tone of depression, guilt, and underlying hostility.

RORSCHACH ANALYSIS. Mrs. W.'s Rorschach (Test Summary C) reveals her evasiveness and the barrenness of her emotional life. She virtually rejects four of the cards, II, III, VI, and X, giving only "don't know" responses tempered by some color naming and such primitive responses as "ink" and "water."

Although there are in evidence some sporadic and ineffectual attempts at impulse control through anatomy, geography, and X-ray responses, raw sexual responses break through on cards I and VII where she sees female sex organs.

PERSONALITY EVALUATION

The patient's problem appears to be pervasive, involving personal, emotional, and social areas of adjustment. Her difficulties seem more an outgrowth of inadequate preparation in early childhood than deterioration of once-adequate personality defenses.

Poorly equipped for adjustment in a complex competitive society by her inadequate training and unwholesome environment, a constant feeling of being lost, helpless, and chronically insecure plagues her. Impulses are acted out to afford relief from her oppressive tensions. In her persistent gropings she attaches herself parasitically to anyone with whom she can gain some small measure of support and affection. The price to be paid is of little consequence. To her the important factor is not to be alone—to be protected rather than having to face the life of a social isolate.

The psychological test data highlight the main feelings from which she seeks escape and her means of defending herself from them. These are feelings of being alone and rejected. Her life thema as displayed in her expressive behavior and test data is: "Nobody loves me, I am the rejected child." With her inadequately developed facilities she tries in vain to defend herself against her basic feelings of insecurity.

When faced with conflict, Mrs. W. becomes guarded and evasive. The inadequacy of her defenses adds to her frustration, but she dares not express her resentment openly toward her mother on whom she blames her difficulties. Lacking a direct outlet for her hostility, she turns it on herself where it may be expressed as morbid apprehension of bodily harm or in repeated suicidal attempts.

The effort to deny her hostile impulses at times results in dissociative reactions. She reports attacks of numbness on the entire right side of her body. She is convinced that this is not imaginary as she is able to insert pins into her skin without any felt sensation! This sensory impairment occurs intermittently and lasts varying periods of time. On a few occasions she has had lapses of memory, such as occurred during the fire, when she cannot definitely recall what she has been doing. It is during these times when ". . . my mind leaves me and I do things I don't remember though I must have done them." Oddly enough these periods are both efforts at denial of her destructive and sadistic impulses and an opportune occasion for their expression. In essence it gives her an excuse to give vent to them since she is not aware of, and thus not responsible for, their occurrence.

TREATMENT PLAN

In planning treatment for Mrs. W., her high motivation had to be balanced against her emotional instability and her negativism toward being hospitalized. All things considered, it was felt that she would have a better chance for rehabilitation on an out-patient basis than if she were committed.

PSYCHOTHERAPY

GOALS. Preparation for psychotherapy actually commenced at the time of the initial contact with Mrs. W. during her psychodiagnostic examination. It began with deep empathy on the part of the therapist for this woman who represented for him, not just one, but a large group of persons in our society, forced to face relentless social obstacles throughout their lives. As a member of the Negro minority himself, the therapist's empathy was heightened by his own anger as a first-hand witness to the frustrations and self-hatred of these people. Their self-hatred appeared in the triadic pattern: conviction of unlovability, diminution of affectivity, and deep hostility, which stemmed from their restricting environment.

In her turn, Mrs. W. accepted the therapeutic relationship, expressing a need to disentangle her troublesome past from her present aspirations by pledging her wholehearted cooperation in any proposed psychotherapeutic venture. She was apparently at ease with the therapist, feeling that her colloquialisms, profanity, and unusual behavior were understood in terms of her sociocultural matrix and not merely as personal deviations from normality. She looked hopefully toward therapy as a socially acceptable channel for satisfying her frustrated dependency needs. At last, someone really "cared."

The therapeutic goal was to help Mrs. W. build up a sense of personal worth so that she might realize her potential for becoming a good mother and an effective member of society.

To achieve this goal, a corrective father-daughter relationship was established between therapist and patient, on the strength of which supportive, directive guidance was given in certain problem areas where she was having difficulty.

FATHER-DAUGHTER RELATIONSHIP. Her main social relationships seemed to be singularly with transient father-figures in a sado-masochistic framework. To nullify the negative parental influences, the goal of the first phase was the establishment of an enduring father-daughter relationship between therapist and patient. This was done by the therapist's maintaining the accepting and flexible role of an ever-present, protecting, and patient father-substitute. Mrs. W. was allowed access to the therapist as she felt the need and with any means at her disposal to test his sincerity. This she did by engaging in repeated drinking sprees and by initiating more masochistic relationships with older men toward whom she had become obligated through their bestowed gratuities.

Face-to-face transactions initially consisted of brief ten to fifteen minute meetings during which she consistently began with the phrase, "I ain't got nothing to talk about." Reassured that this behavior was acceptable she gradually began to relate in diary-like fashion recordings of her daily activities with no reference to her feelings or thoughts. Occasionally she would express a summary emotionally toned statement, "I'm mad!" At these times the therapist would explore from the periphery inward all the situations which served to arouse her anger, to the point where a "mad headache" developed from her pent-up anger. When this point was reached her angry feelings were verbally expressed for her in her own unique language if she did not do so herself.

Since the patient had to commute more than twenty-five miles by bus for her weekly appointments, which were paid for out of her meager public assistance allowance, an alternative to the conventional interview was arranged. She was permitted to telephone her therapist once a week and at any other time she felt the need or had a "mad headache" coming on. On the basis of the phone check-ups, verbal progress reports were made which were added to the written probation reports that she herself submitted. This phase continued for approximately a one and one-half year period, with hospital and home visitation during her terminal stages of pregnancy and post-partum convalescent period.

SOCIAL RELATIONSHIPS. The second phase formally commenced after her six months' post-partum check-up. This period was largely devoted to education regarding sexual physiology, social relationships, and cultural mores. These instructional sessions were executed on a very concrete everyday level, using her own current sexual and social experiences as well as her apparently psychogenic illnesses as subject matter. In other words, whenever some behavioral act or question arose about which she manifested some tension or anxiety, practical instruction with hints at prophylaxis were instituted. During this phase of therapy, the patient expressed a desire for a private physician since she had acquired a health and accident insurance policy covering her children and herself. She was referred to a fatherly physician who started her on a preventive program of health.

Unfortunately, this constructive development was nullified by the return of her mother who chided her about having to call up a "crazy doctor" every time she wished "to have some fun" or had some problem or question about her daily living. Her mother also criticized her following the advice of "a old fogy pill pusher." The result was resistance toward the therapist and termination of work with her physician. She asked many questions about what would happen to her condition, her probationary status, and her future adjustment if she stopped her appointments and withdrew from therapy. Soon after this questioning period she telephoned one night to inform the therapist that she was pregnant by a man whose wife had just been released from the state hospital. The reason for the pregnancy was given in terms of her anger at her mother for selling her unpaid-for furniture in order to pay gambling debts. She had become so infuriated with her mother that she went out on a drinking party with this man and "went to bed with him without my button." Again, visitation during the antepartum ensued and continued through the post-partum period until she was discharged from the hospital.

After discharge she was seen twice weekly with the aim of effecting a separation from her mother and brother by obtaining an apartment of her own in a respectable neighborhood. Following the long-discussed move, a period for working through her guilt feelings about leaving her mother stranded was necessary. These guilt feelings were found to be repetitions of earlier ones which had led her to chronic self-disparagement. Mrs. W. was now able to express the insight, "It's me and my damned mad spells that keep me always getting into more and more trouble and then feeling guilty and punishing myself by having more babies."

With her new-found feelings of independence and determination to improve her social status, she resolved to secure a divorce from her estranged husband and the custody of the children. Steps were taken to help her secure adequate legal aid, Red Cross investigation, and probation clearance in order to expedite her divorce proceedings. However, when informed of her proposed actions, her husband threatened her and made repeated efforts to obstruct her.

During this turbulent period, Mrs. W. attempted suicide by ingesting ant poison when her husband, as a last gesture, claimed to have evidence which would result in his taking the children away from her. At this time the psychotherapeutic transactions were concerned with helping her ventilate her pent-up feelings and with confronting her with the manipulative motive behind her behavior. Subsequently, supportive-directive guidance was continued until the divorce proceedings had ended in her favor.

PERSONAL GOALS. The third phase of therapy has started with an attempt to aid Mrs. W. in establishing long-range, socially acceptable goals for self-enhancement. She has been encouraged to move into a more respectable neighborhood, and to enter into community activities. She has also been urged to complete her education and acquire adequate preparation for a sound vocation. Along with these efforts, her appearance and health have been presented to her as important assets to be developed. As a result, she has been trying to reduce her corpulent figure and to maintain good health without relapses into drinking sprees.

The terminal steps of her therapy have not been thoroughly explored or discussed, but will be directed toward her critical readjustment following the expiration of probation which has served as a brake on her impulsive acting out. Last and most important is the consideration to be given to preparation for her middle age with prospects for marriage and a secure future.

THE SUMMING UP

Mrs. W.'s life began in a minor key with her entrance into a world submerged in an economic depression. Her status as an unwanted dark-skinned Negro girl in a Midwestern substandard community could hardly have been lower. In the prevailing social climate, her working-class Negro family suffered from collective insecurity, low morale, and low morals. Daily accumulations of tension were dissipated through living for the moment, and displacing hostility onto the weaker members of the group who thus served as scapegoats. Such was the way of life of the particular subculture to which our patient was introduced.

In terms of her own family, she was the dark-skinned daughter of a promiscuous light-brown-skinned mother who was uncertain of the child's paternity. The mother expressed her lack of affection for the little girl early and repeatedly by calling her a "millstone" and treating her in kind. She showed marked preference for her lighter-skinned son. Obviously this was a mother on whom the growing girl could place little dependence for the gratification of either material or emotional needs. The resultant impact on her developing self-esteem was clearly seen in the patient's self-depreciatory behavior in her relationships with older men with whom she tried to rival her mother. Sex early became for her a sado-masochistic maneuver to gain affection or to escape from frustrations.

Little is known of the alleged father's background other than that he was reputed to have been a light-brown-skinned, irresponsible man with a meager education and a menial work history. He also had little regard for his daughter. He left the picture as he had entered it, a relatively unknown entity who contributed nothing to his child's welfare and was never available in time of need. The parental role was made even more shadowy by the variety of transient "Daddies" who followed in his wake whenever the mother was in town and the variety of transient "homes" to which she was farmed out whenever the mother was off on one of her frequent sprees.

In spite of the grim general picture, all was not on the negative side in Mrs. W.'s background. Among the few assets were the strong feminine models represented by the aunts, grandmothers, and school teachers from whom she acquired her social ideals and personal conscience. Unfortunately, however, exposure to each of these influences was of brief duration, and presumably incorporated only in a fragmentary way.

The unfavorable environmental conditions provided fertile soil for the development of the fear and distrust of men, the sexual hedonism, and the insecurity that were to characterize the patient's later behavior. What few early peer relationships she had were fraught with insecurity and embarrassment. She had no confidence in her status with her brother since he remained abusive, rejecting, and exploitative like his mother. With her schoolmates, she felt accepted only on an academic level. Socially they did not accept her because of her shabby clothing. Other early relationships were on an exclusively sexual basis, thus setting the pattern for circuitous gratification of her need for love —a pattern quite normal in her social group.

Mrs. W.'s central problem appears to have resulted from her rejection as an unwanted dark girl in an unstable Negro family. The unpleasant images of herself constantly reflected in the attitudes of those closest to her have prevented the development of healthy self-esteem. In order to maintain internal balance in the face of the catastrophic ego threats to which she was exposed, she initiated restitutive maneuvers and built a social façade which required her constant preoccupation. The ego defenses resorted to included denial, affective withdrawal, dissociative and psychophysiological reactions. When things got too much for her, these defenses failed and she acted out her impulses in illegitimate pregnancies or in suicidal attempts.

In a situation with so many odds against her, she has handled the blows with the only means she had learned from her parents and subculture. Throughout the uneven struggle, her stamina has been apparent in her maternal interests, in her academic success, and in her striving for self-enhancement.

At present, as the poignant memories of her unsavory past experiences fade, she is able to take a firmer hold on the present and to plan a better future for herself and her children.

Test Summary

A. Draw-A-Person Test Inquiry

Mrs. W. first drew a nondescript stick figure (Fig. 4–1), followed by the female (Fig. 4–2), and then the male (Fig. 4–3). She made these figures very methodically, drawing with slow, deliberate, light strokes of the pencil. During the initial as well as the terminal phases of drawing she made many remarks, and expressed embarrassment that she did not know what people looked like sufficiently to depict them graphically.

Inquiry

(Best Part?) Her face. (Why?) For looks (laughter).

(Worst Part?) Her leg. (Why?) Because it's burnt.

(Part Trouble?) No parts. (However, Mrs. W. continued to talk about her burned leg.)

(Think?) Getting out of this jail house, being a mother to her children and what's going to become of her children when they get grown. She's got five babies.

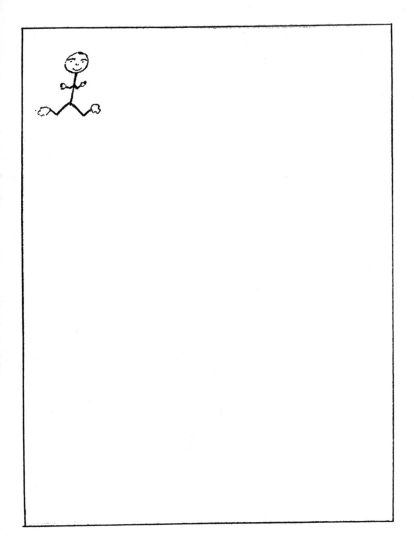

FIGURE 4–1. Draw-A-Person Test (Stick Figure).

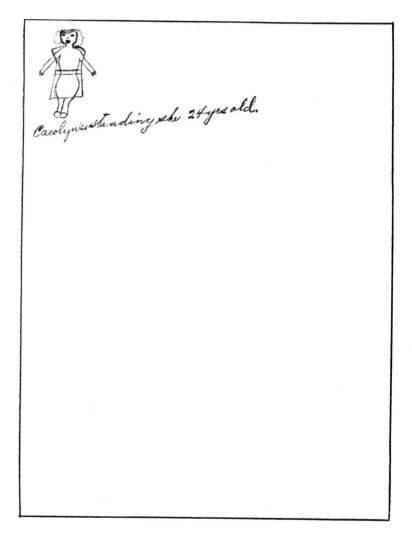

Caolyn is standing she 24 yrs old.

FIGURE 4–2. Draw-A-Person Test (Female).

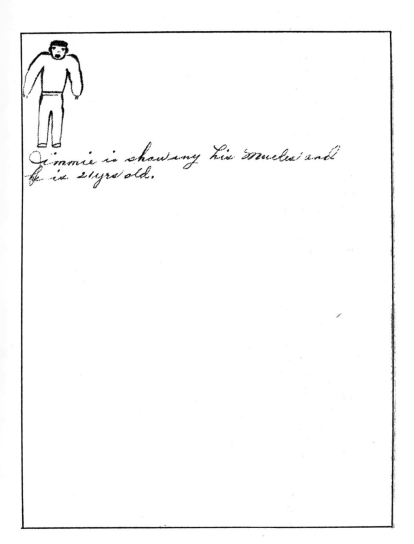

FIGURE 4–3. Draw-A-Person Test (Male).

(Feel?) Most of the time she feels all right . . . has some headaches. Every day you see her she is the same way.

(Happy?) Uh huh . . . by the expression on her face. She seems to have a smile on her face at times . . . no cares and no worries.

(Well?) To look at her she is. Never can tell what's wrong on the inside by looking on the outside.

(Need?) Her five babies.

(Feel People?) Same way. Always treats them the same. Always expects people to treat her nice because she treats them nice.

(You Feel Her?) I feel . . . no way. I could feel . . . she's just a nice person to my idea.

(Feel Most People?) Uh huh, because if people treat me the same way every time I see them, they're just nice people to me.

(How Describe Person?) Well, through all of her childhood up to her twenty-four years old she tried to be a lady. She has never been a bad girl and doesn't run around. She's not a perfect girl . . . but almost to the perfect (laughter).

Test Summary

B. Sentence Completion Test

1. *When she was completely on her own,* she left home.
2. *She often wished she could* go to a movie.
3. *It looked impossible so she* must stay home.
4. *I used to feel I was being held back by* my mother.
5. *She felt proud that she* could get out sometime.
6. *Her father always* was nice to her.
7. *A person who falls in love* never have a happy life.
8. *My first reaction to him was* when I first met him.
9. *Sometimes she wished she* was out of town.
10. *Usually she felt that sex* was just another adventure in life.
11. *I could hate a person who* thinks they are cute.
12. *Her earliest memory of her mother was* when she was a child.
13. *When people made fun of her, she* just cried.
14. *When I think back I am ashamed that* I have been wrong in life.
15. *When I have a decision to make* I make up my mind then.
16. *Love is* a wonderful thing if they love you.
17. *I dislike to* hate other people.
18. *I feel that people* should be the same, equal.
19. *After he made love to her, she* was very happy.
20. *If I can't get what I want* I have to do without.

21. *When I am criticized,* I think people should not.
22. *She felt she had done wrong when she* left home.
23. *She felt she could not succeed unless* she got her a job.
24. *I used to feel down in the dumps when* I had to let my kids go.
25. *Most of all I want* is for my 5 children to come home to me.
26. *My sexual desires* is to be with the man I love.
27. *At times she worried about* her children.
28. *She did a poor job because* she didn't know better.
29. *Most marriages* are not successful.
30. *When she does a poor job she* is just lazy.
31. *She felt blue when* her man left her.
32. *When I meet people I generally feel* good to see them.
33. *My first reaction to him was* when I first met him.
34. *I feel guilty about* this trouble because I done it.
35. *People in authority are* suppose to do there job.
36. *I felt happiest when* I was out on the outside.
37. *She boiled up when* she heard he had left her.
38. *When they told her what to do, she* just cried.
39. *Her greatest worry was* how she was going to make ends meet.
40. *Most women act as though* they are man crazy.
41. *When I feel that others don't like me* because I am not like them.
42. *More than anything else she needed* is her 5 children.
43. *I could lose my temper if* someone made me mad.
44. *I am afraid of* nothing.
45. *Whenever she was with her father she felt* the same as with her mother.
46. *When they told her to get out she* just pack up and left.
47. *When I think of marriage* it is not for me, I have learn my lesson.
48. *When she was with her mother she felt* like any other daughter.
49. *Most men act as though* they are woman crazy.
50. *I feel sad about* being here in jail.

Test Summary

C. RORSCHACH PROTOCOL

Response	*Inquiry*
CARD I. 24″ (A girl told me this was coming up.) 1. Could that be some water? Don't know what it looks like. To me it looks like some land on some water.	1. All around in here is land and on the sides starting from the white is water. (Q) From maps and things I've seen. As a map from pictures in books. (Q) Land and water combined. Shadings all blend in together.

Response	*Inquiry*
2. Then again, it looks like the form of the inside of a woman's body. Neck, arm, body and then on down in here. Stomach right in here. I don't know if this is a man or woman . . . lower part . . . insides of a man or woman . . . private parts. Up here is the lungs.	2. Well the shape . . . the way it's sloped out. Line is backbone going all the way through. X-ray of a person I guess because it's on this white board and grey and black color and see the shape and how it's made. A woman's private parts.

CARD II. 48″
I don't know what this is . . . I don't know what it looks like. That's one on me. It doesn't remind me of nothing.

(Q) Black and red ink.

CARD III. 29″
That don't either. I ain't never seen nothing that looks like this. Yet and still there is something in the world that looks like this.

I see some black ink and some red ink and some grey ink.

CARD IV. 18″
1. This looks like a flower . . . an orchid.

1. This up here and petals on the orchid. Shaped just like an orchid . . . and greyish black.

CARD V. 8″
1. And that looks like a bat.

1. The wings, head, and feet. (Q) As a picture . . . maybe because it was black.

2. And upside down it looks like a butterfly.

2. Comes out this way and wings are shaped like that and wings shaped like this. (Q) Picture of a butterfly. A black butterfly with grey fringes.

CARD VI. 30″
I don't see nothing in this one . . . I still don't see nothing.

It's just a black through the middle and greyish black on the sides.

CARD VII. 9″
1. You want to know the truth? This looks like a woman's vagina . . . vagina . . . to my eyesight. I don't know what that is around the sides.

1. The split and to tell you the truth that looks like the purl tongue up there. Women's legs and buttocks and she's got her legs open.

Response	*Inquiry*

CARD VIII. 12″
1. This looks like somebody's back . . . their spine . . . right in here.

2. That looks like a rat there . . . on both sides . . . that looks like rats.

1. Spine and backbone of a person . . . an X-ray. Small lines that you can see the bones coming out.
2. Head, tail, and legs. Looks like the rat on my little nephew's birthmark. (Q) As a picture . . . where the color blends into it . . . it looks like hair.

CARD IX. 32″
1. These here look like two men's heads in here.

1. Big heads and a mustache. Just a picture . . . mustache stands out . . . fringes for the hair.

CARD X. 35″
I don't see nothing on here . . . just a blank but different colors.

I don't see nothing on that but different colors: blue, yellow, orange, pink, green, and then a sort of purple.

5

"Color Conflict" as a Defense

Howard E. Mitchell

AN INTRODUCTION TO EDDIE

There appears to be merit in introducing Eddie in the same sequence that we met him at the clinic where he sought treatment. The content of his initial contact points up the conflict over his ethnic group identification. It also gives us the first clue to the relationship between his color conflict and certain unconscious personality dynamics; namely, the relatedness of his color conflict to his dependency-independency problem manifested in his need to be different, to be "an individual," and to achieve.

FIRST IMPRESSION. In February 1947, Eddie, a tall, lean, dark-skinned, twenty-three-year-old Negro, appeared in the clinic without an appointment and demanded to be seen immediately by the intake social worker. Although receiving compensation for a service-connected psychoneurotic condition, he requested medical attention, stating that he did not understand why the physician had referred him to a psychiatric service. He also told the intake worker that he was attending school and had absented himself because of his illness and would not be able to keep an appointment the following week. In order to clarify the type of treatment offered by the clinic and to better understand what Eddie was seeking, he was seen as soon as possible.

When it was pointed out to him that the clinic offered psychological help to which he was entitled, he stated bluntly that what he wanted was medical help for his gastritis. He resisted an orientation toward psychological help saying, "My idea of psychiatry is to be treated like an individual. In the Army the psychiatrists just herded the men through." As the intake worker reacted to this with further structuring of the clinic's functioning, he became less defensive and began to listen. He then admitted a problem of nervousness. In eloquent language he spoke of often wondering how much of his problem was due to his basic individuality and how much to a superimposed nervousness. Continuing, he expressed concern over possessing a violent temper and being difficult to get along with. He was going with a young woman and wanted to marry her but wondered if he should, since he did not know if his interpersonal difficulties reflected his illness or were "a part of my basic character."

Just when he was becoming more amenable to psychological help, however, he again mobilized his ego defenses, telling the social worker, "I guess these things aren't too important; I'd just like to see a psychiatrist because I'm curious about them." The intake worker informed Eddie that curiosity was not a sufficient basis on which to make a psychiatric contact. He then decided that he would go back to the Medical Division of the Veterans Administration and seek medical help for his gastric condition. His negativism at this point led him to remark that he was getting "the run around like in the Army." The social worker, perhaps in her own defense, called attention to the fact that he must have felt differently at one time about the military service because she noticed on a biographical data sheet before her that he had enlisted in the service. This triggered considerable feeling.

COLOR SENSITIVITY. He grimaced as he stated how disappointed he had been about his service experience. He went on to say that he had completed high school in 1942 and desired more education. He had had a little training as a civilian worker with the Signal Corps in radio and radar and enlisted because "there were so few Negroes in the field, and I thought I would have a chance to do something constructive." His initial disappointment was his assignment to the field artillery rather than the Signal Corps. A more serious disappointment was that the army destroyed his pride. He could no longer be an individual. He felt unwanted and completely out of place. Eddie commented that people with low-grade intelligence make the best soldiers. He was too aware of what was going on relative to army policy, particularly as it related to Negro troops, to be satisfied with conditions. Therefore, he could not be a good soldier. "Anyway," he remarked, "a good soldier in my outfit was an 'Uncle Tom' Negro—that I could never be!"

The social worker commented upon the intensity of his feeling about color differences. Eddie continued on this theme, stating that he could never learn to be servile to anyone and perhaps this was the reason he had had difficulty "soldiering in the South." "I am an individualist who can never conform to anything which is alien to me or wrong," he declared. His early experiences in the white community had not prepared him for the racial intolerance to which he was subjected in the army: "It was more than I could bear."

Despite considerable ventilation with apparently good affect, he did not decide to accept psychological help at this time. The clinic did not hear from him until twenty-eight months later. Then he called requesting treatment, saying, "I am disgusted with everything."

"Return engagement." A different intake worker saw Eddie at this time. She immediately acknowledged his previous contact. In response he stated that he had been receiving medical help for his gastritis, but he was convinced that he needed additional help of a psychological nature. He had been talking over his problems with friends but this was not satisfactory. In fact he had not found them trustworthy. Since his initial contact he had married the young woman to whom he referred during that interview. She was currently his "sounding board." He alluded here to experiencing some marital discord and without further elaboration blurted out, "I am tired of fighting people and situations, I need help."

From the above content he again began discussing his army career. He spoke of how he had been regarded as a trouble maker, because he had beliefs and ideals "that I stood up for." He wanted to be regarded as a person, not a Negro, in the army. This he had found impossible. The social worker picked this up and led him into his anxiety about being regarded as a distinctive individual needing help, as a patient—not a *Negro* patient. He admitted that this concerned him. He questioned, on the other hand, whether any white therapist could "be so objective as to know what I experience as a Negro?" Following more ventilation and clarification he indirectly returned to the racial theme. His inability to gain employment because of racial discrimination had been the circumstance that had brought him back to the clinic at this time.

Since his last contact Eddie had completed a four-year course in industrial designing. Nevertheless, when he sought employment in the field in which he had been trained, he met rebuff after rebuff "because I'm a Negro," he explained. In desperation he had finally accepted a position as a postal clerk. This job offered no satisfactions—only the security of a weekly pay check. His pay check, however, was smaller than that of his professionally employed wife, and he had misgivings about this. The matter that disturbed him most was that racial discrimination had upset his timetable. He had fantasied rapid advancement in his chosen field and, after gaining experience and financial resources, establishing his own business. He hated being slowed down; after all, he planned to retire from his own business at age fifty!

EDDIE ACCEPTS HELP. Eddie left the above interview still displaying marked ambivalence toward treatment, although he accepted an appointment for a neuropsychiatric screening examination. He kept this appointment but broke the one scheduled for psychological studies recommended by the neuropsychiatrist. When the intake social worker contacted him subsequently about his intentions regarding treatment he kept questioning "whether treatment can help me so long as I can do nothing about the situation." The latter referred to his inability to secure gainful employment in his chosen field because of racial discrimination. With the aid and support of the intake social worker he finally was able to undertake the psychological examination, remaining, however, somewhat fixed upon the racial theme as the source of his difficulties.

DIAGNOSTIC STUDIES

THE NEUROPSYCHIATRIC EXAMINATION. For the most part the neuropsychiatric examination report covered historical material that we shall report in greater detail elsewhere in this paper. The screening neuropsychiatrist saw Eddie as "a slender dark-complexioned, asthenic looking young Negro male who was somewhat uneasy at first, as if unable to take it for granted that we are truly interested in him." The report went on to say, "Later in the hour he relaxed and his guarded sensitive attitude diminished. Intelligence seems better than average. He brought out some objections to psychotherapy, but after a short discussion readily agreed to it. Diagnostic Impression: Anxiety reaction; Recommendations: Individual psychotherapy; prognosis fair."

THE PSYCHOLOGICAL EXAMINATION. The psychological test battery consisted of the Rorschach, Stein Sentence Completion, and Bender Gestalt tests. The examiner had intended to administer additional tests in a later session but Eddie canceled this appointment.

The psychological report summary pointed out that his capacity for intellectual functioning was superior, although emotional disturbances tended to reduce his efficiency to average. This is evidenced by his Rorschach variable form-level, his good "originals," and the variety of content (Test Summary A). It was also indicated by his generally good achievement on the Bender Gestalt, marred only by over-stroking of lines and erasures (Fig. 5–1). Moreover, in the words of the examiner, "One of Eddie's crucial problems is his desire for status which leads to over-intellectualizing and being unrealistically ambitious and grandiose in his undertakings." Concerning the latter, witness response I—1 on the Rorschach, a "gymnastic pyramid," and the disproportionate W to M ratio, which is 33:7. Also note the large numbers of Sentence Completion responses (Test Summary B) referring to being successful, items 50, 56, 96; having high standards, items 59, 75, 83; and working and striving to achieve, items 1, 5, 17, 26, 27, 33, 44, 45, 49, 50, 64, 66, 69, 71. Moreover, the frequent reference to clothing percepts and art forms in his Rorschach protocol responses I—4, II—5, IV—5, VII—5, VIII—6, IX—2, X—2, 8, suggest an effeminately oriented sensitivity to external social phenomena in general.

An apparent reality factor seems to be that such sense of status that he has been able to achieve is frequently destroyed. This is evidenced in Sentence Completion responses 9, 30, and 32 which point up his sensitivity to racial discrimination. Hence, he aspires to be his own boss, work independently, and make a unique contribution. His protocols reveal considerable anxiety, tension, and hostility, some of which is attached to his own problem of status and some of which is free-floating. The latter seems to stem from two sources, rejection in early life with a sense of isolation and coldness, and severe sex role difficulty with women over his own potency.

His interpersonal difficulties are pointed up in the frequent use of distance mechanisms in the Rorschach such as a ceremonial mask, IX—2, comics, IX—3, cartoons, VII—1, and silhouettes, IX—5. The hostility he feels when his narcissistic needs are not satisfied in human relationships is suggested by the fighting buffalos, V—5, the turkeys pecking at each other, V—4, as well as the three anxiety-laden references to fire, II—7, IV—3, V—3.

The patient's sex role difficulties are not only apparent in the aforementioned references to women's clothing but are manifested generously in other Rorschach responses.

For example, in II–7, he perceives the female in the lower red detail; in II–4 the animal has its hind legs cut off; in VII–6, the snow is dirty; and in VII–5 he sees a zipper in the "vaginal" area.

Drawing heavily upon the patient's behavior in the testing situation, the examiner stated further in the psychological report:

> He is dependent, but fears rejection to the extent that he has difficulty entering relationships. However, his ability for rapport is good; some insight is present and one may look for improvement if a good relationship can be established. Clearly this man requires a great deal of acceptance. He must feel sure of the interest of the therapist before such a relationship can be established. Uncovering therapy if begun slowly should be beneficial.

HIS EARLY ENVIRONMENT

FROM SHELTER TO "JUNGLE." As early as the second therapy hour one began to appreciate the derivation of Eddie's marked status striving and its relationship to his color conflict. However, one began to appreciate the bearing of cultural factors upon his emotional problems in listening to his account of the character of his environment during his formative years.

The patient, an only son and the younger of two siblings, was born in Philadelphia in 1924. Eddie's home up to age ten was in an apartment provided by a large hospital where his father served as custodian. His memories of this environment are mostly of his running errands for the professional personnel of the hospital, being given gratuities by them, observing the important contribution they were making to humanity, and becoming determined that he too would "amount to something." These accounts of his early life reflect isolation from the Negro community. He attended a school in which the majority of the pupils were white, as well as all the teachers. There was little contact with the Negro community. On infrequent occasions his family attended a Negro protestant church although he described his mother as being "as religious as they come."

There was little time for play; in Eddie's words, "There were too many interesting things going on in the hospital that I could look at and learn from, to be worrying about playing around—besides I was interested in making a buck when I could." This life he professed was satisfying to him. From it he learned those typically middle-class values and aspirations which he holds in high esteem. Suddenly at age ten this world came to an end. He was thrust into the strange, foreign world of a Negro ghetto. "Into a jungle," was the phrase he used to describe this new environment.

His father had bought a restaurant on a highly commercialized street in a thickly populated Negro community. He moved his family from the protective custody of the hospital to an apartment above his eating establishment. Eddie recalled being terrified by his Negro classmates. He had to pay for his safe custody to and from school with pastry from his father's restaurant. He also recalled having the onset of his stomach symptoms at this time. For relief he would return to the hospital and some of the doctors would give him free medication and attention.

His mother had objected to their moving from the hospital and after one year, "sent us to live with her sister in New Jersey while she went to work." "Mom was not going to see us kicked around," Eddie said. His mother after one year rented a house in a respectable, lower-middle-class Negro community and sent for Eddie and his sister. It is significant in terms of the fund of hostility built up toward the father that the patient stated in unfolding this part of his history, "My father came to live with us after he decided he was no good in business. Everyone but himself could have told him he was going to flop." There followed a tirade of feeling that a Negro is foolish in establishing any business in a Northern urban community that is totally dependent upon Negro consumers because they are unreliable, unpredictable, and economically unstable since the white boss controls their purse-strings.

Eddie lived with his parents in his new home until he enlisted in the army in 1944 at age twenty. He completed high school satisfactorily, participating on the track team and the debating club. Humorously, he remarked that he got his first track work running from "those guys in that place where we used to live." Debating was interesting to him because "I get pleasure from challenging the accepted point of view." It was this kind of thinking that got him branded a radical in the army. His sister, the recipient of a scholarship to a teachers' college, was away attending school during this period. Eddie missed her companionship and counsel although he had many friends. Closer scrutiny revealed that, although he had many friends, these relationships were maintained at a distance. He spent the major part of his leisure time manipulating mechanical objects in a shop in the basement of his home.

MATERNAL DOMINATION.   Eddie described his family constellation as a matriarchy, with his mother in the dominant role as its moral backbone, reliable provider, and final judge. In fact, the only major decision he could recall "that she did not really make" had to do with his father's buying the restaurant and their moving. Even here she was ultimate judge and victor. And he never questioned that it might have been otherwise.

Throughout treatment Eddie was unable to admit that his mother had any human frailties. He spoke in glowing terms about her many sacrifices for him and his sister. She worked hard after the family's separation "to give us the best of things." Eddie recalled his mother staying awake all night to finish making a dress for his sister after working all day outside the home. He recalled her taking extra jobs so that she could buy him a particular tool that he needed for his work shop. He had little recollection of demonstrations of affection in a close manner from his mother toward either him or his sister. By contrast, he recalled being embarrassed by his mother's sister "who was always slobbering over you —I'm glad Mom wasn't like that," he would remark. Psychodynamically he felt a sense of deprivation here with some resultant resentment. On the other hand, the strict discipline and firm hold that his mother exerted developed a rigid superego that would not tolerate any criticism of her.

It is significant that misbehavior was continually interpreted by his mother in racial terms. When either he or his sister did anything wrong they were told they were acting according to the white man's stereotype of the Negro. This was often carried to extremes. He told of an occasion on which he received a birthday gift from one of the white physicians at the hospital. The gift was a kite which he assembled and enjoyed flying the afternoon it was given to him. When his mother came home from work, she severely criticized him for not having immediately written a note of appreciation in his best fourth-grade penmanship. According to her, Eddie was acting "just like a nigger" in being so ungrateful.

WEAK FATHER.   Eddie's father was described as a slightly built, dark-skinned man who was largely self-taught, with little formal schooling. "He attempted to be strong willed," Eddie stated, "but was always yielding to some temptation." By this Eddie meant that his father could be easily tempted by the dictates of others and "always owed somebody something." This fact had a marked impact on Eddie's feelings about his interpersonal relationships. In treatment he had difficulty accepting the concept of "a normal amount of dependency" on others. Being dependent meant "being weak and I've seen what that did to Dad . . . I'll never be satisfied until I'm my own boss."

Apparently the father was only remotely sensitive to his son's growing needs. For the most part he was busily engaged in fighting for his own autonomy from his wife, who adopted the dominant role in the family. Once his independent business venture failed, he returned to the family a beaten man. He turned almost completely to activities outside the home. When infrequently home he sternly reprimanded Eddie for the slightest transgression. By such criticism he offered little chance for his son to develop a good identification with him and helped instill a deep feeling of inadequacy in the boy.

From Eddie's fourteenth to eighteenth year his father contributed less and less to the financial support of the family. His parents began to have frequent arguments in the presence of Eddie and his sister. His mother finally openly accused her husband of supporting other women which he first denied but later admitted. During this time the father was employed as a chauffeur by the owner of an exclusive women's apparel shop. A few months before Eddie's enlistment in the service his father was apprehended for stealing clothing and giving it to one of his mistresses. When he would not disclose the woman's identity, charges were pressed. He was found guilty and served two years of his six-year sentence. It would appear that this criminal behavior served to focus the hostility Eddie felt toward his father.

Eddie made it clear that his father changed a great deal on his return home from prison. He was more appreciative of his son's needs and interested himself in some of his activities, attempting to make up for lost ground. Moreover, he was no longer brusque, stern, and critical of Eddie.

SISTER'S COMPANIONSHIP. If there was any one member of his family toward whom Eddie felt a close emotional relationship, it was his sister, Rebecca, who was four years his senior. She was his confidante, supporter, ego ideal, and protector during childhood. In a number of ways she also assumed the maternal role in the mother's absence. He frequently recalled Rebecca's "keeping me from getting mauled that year we lived above the restaurant."

He had some envy of her academic attainments, but for the most part her scholastic success only served to heighten his already lofty aspirations. His mother used his sister's accomplishments as a yardstick to measure the boy's attainments.

Eddie missed Rebecca's companionship when she left home to attend a teachers' college after receiving a scholarship. He particularly missed her counsel during those trying days when their father got into difficulty, and Eddie subsequently decided to leave home and enlist in the service. Toward the end of therapy he often wondered "whether I would have run away if Becky had been around."

MILITARY SERVICE

INITIAL DISAPPOINTMENT. For Eddie, leaving home and going into the service represented running from one hostile, threatening environment into another. When his father was apprehended and convicted it was a tremendous blow to his pride. He felt socially disgraced. He was more consciously concerned with the probable effect of these events upon his further education and the achievement of already fixed vocational goals than upon any other aspect of his living. Therefore, he joined the Signal Corps because it promised rapid advancement "without questions being asked as to what my father did, or the kind of work he was in, as I'd have to state on a college application blank."

It was true "Uncle Sam" did not ask Eddie many questions when he enlisted. He was not even asked whether he wanted to remain in the Signal Corps but was immediately shipped to the artillery! As with most disappointments, he interpreted this assignment in racial terms—"No Negro got what he asked for in the army . . . they sent all of us to do the menial jobs, then couldn't understand when we would object. You had to be a dumb, ignorant Negro reared in Mississippi or Georgia to take the crap they dished out."

LATER RESENTMENT. He resented his assignment to a Negro outfit and he resented being stationed in the deep South. In many ways he relived his experiences of the year above the restaurant. He felt out of place, misunderstood, and unable to communicate with other Negro soldiers. Increasingly, he withdrew to himself and exerted a great deal of effort to achieve sergeants' stripes in the communications section of his artillery unit. His principal motivation was that sergeant status would permit him to have private quarters in the barracks away from the "constant swearing, playing-the-dozens, and gambling of those Uncle-Toms." He eventually lost his stripes after a series of run-ins with his company commander. It was significant that he talked about this officer in much the same terms as he talked about his father. They both represented inadequate authoritative figures who leaned too heavily on others and when they tried to act independently, failed miserably. His service experience not only frustrated his aspirations (hence his repressed dependency needs) but served to focus his hostility toward male authority and heighten his anxiety about his color problem.

After losing his stripes in September 1944, he gained the reputation of being a "guard-house lawyer" as he advised the other soldiers of their rights. With some pride he stated, "It got to be poison to be seen talking with me." His gastric symptoms became prominent and he was hospitalized on two occasions for gastro-intestinal studies. He happily returned to civilian life with an honorary discharge on October 22, 1944.

POST SERVICE

Eddie returned home to live with his parents following service. His mother made every effort to give him all that he had missed in the two years he had been away from her in the service. His father, then on parole, stayed around home "more often than I could ever recall, worked hard, and stayed out of trouble." His sister had completed graduate work and was teaching in a Negro secondary school in another Eastern city. After a few weeks of taking things easy, he took a civilian job with the Signal Corps. "Mom kept after me to use the G. I. Bill so I enrolled in a course in industrial designing." He completed this four-year course before entering treatment in 1949. After completing school he married a young woman he had known since high school, following a brief engagement.

Unable to find employment in industrial designing he took a job as a postal clerk. At the time he began psychotherapy he would have recurrent anxiety attacks every time he had to take the periodic postal schema examinations. One of his first steps toward realistic vocational adjustment followed the uncovering that he had an unconscious need to fail these postal examinations. He could not quit the job for fear of retaliation and ridicule from both his wife and his mother. Prior to the above disclosure he defensively expressed his difficulties at the post office in racial terms. "What's the use of trying to get ahead, only the white guys get the breaks," he would remark. The continued pressure from his mother to get ahead, combined with the fact that his wife enjoyed professional employment, enhanced his fantasies about attaining distant and unrealistic personal and vocational goals. He rationalized that all his dreams would come true if he were not a Negro!

COLOR, AND CONFLICT WITH WIFE. Increasingly, his wife became the focus of displaced hostility felt toward his mother. He resented the fact that she did not compulsively plan for their future as he did. Finally he asked her to leave him in March, 1951. He projected that she obviously did not need him because she was not going along with the plans he had made. For the most part she was not dependable "because like so many Negroes her parents didn't teach her a damn thing about planning for the future." One bone of contention between Eddie and his wife was that she did not enthusiastically endorse his plans to build a home in a somewhat remote and undeveloped suburb about which he excitedly remarked, "there are no Negroes for five miles." No matter what the issue in his marriage or in his work, it was colored by his defensiveness over his minority group status.

STRATEGY OF HANDLING EDDIE'S COLOR CONFLICT

Prior to Eddie's assignment to the writer for psychotherapy he had been treated for six interviews by a neuropsychiatric resident who, to both professional colleagues and patients, proudly professed his Southern heritage in a marked Southern drawl. When this resident left the clinic, the writer volunteered to treat Eddie. Although the resident reported that his brief contact with Eddie had yielded an amicable relationship, the writer disagreed with his concentration upon Eddie's racial conflict as he attempted to "sell himself" to the patient. It seemed probable that his emotional disturbance was not caused by his color conflict. His color conflict represented a medium through which he identified with his mother and expressed deep resentment toward his rather inadequate father. It seemed best to deal with his color problem in the context of his other ego defenses.

Other team members readily agreed with this assignment. They expressed the opinion that "Eddie needs a Negro therapist who he feels can empathize with him." There was little apparent realization of other salient factors warranting consideration. For example, the factor of intra-color conflict among Negroes might have argued against such an assignment. This dark-skinned Negro might have been more resistant to being treated by a light-skinned Negro therapist than by a white therapist.

Contrary to his initial ambivalence he was a faithful and meaningful participant in the therapeutic relationship. He was seen for a total of one hundred and four treatment hours from January, 1950 to August, 1953. Until April, 1952 these treatments were on a weekly basis; then he was seen every three or four weeks. The patient's wife was seen by the team social worker for twenty hours during 1951 when the focus of his problem centered upon his relationship with his spouse.

THERAPEUTIC CHANGES. As therapy progressed and centered upon his basic dependency-independency conflicts significant changes occurred in his personal living. As he became cognizant of his deeper problems he began to take realistic steps toward his goals and aspirations. There was increasingly less about his color conflict as he learned to transfer his dependency from his mother to his wife. With her approval he quit the postal job again, looked for a job in industrial designing and was immediately hired. He had not been on the job many weeks before another concern offered him employment directly in the area of his interest and skill.

His characterological pattern was not altered relative to his compulsive traits, for he worked week ends and holidays to build his home. To his surprise his spouse suddenly became dependable and shared the labor and frustrations of their mutual enterprise.

When Eddie was last contacted, in October, 1956, he and his wife were living comfortably in their new home, were the proud parents of a seven-months-old son, and Eddie had begun his own business which he operated on week ends. To a joking inquiry whether he still planned on retiring at age fifty, he replied, "I don't think so, I'm having too much fun at my work."

AFTERTHOUGHT

In working up this case, the writer was able to find no reference to Eddie's color conflict in the closing summary of notes covering the last forty treatment hours, in marked contrast to the content of his initial contacts. This left him with the feeling that to some extent the strategy conceptualized had proved effective in handling Eddie. It also left him wondering whether color conflict is ever a *basic* determiner of emotional disorders.

Test Summary

A. RORSCHACH PROTOCOL

CARD I. 9″

Response	*Inquiry*
1. ∧ Looks like a gymnastic pyramid to me. An inverted V. W M H O	1. Location: Whole Seems as though the 2 basic figures standing on one leg. Persons on shoulders doing hand stands. On top, 2 more.

Response	*Inquiry*

2. ∧∨ Possibly a monument of some sort.

W   F   Arch

2. Location: Whole
Two perspectives. Cantilever ledge. These levels with flowers of green and archways. Has loose form.

3. ∧ > Reflection of a dog looking at himself in the water.

W   Fk,FM   A

3. Location: Whole
Ear, back haunched. Nose here. Probably has mouth open. Background of foliage.
(Q. What suggests foliage?) Difference in color suggests it.

4. ∧∨ <∧ >∨∧ A headpiece—costume headpiece.

W,S   F   Cg

4. Location: Whole
Around forehead. Stones or sequins.
(Q. Where are stones?) They are these spaces.

CARD II. 5″

1. ∧ Two bears—even two dogs smelling one another.

WX   FM   A   P

1. Location: All except upper and lower red detail.
Shape. Front curved like dog's paw.

2. ∨ Butterfly.

W   FC   A

2. Location: Whole
Antennae. General shape of wing.
(Q. Anything else about it?) The shape and the color.

3. ∧∨ > Scared cat—frightened cat.

D   FM   A

3. Location: Right half of main detail.
Way the back is arched. Front paws forward gives impression scared.

4. > Animal with head, looks like hind legs been cut off or something.

dr   CF   A, Blood

4. Location: Rare detail encompassing large portion of main detail and red portions.
Color of red suggests blood. Upper part of leg and again color suggests blood.

5. ∧∨ Possibly could be a print on a fabric.

W   F   Art

5. Location: Whole
What we call in art a "free-form." Rough outline.

Response	*Inquiry*

6. ∧ Part in here a geometric form with a black background or . . .

S   FC′   Art

6. Location: Center white space; the color.

7. ∨ One of those old oil lamps with flame coming out the top.

S,D   mF,CF   Fire

7. Location: Center white space and lower red detail.
Shape of lamp. Different hues of red and around top perfect variations in the color of the flame and shape.

8. ∧ Possibly idea for redesigning water tank on top of building.

S   F   Arch

8. Location: Center white space. Shape.

CARD III. 24″

1. ∨ < ∨ Picture of fortune teller looking in crystal.

Ｗ×   M,Fc   H   P

1. Location: All grey-black portions.
Arms raised. Reflection of sunlight making this glow. Have on headdress.
(Q. Why fortune tellers?) Because of clothing. Color and detail in garments can't be seen.

2. ∨ A fly, face of a fly.

D   F   Ad

2. Location: Large, black detail of lower middle.
Large eyes, way they bulge on side of head.

3. ∧ Piece of crockery. Pottery. A free design on it.

W   F   Obj

3. Location: All grey-black portions.
Shape and free design. No color.

4. > Possibly a reflection of water in the lower half.

Ｗ×   Fk,C′   Ls

4. Location: All grey-black portions.
Like a mountain with snow on it.
(Q. You said snow?) The white suggests it and the variations in color gives 3 dimensions in shadows.

CARD IV. 6″

1. ∧ A big shaggy dog lying down. Ears flopping on one side.

W   FM   A

1. Location: Whole
Top of head and ears. Sides. Impression of upper part of legs. Front paws together.

Response	Inquiry

2. ⋁ Looks like head of a dog here.

W   F   A

2. Location: Whole
Ears, top of head.

3. ⟩ One half looks like big fire with smoke going up.

dr   mF,cF   Fire

3. Location: Left half of blot.
Smoke drifting in columns. Color gives feeling of gas or smoke, gets lighter and darker.

4. ⋀ Looks like person in elaborate costume, gown, or robe of some

W   M   H

4. Location: Whole
Head here, arms outstretched. As if in embroidery.
(Q. Why in embroidery?) It's the shape mainly.

5. ⋁ Again look like coat or garment being ripped apart. Split down center.

W   Fc   Cg

5. Location: Whole
Sleeves. Impression of inside the way it's lighter here and darker other places.

CARD V. 5″

1. ⋀⋁ Like a butterfly.

W   F   A   P

1. Location: Whole
Wings and antennae.

2. ⋀⟩⋀ Then top looks like one of those dancing costumes with heavy puff sleeves or fuzzy sleeves. A girl with headdress on.

W   F   H

2. Location: Whole
Sleeves, part of arm. Head and headdress.
(Q. You said puffed or fuzzy sleeves?) Shaped like that.

3. ⟩ This looks like fire and smoke.

dr   mF,cF   Fire

3. Location: Left half of blot turned sideways.
Flame licking up. Difference in density of color.

4. ⋁ Two turkeys or birds, one on each side, pecking at each other.

W   FM   A

4. Location: Whole
Fan tail, long neck. Mantle from chin not seen. Head arched to side.

5. ⋀ Buffalo been fighting and comes together. Two rams or deer or bulls.

W   FM   A

5. Location: Whole
It's the hind legs, front legs, hump in back and tail.

Response   *Inquiry*

CARD VI. 32″

I really don't get anything out of
this. Top could be design . . .

1. ❯∨❮ Then too, top part of bro-   1. Location: Whole
ken street light, gas light.   Outrigger for ladder, made of
                                        cast iron. Wick in cup like effect.
W   F   Obj   O   (Q. What helps to give impression
                                        of being made of cast iron and hav-
                                        ing a wick?) The general shape.

CARD VII. 8″

1. ∧ Like a cartoon of two kids   1. Location: Left half of blot.
dressed as Indians.   Feathers in heavy cropped hair,
                                        chins out. Holding their hands back
D   M   (H)   of body.

2. ∨ Here looks like two girls danc- 2. Location: Whole
ing. Holding something up. Idea   Shoulders, small wrist and has
they are doing modern, interpre-   wide, short skirt.
tive dancing.

W   M   H

3. ❯ Half of card looks like a cluster 3. Location: Left half of blot.
of clouds.   Variations in color give impres-
                                        sion of three dimensions or gas. And
D   KF   Cl   the shape helps.

4. ∧ Looks like two teen agers do-   4. Location: Whole
ing modern dance. Jitterbug or   Arms out, hair and body.
something.   (Q. What gives idea of hair?) The
                                        shape, swooped up.
W   M   H

5. ∨ Piece in here looks like zipper 5. Location: Dark center of bottom
off of a sweater.   D.
                                         Looks like the shape of a track
d   F   Cg   and slide with a hook.

6. ❮ Also looks like snow. Patches   6. Location: Whole
of snow on water. In gutter   Shape and variations in color sug-
somewhere, dirty, been laying on   gests dirt and three dimensions.
ground.

W   cF   Ls

7. ∨ Heavy shadows give form of   7. Location: Whole
three dimensions. That's the feel-

Response	*Inquiry*

ing I get—heavy shadows.

W   K   Cl

CARD VIII. 5"

1. ∧∨∧ Looks like head of some kind of an insect.	1. Location: Whole Impression mainly from eyes and nose.
W F Ad	
2. ∨ Like an orchid, probably coming apart.	2. Location: Whole Color and shape. Orchid color and forms.
W CF Pl	
3. < Looks like reflection of an animal crawling or walking on stones at the water side. Can see reflection.	3. Location: Whole Stones and animal here. Shape again and almost the direct same thing in reverse.
W FM,FK A P	
4. < Peach and strawberry ice cream. The coloring.	4. Location: Right half of lower red-orange detail. Color and shape.
D CF Food	
5. ∨ Some type of wild flower.	5. Location: Whole Color and shape.
W CF Pl	
6. ∧ Costume or some kind of headdress, like ladies' fabric, soft.	6. Location: Whole Comes to peak, shape. The color and shape.
W FC Cg	

CARD IX. 9"

1. ∧∨ Portion of a water coloring, colors run together and blend.	1. Location: Whole As if artist unable to control flow and amount of water—the way colors run together.
W CF Art	
2. ∧ Might look like ceremonial mask. Just head and shoulders of person wearing it.	2. Location: Whole Head piece over eyes. Light and dark variations suggest it.
W M,FC Hd, Mask	

Response	*Inquiry*

3. < Something from comics.

 ·D   F   (H)

3. Location: Right green detail.
Suggests cartoon shapes.

4. V > Here is a composite photo.
Eyes of an animal, herd of cat-
tle or sheep. Natural bridge.

  dr   FM,cF,FK A, N

4. Location: Inner center detail.
Spots like eyes. Darker part is
photo of bridge in shadow. The
color helps and the reflection in water. Herd going over bridge.

5. > Section here silhouette of man
with heavy mustache.

  D   F   Hd

5. Shape

CARD X. 6"

1. V Lot of wild flowers growing.

  W   CF   Pl

1. Location: Whole
Color and form of the whole card.

2. V Part of a musical show costume.

  D   Fc   Cg

2. Location: Left half of pink portion.
Shape and color.

3. ∧ Looks like nightmare to me.

  W   FC   A

3. Location: Whole
Shape and color. Bugs in a nightmare.

4. > A spider in here.

  D   F   A   P

4. Location: Outer blue detail.
Shape more than anything.

5. > Impression of a canary. The
yellow.

  D   CF   A

5. Location: Outer yellow detail.
Color. and the form.

6. V Also a caterpillar.

  D   FC   A   P

6. Location: Left half of lower
green.
Shape and color.

7. V A fantasy. Bugs are holding
all this up.

  D   FM   A

7. Location: The top middle portion and the pink detail.
Bugs standing on pole holding up
pink things.

8. ∧ Good print for woman's dress.

  W   CF   Art

8. Location: Whole
Color and shape.

RORSCHACH PROFILE

Total R = 53

W	33	M	7	H	6	F%	28
D	12	FM	8	Hd	2	A%	36
d	1	m	3	(H)	2	P	6
DdS	7	k	2	A	17	S	3
App:		K	2	Ad	2	Orig	2
W(D d DdS)							
				Art	4	SUM C	10
Seq:	Orderly			Arch	2	M:C	7:10
		F	15	Pl	3	W:M	33:7
		Fc	2	Cg	5		
		c	1	Fire	3		
		C¹	1	Ls	2		
		FC	4	Cl	2		
		CF	8	Food	1		
				Obj	2		

Test Summary

B. STEIN SENTENCE COMPLETION TEST

PART I

1. *Charlie was happiest when* he was busy.
2. *He liked nothing better than to* work with machines.
3. *John's wife* is a very nice person.
4. *Nothing annoyed Bob more than* a lot of people.
5. *Mike's fondest ambition* to work on a big construction job.
6. *When Frank saw his boss coming, he* stopped work.
7. *Bill got irritated when they* told him he didn't know what he was talking about.
8. *My greatest fear is* poverty.
9. *When told to keep in his place, Henry* moved.
10. *What Tom regretted most was* he left the job.
11. *I admire* a person who will try to create something different.
12. *Nothing made Harry more furious than* to be . . .
13. *Joe was uneasy because* he could help.
14. *John thought that his future* looked black.
15. *The fact that he failed* didn't stop him.
16. *A person's life* is his own to live.
17. *When he saw that the others were doing better than he, John* tried harder.
18. *Every time he wasn't invited, Ralph* laughed it off.

19. *As a child he* loved tools, machinery and drawing.
20. *I try hard* to make good.
21. *The war interfered with his plans for* going to school.
22. *Finding no one who could help him, Will* became disgusted.
23. *The main driving force in my life is* peace of mind.
24. *The thing which bothered Harry's conscience was* failure.
25. *Bud's family* is a grand group.
26. *On his evening off, Paul* liked to work on his hobby.
27. *Bob's defeat made him* work harder.
28. *I usually feel awkward when* praised.
29. *My standards are* too high.
30. *Nothing is so frustrating as* be refused a job.
31. *My lot in life* belong to Elaine.
32. *He was confused about* discrimination.
33. *Fred would do anything in order to* get that job.
34. *Joe feels that he suffers most from* frustration.
35. *The men under me* should always be considered.
36. *Bud would rather do without* than steal.
37. *After Bob left the interview, he thought* there was no problem.
38. *His father* was basically good.
39. *George was sorry after he* got angry with her.
40. *What they liked about him most was* his gift of gab.
41. *Whenever there was overtime work to be done, Bob felt* good.
42. *People think of me as* a darn fool.
43. *They made fun of his accent so Tom* never spoke in public.
44. *Bud could work best at* his own shop.
45. *I always wanted to be* my own boss.
46. *He is often at a loss when* Elaine is gone.
47. *He often thinks of himself as* too radical.
48. *When they said that it was dangerous, Bert* tried anyway.
49. *From past experience Bill learned that he* could work better alone.
50. *I take pains* with my work.

PART II

51. *John prefers the company of* a very few people.
52. *He didn't like Bill because he was* two faced and gushy.
53. *Dave felt that the men over him were* all right on a whole.
54. *The thing which got him into trouble was* the fact he questioned commands.
55. *It was irritating to be* questioned when right.
56. *Bill is afraid of* not being successful.
57. *His younger days* were happy.
58. *Roger would have done anything to forget the time he* spent in the Army.

59. *Others think my standards are* too high.
60. *What bothered Jack was their* false values.
61. *Jack really became angry when* she was stubborn.
62. *Charlie felt his acquaintances* cold.
63. *My family* is nice to me.
64. *When Dick failed the course he* took it over.
65. *My greatest worry is* failure.
66. *When luck turned against him Joe* kept trying.
67. *If I would only* . . .
68. *He went mad when* he failed.
69. *I often* dreamed of being my own boss.
70. *He is apt to complain about* carelessness.
71. *I dream a great deal about* my own business.
72. *His mother* work hard and need a rest.
73. *Discouragement made him* blue.
74. *Joe is most troubled by* failure.
75. *He made a point of* being first.
76. *If Fred could only* go.
77. *My philosophy of life is* a plain & simple life.
78. *The people who worked in Jerry's department* are good.
79. *Most of the time* there is nothing to do.
80. *He was dominated by* no one.
81. *My worst fault* wanted add things.
82. *When I have something to say and others are around* be considerate.
83. *I enjoy* finishing a good job.
84. *When they turned him down for the job, Bill* was depressed.
85. *Most people do not know that I* can do it.
86. *It is embarrassing* to her as well as myself.
87. *When they told him that the job may be too much for him, Donald* try anyway.
88. *The main thing in my life* is my wife.
89. *He thinks of himself as* being fair.
90. *When they laughed at Fred, he* laughed too.
91. *When they decided to put him under pressure, Frank* said nothing.
92. *I would rather* try than anything else.
93. *When the other men avoided him, Bob* ignored it.
94. *My greatest ambition is* research studio.
95. *I suffer most from* depression.
96. *I often think about how I* can succeed.
97. *The worst thing was* no money.
98. *I was happiest when* Elaine was happy.
99. *When he thought that the odds were against him, Bill* kept try.
100. *My goals* are a small home, two kids, and my own studio in the country.

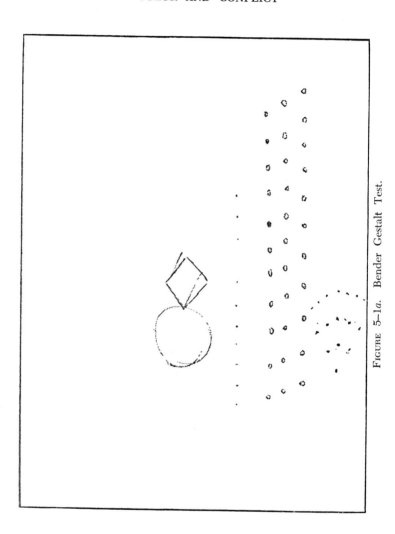

FIGURE 5–1a. Bender Gestalt Test.

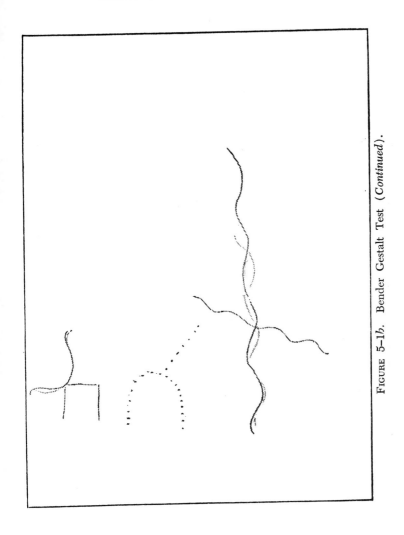

FIGURE 5-1b. Bender Gestalt Test (*Continued*).

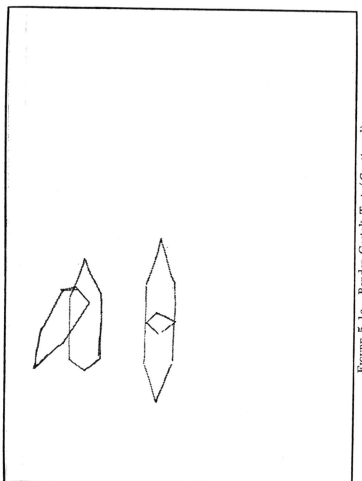

FIGURE 5-1c. Bender Gestalt Test (*Continued*).

Negro Postscript

In all three cases that we have studied, membership in the Negro minority has contributed to their difficulties, but in different ways. In Wendell, his original white identity, which was realistic in terms of the peculiar circumstances of his life, proved to be his mainstay through vicissitudes which would have disorganized a weaker ego. In Mrs. W. the situation was reversed insofar as she started out unwanted and was doubly rejected on account of having darker skin than the others in her family. In both cases, disciplinary and moral inconsistencies prevented the development of a consistent pattern of superego control. They depended heavily on denial as a defense, resorting to acting out when denial failed to hold their unruly impulses in check. Guilt feelings and intropunitive behavior also played an important part in Mrs. W.'s personality. The therapeutic problem for both was to improve the self concept so that the individual might develop more effective coping mechanisms and assume adequate social responsibility. For the boy an essentially intact but weakened ego needed to be shored up by helping him find a strong identity in his own ethnic ingroup. For the woman the task was the same, but there was less to build on in view of her negative core identification.

In Eddie's case, color conflict does not play the central role it does in the other two. His early experience, like that of Wendell, was in a protective Caucasian environment. Later, when he encountered discrimination, he did not internalize it but projected it instead, using "color" as a rationalization for failure of any kind. Therapy was directed toward uncovering this defensive mechanism and getting at the deeper problems of his ambivalent dependency on his dominating mother and his hostility toward his weak father. Even these "deeper" problems were to a certain extent a reflection of the ethnic subgrouping, inasmuch as the parents' partial sex role reversal is still a prevailing pattern among Negroes.

Although both Mrs. W. and Eddie have worked successfully with Negro therapists, the factor of ethnic similarity as such was not the most significant aspect of therapy. In fact, as Dr. Mitchell indicates, it can complicate such a situation by introducing *intra*racial tensions regarding skin color. It is the therapist's ability to get *under* the skin that is crucial to the success of the therapy! It was only in the case of Wendell that a Negro therapist seemed especially indicated because of his great need for good models to help him achieve his belated Negro identification.

PART III

AMERICA'S FIRST FAMILIES

Preview

America's "First Families" represent a wide cultural diversity alien to the American way of life! The vicissitudes of their tribal integrity have followed the vicissitudes of political change in the United States. Some Indian cultures have survived better than others and present their members with more consistent patterns to follow in modeling their personalities. Where the individual has found a good identity in his original culture, he is capable of articulating with the dominant one without feeling threatened by it. Where his basic identity is ambivalent, however, his integration with the main cultural stream is likely to be less smooth.

The three cases in this part—Ella, a woman of Negro-Indian mixture, Lola, a full-blooded Hopi girl, and John, a Navajo—point up some of these differences.[1]

---

[1] Some further discussion of Hopi and Navajo differences may be found in Georgene Seward, *Psychotherapy and culture conflict* (New York: The Ronald Press Co., 1956).

6

Role Confusion in a Negro–Indian Woman

Channing H. Orbach and *Carl H. Saxe*

Ella was born of a Negro father and an American Indian mother. In this mixed background and with the particular set of developmental experiences to which she was exposed, she found herself facing insoluble conflicts. In 1955 Ella recognized her need for professional help and came to a mental hospital.

All her life Ella had sought to acquire an identity, to achieve some sense of wholeness in her personality, but in 1955 the fragile boundaries of her ego gave way and what little identity she had was consumed in a schizophrenic holocaust.

THE ILLNESS

FIRST SIGNS. At the time of her admission to the hospital Ella was twenty-five years old. She had been struggling to hold herself together for two years prior to her hospitalization. Ella has always been a seclusive, withdrawn person who considers herself quite different from other people, especially her siblings. When she was not able to get along with others, she was inclined to blame herself. She has tended to be overconscientious in her work because of her feeling of racial inferiority and her need to prove that she is as good as white people in order to win their acceptance.

These personality traits were combined with a prominent ego-alien symptom—a lifelong darkness phobia, especially interesting in view of her uncomfortable identification with her Negro father.

Two years before her current hospitalization, while she was in the armed forces, she learned that her mother had been burned to death in an explosion of an oil stove. Following this event she developed a compulsion to count her fingers and other objects, and she began to have depressive feelings. She spent the final four months of her service career in a navy hospital. Following her discharge from the navy her symptoms gradually became more severe, and she toyed with the idea of doing away with herself by jumping in the ocean. Finally, she was admitted to a hospital on a voluntary basis.

IN THE HOSPITAL. Ella is a slender young woman with light brown skin. On superficial glance, one might easily mistake her for a Negro. However, she has the aquiline nose, high cheek bones, and straight black hair of her Indian forebears. Her face bears the scars of frequent bouts with acne, and she has a tendency to pick at it absentmindedly as she talks. Very soft spoken, she has a well-modulated voice and a vocabulary that shows her to be a person of above average intelligence. She is more literate than an abbreviated formal education would lead one to surmise. With the ward personnel who attempted to get to know her, she discussed "the meaning of life," the possibility of reincarnation, and other broad philosophical questions, all of which she recited in a somewhat dreamy, preoccupied manner.

Ella was invited to join a therapy group. She was quite fearful at first, needing much encouragement and reassurance. She sat tensely and rigidly in a chair next to the door but was extremely attentive to what was going on, occasionally startling the other members with a pungently pertinent comment. When the conversation became too upsetting for her, she would flee to the safety of her ward. After a while, she gave up the group entirely.

On the ward one would be most apt to find Ella sitting near the entry. She was not prone to initiate any contacts with the other patients, but she was responsive, articulate, and cordial when others talked to her. She would have nothing to do with ward activities, but other than this she presented no great problem of ward management. She told her doctor that she had a recurrent dream of riding in an elevator, the door of which would always shut before she could get out. She also told him about her compulsion to count her fingers, the squares in the linoleum, the number of chairs in the room, the days on the calendar, and anything else that came to her attention.

Unlike many mental patients, Ella recognized that she was mentally ill and needed help and protection. But she also had a need to run away from the discomfort of facing her problems. Her behavior toward the doctor, much like her behavior in group therapy, pointed up the two horns of her dilemma. She would make angry demands of him that he make her well, while at the same time demanding that he discharge her from the hospital. Much as she wanted freedom, she paradoxically refused to be transferred from the maximum observation ward (to which all newly admitted patients go) to a ward where she could have had considerably more freedom as well as more responsibility for her own care. After four months of wavering, she left the hospital without permission. Three months later it was learned that she had been admitted to another hospital in a state nearer her home.

THE FAMILY BACKGROUND

Information regarding her parents and her own early history was obtained from Ella herself. We may regard it as reasonably reliable, albeit sketchy.

NEGRO FATHER. Ella's father was a Negro from New Orleans who can also claim French blood in his background. He was only semiliterate, having but a third-grade education. He has worked hard and steadily as an unskilled la-

borer in the same cement plant for most of his working life
and even during the Depression succeeded in making an
adequate living. He spent his own early life in the deep
South, moving North presumably to find work. Here he
met Ella's mother and married her, in the face of serious
opposition between the two families over the marriage.

INDIAN MOTHER. Ella's mother as a member of one of
the Iroquois nations spent most of her early life on an Indian reservation where the primary occupational activity
was farming. In contrast to the father, she had attended
college and tended to look down her nose at her husband,
both for his ethnic background and for his lack of education. Her own education, however, did not free her entirely from the superstitions of her ancestors, and she told
Ella stories of magical rites and of spirits, good and evil.
While Ella feels that she rejected these ideas, the magical
thought processes involved in the ideas may well have provided the groundwork for her own pathological thinking.

Both parents drank excessively. Ella recalls week-end-
long drunken parties at their house which often disturbed
her. Despite the drinking and the ethnic, socioeconomic,
and educational tensions between her parents, the marriage
must have established some sort of equilibrium, because it
lasted for twenty-five years until the mother's death in 1953.

PERSONAL HISTORY

LONELINESS. Ella stated that she was the youngest of
five children, having one sister and three brothers. At an
early age she found herself estranged from her siblings who
used to tease her and call her an "orphan" because she was
the only one who resembled their father. All through her
childhood she had the feeling that she was "outside the
family" and that she did not know who she was. She was
unhappy a good deal of the time and even as a child often
wished for death. During girlhood, her favorite activity was
that of going off into the woods by herself and absorbing

the atmosphere of the trees, wind, and flowers. In lieu of human companionship she would take her dog along for company, and it would seem that she related to him as if he were human. In her loneliness and bewilderment she turned to reading, and also to religion, making a real effort to accept the church completely. With her brothers and sister, she attended parochial school and got along very well with the nuns, whose favor she curried by being obliging and ingratiating.

While she was apparently successful in gaining limited amounts of affection from the nuns, she was unsuccessful where her mother was concerned. She vividly recalls one occasion when her mother attempted to be affectionate. During one of the week-end drinking parties her mother got drunk and then became sick, a rather common occurrence in the household, and one which disgusted Ella. On this occasion she had to take care of her mother who wanted to put a "hand on her" and caress her. Ella ran away in terror and hid. She still recalls this event with anger and disgust.

ALLIANCE WITH FATHER. Partly because of her physical resemblance to her father's side of the family, Ella found herself forced into an alliance with her father.[1] He grew to depend on her to help him with reading and "figuring things out." Ella was sufficiently identified with her mother's educational values to resent him for his meager schooling, but despite this feeling she sided with him against her mother and her siblings in family arguments. It is probable that she experienced more warmth in this relationship than in any other, but the price she had to pay was a stiff one. She could no longer make even a pretense at claiming any status in the family, but had to occupy the same lowly position that her father did. She was ostracized, frozen out of the select inner circle of the family.

---

[1] This alliance with her father occurred despite the traditional dominance of the woman in Iroquois society.

Although Ella never completely renounced her educational values, she left high school before graduation and obtained a job in a factory. In this capacity, too, she felt that she was only a second-class citizen in the family. While her siblings were free to work or not as they saw fit, her mother expected her to contribute to the support of the family, as her father did.

ESCAPES FROM HOME. Ella made two abortive attempts to carve out her own destiny in her earlier years. At age twelve she ran away from home. The exact reason for this is not known, although according to the patient, it was an attempt to get away from her father particularly. At sixteen she ran away again. This time it was because she was afraid her father would find out about her relationship with a boy. She found a job as a nurse in a family where there were children. Her father called the police to search for her. She was found and brought back, but she said she felt like a criminal thereafter.

For the next seven years Ella worked steadily at the factory job mentioned above, resenting her mother all the while for her preferential treatment of the siblings in the matter of contributing to the family support. Finally she saw another opportunity to get away from home. She joined the navy and made a fair adjustment for the first three months until her mother's untimely and violent death.

RETURN TO FATHER. After her medical discharge from the navy, Ella came to California to live with her sister, who had married a Negro and had five children. While she was living with her sister, her brother-in-law introduced her to a Negro friend of his. He was ten years her senior and had been married previously. After a one-month courtship they were married, but the marriage lasted only fifteen stormy days. They bickered constantly over the question of who should handle the money. Her husband had had his "fingers burned" in his previous marriage when his first wife had absconded with all their common funds, and he was determined that this time he would remain in control of the finances. Ella on the other hand, was just as determined that she would be the manager, and resented being punished for her predecessor's behavior. She had hoped that this marriage would settle once and for all the question as to whether she was Negro or Indian. She found, however, that her husband would not accept her as a Negro, and she was again confronted with her lifelong dilemma.

The marriage ended on New Year's Eve when they went out with her sister and brother-in-law. Her husband got drunk and insisted that they "do the town" together. She refused and he slapped her. Her brother-in-law stepped into the argument, whereupon her husband became so angry that he walked out. The next day Ella left California to return to her father in the East.

BACK IN CALIFORNIA. She kept house for her father for a brief period until her sister, who was about to give birth to her sixth child, called upon Ella to come back to California to help her with the other children. She obtained a job in an aircraft plant where her feelings of racial inferiority and her compulsive character traits drove her to make an outstanding work record. She volunteered for all sorts of extra work and was extremely meticulous in the performance of her duties.

HOSPITAL AGAIN. During the five days of her sister's hospitalization, Ella stayed home from work and had complete responsibility for the children. She was profoundly apprehensive about their care, attempting to control her own anxiety by keeping them confined to the house for the entire interval. After her sister's return home from the hospital, she resumed her job, but found that now she could neither concentrate on her work by day nor sleep by night. Feeling more insecure than ever, during one attack of insomnia, she got out of bed to walk down to the ocean where she contemplated suicide. It was at this point that she recognized that she needed help. She went to the nearest hospital where the psychiatrists advised immediate hospitalization. She rejected this idea at first but, as her difficulties increased, she finally requested admission.

DIAGNOSTIC PICTURE

To say that Ella "responded" to the test material would be to rob her performance of its flavor. It would be more appropriate to say that she lived or relived the tests. Her TAT stories were frankly autobiographical, and she poured out her resentments, frustrations, and longings as if she were making entries in her diary. The things she saw in the ink blots terrified her because they seemed so real and so close to the way she actually saw herself and the world. It was as if she were looking into a mirror. Could not the examiner see what she was seeing?

TAT FANTASIES. Ella's TAT stories are a chronicle of inner turmoil, of Oedipal love and rivalry, of sadism and masochism, of frustration, injustice, self-sacrifice, self-pity, and self-hate (see Test Summary A).

In response to Card 2 she tells us the meaning of her feeling "outside of the family." In the story the girl does not "want to go to school." She does not want to accept her mother's values, so under the guise of "helping her father," the girl makes herself into a work horse. She manipulates the situation in such a way that her mother has to be punitive toward her in order to provide a legitimate reason for "resenting her mother." She knows that her alliance with the father "would make her mother mad." It insures her continuing to get the satisfaction of being abused. This is the role she enjoys and perpetuates by stacking the cards against herself. Finally in the story she knuckles under to her mother's domination—she goes to school and grudgingly identifies with the aggressor. As she says in her story to Card 1, "You can lead a horse to water but you can't make him drink it." Ella is really saying, "You can make me do it but you can't make me like it."

In Card 8BM she develops the sado-masochistic theme further and shows us how it has been expressed in her occupational adjustment. Freely translated it reads, "Mother forces me to be something I do not want to be. This makes me angry enough to kill her." The boy is "thinking of himself as a doctor and with that knife in his hand, he would take it and rip the man's chest wide open." But instead the boy becomes "a real good surgeon—he puts his heart and everything in his work." The story is paradoxically entitled "Rebellion." For Ella "rebellion" means to do more than is expected of her and to enjoy suffering every minute of it.

Ambivalence has been Ella's undoing. Perhaps if she had ceased to look for dependency gratification from her mother, the resolution of her identification conflict would not have been so difficult. Along with the hate and resentment, however, there is the hope of some affection and love to be obtained from mother. In Card 7BM she says that mother was not always "crabby." Maybe there is some love to be obtained from her if she waits long enough, if she "perseveres." In Card 10 she tells us how it might have been. The parents "love each other." There is closeness, warmth, and affection but, alas, not for her! Such happiness is only to be found in story books.

"Making her mother mad" apparently has the meaning of incestuous love for father according to Card 4. In fantasy, Ella lives in sin with the father figure. "They're not legally married, just common law." In Card 13MF she falls into the trap that her ambivalence toward her mother has set for her. In spite of her efforts to cast out the internalized image of her mother, she has identified with her mother's social values. Ella is the "rich society girl," the socially superior member of the alliance. She has thrown her life away on her worthless dolt of a father, and now she must pay for her hostile and incestuous wishes. She has sacrificed her life for him, given up her cultural birthright, and all she has to show for her sacrifice is pain, suffering, and death.

In Card 12M she perceives the "blackness" of her father. Here "black" seems to have a two-edged meaning. Not only does it pertain to the color of his skin, but to Ella it also means wickedness and evil. He is the "devil," the serpent, who tempted her with the forbidden fruit, the "apple," and destroyed her innocence. Now she herself is "black" and "evil" like her father. She feels that his blackness somehow rubbed off on her.

Ella toys with the idea of suicide as a possible solution to her dilemma. Her death on Card 13MF causes those who have wronged her to suffer. Moreover it means a balancing of the books, an eye for an eye. She has wished and magically caused her mother's death, so she must die. It also promises a surcease of pain and suffering for herself and a chance for "rebirth" (3BM), a chance to begin all over again with the idealized parents of Card 10. Perhaps in the back of her mind lurks the fantasy of being reborn as a white person with white parents.

Ella's fantasy productions, for all their personalized meanings, cannot be divorced from their cultural matrix. Her perception of the weak, shiftless, inadequate male is quite consistent with the picture of the passive Negro male of the deep South from which her father came. When she sees the couple in Card 4 as living in a "common law" relationship she is accurately describing the casual attitude toward marriage which is prevalent in her father's cultural background. In 13MF the male figure keeps "quitting or getting fired—he'll wander around like a hobo." Here again is the situation that is forced on the Southern Negro by his lack of status and opportunity, while the woman assumes the dominant and responsible role out of necessity. When she says that the man "hates himself" she perceives the ambivalent identification of the Negro male with his white oppressor, where the hate of the white man is internalized and turned against the self, resulting in feelings of degradation and lowered self-esteem.

RORSCHACH. Ella's Rorschach also bears the imprint of her cultural background (see Test Summary B). The frequent allusions to darkness and blackness show how intimately her identification problem is involved with skin color. The black lambs on Card II have at least two levels of meaning. On the one hand she perceives herself as being "outside the family," the black sheep, so to speak.

She also sees herself, however, as the outcast because of her alliance with her father, who is black and whom she resembles physically.

Mutilation fantasies are represented in such responses as "the hand that's torn apart" on Card II; the two figures on Card III pulling apart the head of a third figure; the hands about the neck on Card I, which possibly refers to a fear of lynching. Concepts of this sort are prevalent in the records of Negro subjects. They point up the Negro's anxiety about expressing hostility for fear of retaliation. Ella is no exception in this regard. Her masochistic way of life is perhaps the watered-down behavioral counterpart of her mutilation fantasies. Her facial excoriations, however, are perhaps more directly symbolic of her tendency to mutilate herself. Perhaps this represents an attempt to tear off her dark skin. The scaly lizards on Card VIII could represent the ugly, acne-scarred, repulsive creature which in her guilt-ridden fantasy she pictures herself to be.

While the more formal aspects of her Rorschach productions give no sign of ongoing psychopathological process, Ella's culture conflict presumably contributed to her underlying ego split. Her inability either to accept one aspect of herself and renounce the other or to find a satisfactory compromise solution has built up intolerable internal pressure. The splitting and tearing which she attributes to the ink blots represent an ego that is "coming apart at the seams." Her thinking has become fluid to the extent that the stationary ink blots become forms which change in kaleidoscopic fashion before her very eyes. Sometimes the forms fuse together and appear in inappropriate and arbitrary combination. Her thinking shows signs of becoming primitive, archaic, and magical. All these features point to impending intellectual confusion and attempt at psychotic restitution. Yet her ego breakdown is as yet incomplete, and she still maintains a tenuous hold on reality.

Interspersed with the raw psychopathology are islets of strength. It is true that she perceives hate, savagery, bleakness, and evil, but she has not ceased to reach out for tenderness and love. She is not a totally deprived and barren person. On the contrary, she is a highly intelligent, richly endowed, and gifted person, the "rich society girl" on Card 13MF of the TAT. She has the potential capacity, insight, and integration which comes from being close, in fact, too close, to her unconscious.

RECONSTRUCTION OF DYNAMICS

THE CINDERELLA ROLE. As nearly as can be pieced together from history, tests, and personal impressions, this is what seems to have happened to Ella: Her mother frustrated her dependency needs sufficiently to cause her both anger and anguish but not enough to prevent her from partially identifying with her. Her mother's coolness drove her into the arms of her seductive father who gave her affection tinged with eroticism. He also frustrated her dependency longings but in a different way: Instead of being a pillar of strength he leaned on her and exploited her. His sexual behavior, while arousing her own erotic feelings, also frightened her to the point of twice running away from home.

Having failed in her initial attempts to carve out her own destiny, Ella decided to make the best of a bad situation. She settled down and became a drudge, a work horse. This Cinderella role not only appeased her own harsh superego, but also served to spite her mother. It was as if she were saying, "You don't love me . . . look what you've done to me, how you've made me suffer . . . I'll make you suffer with pangs of remorse by suffering myself."

MAGICAL THOUGHTS. Her mother's death by fire was in all likelihood seen in magical fashion by Ella as having resulted from her own murderous thoughts. Surely she would burn in hell for having caused her mother to burn. Her strict Catholic upbringing made it easier for her to establish this causal relationship. Perhaps the coaching she had received from her mother in Indian superstition added fuel to the "fire." She was indeed a *femme fatale,* a dangerous and evil person who could strike people dead with her powerful murderous thoughts. This is the time when one of the soft spots in her ego gave way and broke out in the form of compulsive symptomatology, namely, the finger counting. It is interesting that she made frequent allusions to hands on the Rorschach. Could this have symbolized that her mother's blood was on her hands?

FATHER VERSUS FATHER-SUBSTITUTE. After her discharge from the navy, Ella found a man who in some ways resembled her father. At least he was Negro and he was considerably older than she was. He turned out to be very different from her father, however, in that he could not be pushed around as had her father. He insisted on being the boss and apparently would not be manipulated into leaning on her and giving her masochistic gratification. She left this man and went back to her first love, her father, a man whom she could manipulate in such fashion.

We can only guess what went on in Ella's mind during the brief period when she was keeping house for her father. However, this was a situation for which she secretly longed. Her hated rival was out of the way and she was in effect living as her father's wife. Thus her sister's call for help may have served a twofold purpose. It extricated her from the incestuous clutches of her father and her own taboo longings, and it gave her a chance again to play the martyr, now as a drudge for her sister.

THE MEANING OF WORK. Her work record at the aircraft plant was more than an effort to overcompensate for her feelings about being Negro, more than merely a bid for acceptance. It was a repetition of her behavior with her mother. She started out with the assumption that she was hated, not only because she was in a minority with reference to the general population, but because she had with her father formed a special "colored" minority group within her own family. She worked literally with a vengeance to make her superiors feel guilty and remorseful.

Similarly she may have assumed the burden of caring for her sister's five children in order to use this against her sister. When her sister went to the hospital and Ella was left completely in charge, the responsibility was more than her defenses could bear since she no longer had a buffer between herself and her own sadistic thoughts. She kept the children confined because something might happen to them which would be her fault. After all when she had previously had murderous thoughts, her mother had died. It could happen again. It was this time that she began to think of suicide.

Even after Ella entered the hospital she played the same masochistic game with her doctor. She denied herself ward privileges, while at the same time demanding immediate discharge from the hospital, in full knowledge, however, that she would be turned down. This gave her the opportunity of pointing an accusing finger at her doctor, turning him into a rejecting, frustrating, parental figure.

ROLE OF CULTURE IN ELLA'S CONFLICTING IDENTITIES

This brings us to the question of the cultural discrepancies in Ella's background and their bearing on her illness. Although many people in white, middle-class culture have to cope with the identification problems inherent in parental sex role reversal, what seems to distinguish Ella's case is that her parents represented the extremes of their respective character types. Her father was a passive dependent person who grew up in a part of the country where the Negro man has a lowly status, lower even than that of the Negro woman. He enjoys little respect or approval either from Caucasians or from his own people. Under such conditions the opportunity for strong male identification is limited, and a passive dependent adjustment is typical.

While in the Negro group the woman attains dominance more or less by default, among the Iroquois female dominance comes from a long-standing matriarchal tradition. The women in Iroquois societies are highly prized and respected and are considered superior to men in certain ways.

Kinship is traced through maternal rather than paternal lineage. Ella's parents thus may be thought of as caricatures of the passive dependent male and the aggressive, domineering female combination often found in middle-class, white society. To a large extent culture was responsible for the personalities displayed by Ella's parents and for the differences between them. Coming from disparate backgrounds and having discordant values they were unable to reconcile the differences between themselves and the over-all culture. Ella reacted to the fact of her parents' internal and external conflict and made it her own personal conflict.

The interpersonal relationships in Ella's family were sufficiently disturbed and distorted to produce pathology. The pattern of rejection and seduction made for chaos and confusion in Ella's emotional life. The basis for rejection may have been, as Ella feels, her physical resemblance to her Negro father. Then again she may have seized on this resemblance to rationalize away the far more frightening feeling that she was unloved and worthless as a human being.

CROSSROADS OF THE FUTURE

What about Ella's struggle for an identity? It seems as though she is at the crossroads. There are at least three roads open to her. The shortest one is the most ominous—suicide. The second possibility, and one that approaches Nirvana, the ethereal state of unfeeling that she fantasies in the TAT, is a complete catatonic withdrawal. She would continue to forge successive layers of the body armor on which she already has a good start. Here she would be safe from the troublesome, frustrating demands of reality and she could safely create a world of her own choosing. Armor (the hard crocodile hide on Card VIII of the Rorschach) has a twofold purpose. Toward the hostile outer world it functions as a shield and barrier. Toward the hostile inner world it functions as a strait jacket to keep her from unleashing her sadistic impulses on the world and destroying it. The third possibility is that she will shed the armor and emerge in a new form; that she will experience a genuine rebirth; and that the healthy, constructive parts of her ego will rally and achieve a new integration. This could be the end of her long search for an identity, an identity of her own, free of the shackles of the past.

Test Summary

A. Thematic Apperception Test

CARD 1. 40″

That looks like me. Well, let's see—let's see. Reminds me of me, of my familiar childhood poses. I guess that's a little boy—this is a little boy who doesn't want to take his violin lessons. It's like he's being forced, like that old maxim, "you can lead a horse to water but you can't make him drink it," so he just sits there staring at it, stubbornly,—he's looking at it and wondering what it's made of,—the string, and what kind of wood it's made of, and what's in there. (Q) Mother made him take the violin lessons and he really didn't want to. He wanted to play out in the sunshine so as long as he's here now he's going to find out all about this violin, about the people who made it, and what makes the music. (Ending?) Oh, he'll sit and wonder and this will go on for hours. Then he'll pick it up and start playing it. (Title?) "Meditation." (Why remind you of you?) Because that's the way I was. Had that pose all the time. Used to meditate and wonder about things and people all the time.

CARD 2. 10″

Oh gee! (Pause 39″) I think that this girl resents her mother. She, the mother, seems like the bossy type. Makes the girl go to school and I don't think she wants to go to school. I think she would rather stay home and help the father plow because I think her mother nags at the father and she really likes to stay home and help—not really to help because she knows that that would make her mother mad. (Q) She'd help him and then they'd be together, and talk about her mother, and in that way she could accomplish a twofold purpose. She wouldn't go to school and that way, she'd whisper to him, and the other might think that they're talking about her and maybe make her feel bad. (How father feel?) He's just like my father. He doesn't care one way or another. He just cares about getting his work done. What the mother says goes in one ear and out the other. (What led up to the situation?) Well, looks to me like this girl didn't want to go to school. She argued, begged, pleaded, bargained, but the mother forced her. Mother has her nose up in the air as if to say, this matter is closed, so I guess she goes to school. This mother is pregnant. Oh, that's why she's so fussy and hard to get along with. The husband understands and won't interfere in the matter. (Title?) (Thinks for a long time) "Confusion," but if that girl was me I'd like to stay home. (Why?) I like the sunshine and air, and horses on the farm.

CARD 3BM. 5″

Oh gee (15″). I don't know about this. Can't think of anything about this picture. (10″) I don't know who this is. Well this is like one of the . . . patients. (Laughs) (What is the patient doing?) Is that a gun? (You tell me) Oh, well, it looks like a gun. Oh yes, I see. This is a mental patient. She wants to commit suicide. I think she went to a lot of trouble to get that gun, then after she got it, she didn't want to use it. (How did she get this way?) She hates herself because she doesn't have the nerve. She was holding it, then let it fall. (Nerve?) She didn't have the nerve, that takes nerve. They say they're cowards, but that's wrong because you really have to have a lot of nerve. Maybe not nerve at all, maybe it takes will. Is that different? (How get in hospital?) (Long pause) She just thought she should be there I guess. If she went there, maybe she'd get this idea out of her mind. (Where get idea?) Well, she feels real weak like she doesn't have any life in her—just dragging along. Eating because she has to. Just living because she has to, because she wouldn't die. (How does it end?) I think she finally believes that she can be helped, that this doctor told her he could make her want to live. She never believed that it was possible, as if all tired out. It's really like a miracle that she'd like to tell everybody about, those who haven't anything to live for and she'd like to pass her good fortune on. Now, as sad as this picture is, I have a very cheery title. (Pause) Let me see—we'll call it "Rebirth."

CARD 4. 20″

Oh gee, this is a—man and his wife. They're not legally married, just common-law. Don't know why, the picture looks like it. (Pause) Is that a picture in the background? (Whatever it means to you) Well, it looks like it could be a mirror. Well, I don't know what he's mad at. She's trying to constrain him. He's trying to go out and inflict physical violence on the person who made him mad. He's very hot tempered. (What person do to make him mad?) Made fun or said something about him living with this woman. She is not concerned about the remark because he knows she's been around and those things don't faze her. Tells him not to pay attention to the remark. Tells him, if these things don't bother me, they shouldn't bother you and she's trying to hold him back. They might have met at a bar so in the end this man sits down, puts his head in his hands and cries. (Q) He cries because—I don't know why he cries, maybe he feels sorry for her because she doesn't feel sorry for herself. (Q) He wants her to get mad, too. (Title? Long pause) Call it "Conflicts."

CARD 7BM. 20″

Why is everybody mad? Nobody is smiling. (Laughs) Do you have any that are smiling? They all look like a rogue's gallery. Gee, I never saw such a bunch of sad people. Old sour grapes. I guess that's me. (Q) I'm sour grapes, that's just the way I am—like all these people. This is the father and son (laughs). Everybody is mad, mad at mother. (Patient laughs long and apologetically.) Well, this boy is mad at his mother again,—oh, why do they make these pictures look like this. He's mad at his mother—doesn't have to be his mother, could be someone else, but that's who I think it is. It's the same old story, something about mother he doesn't like. Father is old. Maybe the mother is old, too. Maybe they had the son when they were real old. And he doesn't understand why his mother is so fussy. He's young and full of life and likes to dance. Father tries to understand, pats him on the back, tells him to try and overlook mother. But the boy feels frustrated and resentful. And the father, he just takes everything, he never says anything, never fusses back because he's lived with her so long and knew her when she was young and not crabby. But the boy, all he sees is the crabby part because he was born when they were old. (Title?) Oh, what's that word—not perseverance—well call it "Perseverance." No, don't put perseverance 'cause that's not it. The way it ends. Father tells him to go along, not to pay attention to mother because that's the way she is. And he promises he'll buy him something real nice.

CARD 8BM. 25″

Now, here's one that's not so sad. This fellow seems to be looking to the future. I guess he's thinking of what he'd like to be when he grows up. He visualizes himself as a doctor. (Why doctor?) I don't know, maybe he likes to help people. People who are sick, you know, in pain. But I don't know how he could have that feeling and be so young. (What is that in the background?) That's what he's thinking. He sees the operating, and that's what he wants to do. He wants to be a big man and there's his assistant back there. (What about the gun?) Is that a gun? I was going to ask you. Oh, I know. Well, if it's a gun, that changes things. His father wants him to be a doctor but he would rather be out in the woods hunting. Father tells him he must be a doctor yet he hates it. He's thinking of himself as a doctor and with that knife in his hand, he would take it and rip that man's chest wide open. That's his way of getting back at his father for making him be a doctor. (End?) I guess he'll be a doctor but he won't like it, and he'll be a real good one too. A real good surgeon. But after he leaves the operating table, he has no more interest in patient. But while he's in there, boy, he's real good! He puts his heart and everything in his work. (Title?) "Rebellion."

CARD 13MF. 25″

Now, let's see. This was a real rich society girl and she fell in love with this fellow—man. He has no ambition. He's a coward. He can never hold a job because he doesn't have self-confidence and he's just barely able to make a living, and this woman sticks by him. She puts up with him, poverty, because she really loves him. They live in the slums and she's used to real fine things, but she never complains, never fusses at him for quitting or getting fired. One day she got sick, went to the doctor, and he told her that she had to have an operation or she'd die. She knew they didn't have money so she never told her husband. And she was in very much pain when it was near her time, but she never said a word to her husband. She dies and he finds out the whole thing. Now it's too late, and now he hates himself for the way he treated her. He wishes he'd die too. He'll never be any good any more. He'll wander around like a hobo. He doesn't have to push himself the little he did when she was alive. He starts drinking. One day they find his body near the tracks. He was probably drunk, wandered near the tracks and the train ran over him. (Title?) Oh, I can't think of that word. It begins with re—not reproach—it's worse than that. He loathes himself. Call it, "To Loathe Oneself."

CARD 10. 30″

Oh gee,—this reminds me of a story book. Like the little girls I used to go to school with, but this looks like the man really loves his wife. Well, it reminds me of the little girl I used to go to school with. That's the way their mother and father was—I never saw my mother and father like that. I used to envy them. (Tell me more about them, their feelings.) Well, they just love each other. And he's holding her. Now, that's a happy picture, don't you think so? (Holds picture away at a distance) This is the way people should be—familiar, husband and wife. (What makes them happy?) Well, they love each other, they're close—not physically. (Title?) (Long pause) "Oblivion, Sweet Oblivion."

CARD 6BM. 2″

Oh gee—tsh, tsh, tsh. Poor mother catches all the heck—oh, no, no, no, oh no. This mother has this son that was in the war and he was missing in action. She's hoped and prayed that he's not dead, but in her heart, she really doesn't believe it, but she tries to believe it. So this young man was a buddy of her son, and he's come to tell her that he was with him when he died and she doesn't want to hear it. She doesn't want to hear it. Although she knows deep down in her heart, she doesn't want to hear from him that he is dead, so she turns her back on him and pretends not to hear what he's talking about. He just walks away leaving her standing there, and she stands there until darkness falls, and that's all she does the rest of her life—stand at the window and look up at the sky. (Title?) "Withdrawn."

CARD 12M. (Shakes head) 30″

Who are these people, doctors or priests? Oh, I know. This is a psychopath, this man, and this little boy is sleeping so nice and he's having good dreams. He's real happy. This man, he's—no, he's not a psychopath, he's black, evil, and he's going to do something to this boy. He's going to put a curse on him because of something this boy's mother did. It's not the little boy's fault, that's why he's so happy and having good dreams. But his mother did something, and he's saying something in a different language, that this boy will never be happy and when he wakes up—oh, I know what—see, this boy took something from this old man, and his mother knew but never said anything about it, and this little boy thought he was right. Instead of getting even with the mother, he takes it out on the little boy because he's so happy. That's what happened to me. (Q) Something my mother did and I had to suffer for it. Same thing happened to mother. (Q) The old man is some kind of devil; the boy took—oh, an apple, and this apple was not an ordinary apple but had some superstition attached to it. (Title?) "The Calm Before the Storm."

CARD 16.

(What is this now?) (Usual instructions) This empty card. (Yes) Oh gee!—Well this is a little girl sitting on top of a hill with her dog. She's looking down into the valley. There are a lot of beautiful trees and some cows grazing in the pasture and she's very happy. She has her arm around her dog and the sun is real bright, and she is just meditating on the beauties of nature and how nice and peaceful it is up there with just her and her dog. That's all. This is called, oh— "Tranquility." (Where'd you get this story?) This is a suppressed desire. I would like to be that little girl. I don't know if that was me once, or if that's the way I'd like to be. It just represents a feeling.

Test Summary

B. RORSCHACH PROTOCOL

Response	*Inquiry*

CARD I. 25″

1. Want me to tell you what it is? Bat, a black bat. He has hands and I guess he's going after somebody, in flight. Don't know whether bats fly or not, but this one does. Put his hands right around her neck, somebody's neck, has hands open so far and fit around somebody's neck. I guess that's—(trails off) (Hold card longer, etc.)

1. (Did you mean an animal or a bat like human when you said hands?) Animal—no, half animal and half man because he has hands like a human and feet like a human. (See any of rest of him) Legs. Looks like woman's form inside there (Was this part of the bat?) Right inside the body is really a woman's form. (Was that part of the bat or just something in there?) Just something in there. (What part of bat is it in?) In his body, you know, you can see it.

2. Could I take parts of it? (If you like) It could be some iceberg, real sharp iceberg.

2. These sharp things here. (Q) Background is white and icebergs should be white against the darker background. I don't know why I thought of icebergs. They look isolated. (Q) I don't know. Gee! I don't know why it looks isolated. (Ice?) Sharp and jagged.

3. Or clouds down here, some real dark clouds.

3. These billows (traces inside with finger), and they're dark too, they're color, like a storm, you know.

CARD II. 60″

1. (Laughs) (Frowns) Well it doesn't look like anything unless you take in the parts. Down here I see a heart, a bleeding heart.

1. (Tell me more about it) Looks like a Valentine heart, when kids. A picture of a bleeding heart of Valentine. (Bleeding?) The color, and then the drops, the drippings.

Response	*Inquiry*
2. Up here is part of the body, one part of the body that was torn apart and laid into two sections.	2. (What part of body?) Could be a hand. A hand that's torn apart. But there's only thumbs on the hand, no fingers. (Torn apart?) Well it looks crude and ragged. You know how you pull chicken joints apart, the skin is ragged and it's not neat like you would take a knife and cut it. One hand with two thumbs and no fingers, that's pulled apart.
3. Two little black lambs on here with noses touching, holding up something. I don't know what it is, their noses. Looks like the tip end of a spear or sword that they're holding up.	3. (You said they were holding up the tip end of a spear?) The tip end of a spear with their noses. (How come?) Might be a circus set or something like that.

CARD III. 10″

1. Well I see two little monkeys hanging upside down.	1. By the tail, yeah. (Describe them?) They're just hanging upside down and their arms are—trying to get balanced to go upright.
2. There's two men, I don't know if they're human. They have their hands on top of—it's a human man. These others aren't. They have their hands on top of his head. He's bald except for a little hair around the edge. He has wrinkles on his brow. They're trying to pull his head apart. One's on this side and one's on the other side. Can you see that? I don't know, I guess that's all. (Arranges cards in neat pile)	2. (Human men) a hat like a Davey Crockett hat. Furry, just goes around. (Fur?) Fuzzy around edge. I changed the hair to a cap. (Why men not human?) Not shaped like humans. (Q) Their head is real long, comes to a peak. The neck is too long. Torso part sort of resembles a human. (Men?) Well they are, aren't they? (Why to you?) They have pants and don't have long hair.

CARD IV. 30″

1. Oh God! (Laughs, shakes head) This over-all picture is a bear rug, you know, laying flat and instead of bear feet he has a man's feet. Real big ones about size 13, they look like to me. And also I see a (trails off).	1. This one that takes the cake. (Impression of bear rug.) Shape, color and these fuzzy-like, like hair or fur all over here. (Points with finger to interior of blot) The dark color.
2. Skull of a dog that is decomposed, the decomposed skull of a dog. Oh Jesus! (Smiles)	2. Oh, right there. No matter how I look at it I can't get away from the dog's staring eyes. You know

Response   *Inquiry*

how they protrude after the flesh —(laughs) Oh God! (Decomposition?) The protruding eyes and I can see the flesh and bones. God! Oh gee! That's terrible. I don't know where I get these ideas. (Laughs) Oh gee! No wonder I'm afraid of the dark.

CARD V. 25"

1. This is some kind of insect, real hairy and furry. That's all I can see.

1. (What kind?) Like a grasshopper or something like that. Not exactly a grasshopper. Has fur on it. Never heard of an insect with fur. (Fur?) These billowy, maybe the color. (How would the color help?) I don't know. (What do you mean by the color?) Dark, dark fur, brown fur. (Impression of brown?) Yes. (Does it look brown?) No but it could be brown, this fur is all brown. (Show me parts) Antennas, head, wings and legs.

CARD VI. 4"

1. This is a fish that has been cleaned, scaled and boned. His head cut off, and this is the—he's flat—split in the middle you know.

1. Skinned, ready for pan. (Skinned?) It's not skinned, it's cleaned (Cleaned?) Well, it's cut open, the backbone's not there. The head is gone, cut off, also the tail and it's laying down in his lap, draining. (Scaled?) I just assumed it was scaled because you usually scale it before you cut it open.

2. That little thing up there is like a totem pole, an Indian totem pole. Has four hands. His head is split in the middle.

2. (Hands come out of totem pole usually?) No, they don't. The wings. Always try to get symbol of thunderbird into art. Somewhere I tried to get thunderbird in. This is one set (of hands), this is the other set. Did you ever see anybody with such a morbid outlook?

CARD VII. 20"

1. These are two little Scotty dogs, their ears standing up in the air

1. Ears, tail, body and legs are all together, neck, little nose, mouth

Response	*Inquiry*
real happy, jumping up and down on a pillow, two pillows.	has little fur, little hair around it. (What about fur-hair?) Color, and gee, his eyes protrude too. Both of these little dogs. I didn't see that before.

CARD VIII. 20"

1. I see two lizards on a branch. (Shakes head, laughs) Oh God! You really want to know?	1. (Branch?) This thing is like a dead leaf. (Lizards?) Just hanging on in air. (Lizards?) They have long tails, beady eyes, and their body is long like a lizard. And they look scaly like a lizard. (Scaly?) This, different colors. Not scaly but you know how. Did you ever see a lizard? Hard like a crocodile hide. (Hardness?) Because their body is rigid and it's not supple. If it was they couldn't hang like that, like those monkeys were different.
2. There's two drops of water leaking through the earth into somebody's casket.	2. Casket, in here. (Soil?) But I can't see it; in other words this water is wearing a space until it gets down there. (Earth?) Just fits in there like a handful of dirt. (What about?) That's where the water is going, that's how I visualize it anyway.
3. I don't know what it is but anyway it's something torn apart. Do they make it like this? (Examiner explains how blots are made) Yes, but they don't make it look like something's torn apart.	3. This blue. I don't know, it could be a piece of meat. Has small bones in it. (Meat?) I don't know, maybe I've seen something like that.

CARD IX. 35"

1. Two babies. They're like Siamese twins stuck together, joined at the bust. One is up and one is down, and let me see.	1. Eyes, a little fuzzy up here. All just like a mass. (One up one down?) Both laying down, if you put one up the other goes down. They have hands too. Red thumb. (What about?) No hair, eyes closed. (Babies?) I've seen babies like that.
2. An Indian riding on a horse, real fast, feathers are blowing back. That's all.	2. That green guy. Just a silhouette. Hands holding on to reins, bent over, going real fast. Can't actually see the horse, can't actually

Response	*Inquiry*
	see anything on here. (Laughs) (Feathers?) Head dress (Indian?) because of the feathers. (Green guy?) (Did you mean that the Indian was green?) (Patient explains that green was just referring to the area) (You said that thumbs of the babies were red. How about the rest of them?) The hands aren't red. (Why not?) Well, look at it.

CARD X. 11″

1. Two caterpillars.	1. These two guys (What about?) You know, the furry kind of caterpillar. (Show me?) (Patient was referring to the edge of the area.)
2. Two crabs.	2. Those blue ones. (Did you mean they were blue crabs?) No. Crabs are red.
3. Some kind of prehistoric monster, dinosaur or something.	3. Oh, this guy right here, this green one, that's his face. (Can you describe it?) Ooh. He has, well there's green smoke coming out of his eyes, big billows of green smoke. His ears stand straight up like a rabbit's—looks like a rabbit. (Is he?) He is a rabbit. (He's not a prehistoric monster any more?) No, my eyes are bad. I didn't look real close but that's just what he is.
4. Three gold balls that signify a pawn shop. That's all.	4. Right here (patient points to blot area). Those caterpillars, they have a man's head—nose, and everything. (Do they still look like caterpillars?) Uh-huh, still caterpillars. (But they have a man's head?) Uh-huh.

TESTING THE LIMITS

(Likes Best)   Card VII. Did you want me to tell you the one that is the prettiest? (Which one did you like the best?) Well, these other things are terrible, and this is nice. (Laughs) (Q) I'm afraid of all these other things and I like dogs, happy dogs. These other things, they scare me, except this one. Well, it's reasonable.

(Likes Least) Card IV. It's the most gruesome. (Q) I don't like hairy, furry things. (Q) I don't know, and then that dog is on there too.

(Sex) Vaginal area, Card IV. A stump where the head is severed. (Of what?) Of the bear. Vaginal area, Card VII. Could be tar holding pillows together.

7

Acute Culture Conflict in a
Hopi Adolescent

Aaron H. Canter

Lola, at fifteen, was a high school freshman, active in school affairs, a pom pom girl, a cheerleader, and a drum majorette. How typically American this sounds! And then, one day, during a heated argument with some of her classmates, Lola suddenly had a seizure, and lay on the floor in a trancelike state, talking to the "breath-spirits" of her deceased parents. How very bizarre *this* sounds—until one is made aware of the fact that Lola, the pom pom girl, is also Lola, member of the esteemed Bear Clan of the Hopi Indian tribe. The study that follows is the story of this girl, caught in the web of these two conflicting cultural patterns, and of how she has fared.

HOME BACKGROUND

The information we have is a condensation of material provided by Lola during a series of therapeutic interviews. It was not possible to obtain a formal history from the Indian Agency, nor to corroborate the patient's statements, except in a general way. The material presented by her has been filled in with socioanthropological data available from previous students of the Hopi Indians and from the scanty data available in Lola's school records.

NATIVE VERSUS CHRISTIAN TRAINING.   Lola was born in the
summer of 1939, on a Hopi Indian reservation in Arizona.
She was the eighth child in the family. At the time of her
birth, her eldest sibling, a brother, was twenty-three and
her nearest was five. Three years later, the ninth and last
child was born. Lola recalls vividly some of her early childhood. The family was poor, and many times was forced to
go hungry. Lola's father, to whom she was very much attached, was a kindly and generous man. "He always tried
to give us everything we wanted, though he couldn't afford
it . . . he was strict with us and would get angry if we
weren't good." Her father was a member of the Bear Clan,
one of the foremost Hopi clans, and went regularly to the
secret tribal rituals and councils. According to Lola, he
never told them anything about the secret rituals and
dances. However, he did want the children to follow "the
Hopi Way." "He always made sure we had our training.
. . . He never smoked or drank, and never would go to my
mother's church meetings, but let us go sometimes."

Lola's mother, who was also a full-blooded Hopi, is described as "more strict" than her father. She was a converted Mennonite, and had been very much influenced by
a sister who had married a Mennonite missionary. She
wanted to raise the children as Christians, and, according
to Lola, "Mother never wanted us to go to the Indian
dances or ceremonials, and wanted us to go to church regularly." Attendance at church, however, was apparently sporadic and seemed to depend upon which parent dominated
the familial scene at a particular period of time. It may
be inferred that the question of religion was the source of
a great deal of conflict and friction between her parents,
though Lola denied any overt quarreling between them.

Four years after Lola's birth, the family moved off the
reservation, under pressure of a cultural–economic crisis,
to an Indian village near the Navajo Ordnance Depot,
where her father secured employment as a truck driver.
The population of the village where the family lived was
both Hopi and Navajo, and apparently the way of life was

a confusing admixture of the folkways of the two tribes and the white man's ways. The tribal languages were not spoken, and the tribal customs and ceremonies were observed only intermittently. However, the cooking and food were, according to Lola, "like the Hopi way." Her father continued to attend the Bear Clan ceremonials, and her mother the Mennonite Church services on Sundays.

Following the move, the family's economic circumstances improved considerably. Lola can recall starting school at the age of six, and the family's being able to afford a new dress and shoes for the occasion.

She and the other children were transported by bus from the village to school, where she attended classes which were predominantly white. She repeated the first grade but thereafter did fairly well in school. "We did well in school for we were afraid to have our father see our report cards."

FAMILY CHANGES.   When Lola was eight, her mother, age forty-nine, became ill and after a few months died of a heart attack. At this point Lola was sent to live with a maternal aunt in Montana. This was the aunt who had married the Christian missionary, and for the next two years Lola was raised as a Christian. Lola was apparently very unhappy living with her aunt and uncle. Her grades at school deteriorated, and when she returned to her father's home for a summer visit at the end of her second year, she prevailed upon him to let her remain with him.

Once again, Lola was enrolled at her old public school. Once again, she experienced difficulties in adjustment, and her grades, reflecting this, were initially poor, though passing. Her chief difficulty during this period was "getting along with the white kids." Toward the end of the semester (seventh grade) Lola's father was suddenly hospitalized and within one month, after some surgery for cancer of the stomach, he died. Lola's reaction to his death was quite intense and her difficulties in adjustment at school and at home increased considerably during this period. Her work at school was completely unsatisfactory, and she was given only a conditional promotion. After some conferences on the problem of Lola's adjustment, the family finally consented to her request that she be sent to a boarding school. In the Fall of the year of her father's death, Lola was enrolled at the Phoenix Indian School.

SCHOOL EXPERIENCES

INITIAL SUCCESS. The Phoenix Indian School is a coeducational institution which is a combination grade and high school for the Indian children of the various tribes in Arizona. The students attend classes and live in dormitories according to their grade placements. There is some informal tribal and clan organization and the school does sponsor some special Indian tribal dances or ceremonials. However, in many respects Lola felt that the Indian School was pretty much "like a school for white people."

Lola made a fairly good adjustment initially and cited the fact that she became a drum majorette, a cheerleader, and a pom pom girl. During her first year, she made a number of friends and got along well with all the students. The school records confirm the story of her various achievements and satisfactory adjustment. However, in her second year (ninth grade) she began to have difficulties with the other Hopi girls "because they were jealous" of her achievements as a cheerleader and drum majorette.

CONFLICT WITH TRIBE MATES. According to Lola, she was approached by the appointed leaders of the Hopi girls in her dormitory and told that her behavior was not proper for a Hopi, particularly one of the Bear Clan. Lola was reminded that she had been remiss in her tribal obligations insofar as she did not attend Hopi council meetings. Lola initially ignored the criticism of her Hopi peers. However, the criticism increased in intensity. After several weeks, there was an increasing attitude of hostility toward her. In addition to her lack of interest in tribal matters, she failed to make any effort to be initiated into or accept her responsibilities as a member of the Bear Clan. "I didn't want to—and they argued with me. They also said it wasn't right for me to go ahead of the other (Hopi) girls. . . . They also said I was paying too much attention to another girl's boy friend."

Her relationship with the other Hopi girls deteriorated to the point where there was open quarreling and actual fighting. It was during one of these fights that Lola had her first ragelike seizure and trance. Lola, in explaining the circumstances surrounding this first seizure said, "I didn't want to pay any attention to their talking (nagging); my mother had taught me not to fight, to be a good Christian." Lola was torn between the Hopi ("peaceful") way and "being a good Christian," on the one hand, and her angry, hostile feelings toward these girls on the other. The quarrels between Lola and the other girls kept increasing in frequency and intensity and Lola had two more seizures. She became increasingly aggressive, and, following her third seizure, she slashed the clothing of some of the Hopi girls, as well as her own apparel. At this point, she was expelled from the Phoenix Indian School for aggressive and destructive behavior.

COMMITMENT

Lola went to live with a married sister in . . . She did poorly at school, was unhappy, and ran away from home. Her sister, unable to manage the girl, appealed to the Juvenile Court, which committed her to a training school for delinquent girls, where she is staying at present.

TRANCE STATES. Lola was referred for psychological examination and evaluation one week after her commitment. Her first week was a stormy one, characterized by fighting at her instigation and destructive behavior. It climaxed in another very dramatic seizure and trance, which raised questions as to her immediate management. Questioning the nurse and sister in charge of Lola's dormitory revealed that Lola did not lose consciousness, that she spoke during the trance, and apparently was talking about or to her deceased parents. The observations of this behavior were noted as follows: "Lola's unusual behavior was certainly not that of an epileptic seizure but represented a very dramatic or bizarre fit." There was no incontinence, biting of the tongue, no clonic or tonic jerking movements. It appeared that following the episode Lola was "not confused" but rather was very angry at several of the girls who tried to restrain her.

When Lola was first seen by the author, she was rather sullen and quite guarded in her approach to him. Her physical appearance and dress were not unusual; she appeared to be a well-developed, somewhat overnourished, sixteen-and-a-half-year-old Hopi Indian girl. Lola was well oriented and answered questions coherently and relevantly, though somewhat reluctantly, during the initial interview. From her responses to the examiner's questions it appeared that the so-called seizure was a hysterical "ragelike" episode. She stated, "If anyone bothers me I'll fight them." She indicated that she often got "very mad" and that she had a "bad temper" which she felt she could not control. She was unable to explain why or how she fell to the floor other than that a "very angry feeling" overcame her and that there might have been a momentary loss of consciousness or control. She was aware of the other girls' trying to help her and talking to her. She recalled resisting their attentions because she wanted to be alone in order to speak to the "spirits" of her dead parents. She would not divulge the nature of the conversation with her parents' spirits and was highly resistant to and angered by efforts to ascertain further information concerning her unusual behavior. However, after several interviews, Lola did divulge the following information.

MESSAGES FROM THE DEAD.   She told the examiner that as she grew angry and upset she was unable to come to any course of action. "I felt I wanted to speak to my parents' 'breath-body' (spirit) so that they could tell me what to do." According to Lola, she did communicate with her parents after she had fainted. During this "unconscious" period she obtained further advice from her father's "breath-body," instructing her to "fight them back." Lola acted on these instructions.

Lola's initial seizures had been the subjects for psychological study when she was at the Phoenix Indian School. In the opinion of the school psychologist they indicated "very disturbed and aggressive behavior accompanied by some periodic hallucinatory experiences which suggest the possibility of epileptic equivalents or the early stages of a psychotic process." A complete neuropsychiatric examination and evaluation were recommended. Unfortunately, Lola had to wait several weeks before an appointment with the neuropsychiatrist could be arranged. During this waiting period her behavior became so aggressive that she was expelled from the school, and the appointment was never kept.

NEUROPSYCHIATRIC EXAMINATION

A neurological and electro-encephalographic examination conducted within two weeks of Lola's commitment revealed "no significant abnormalities." Two weeks later the neuropsychiatric examination was completed by a local psychiatrist. In the summary of the psychiatric report it was noted:

In the psychiatric examination this appears to be a girl who is well oriented in all spheres, shows no overt hallucinatory or delusional ideation, and more or less alternates throughout the interview between passive and overt hostile expression. If the questions in the interview become threatening the patient simply sits still and stares at the wall. Intellectually the child does not appear to be handicapped. I do not feel that the affectual responses in this patient, although appearing dulled, are outside the norms for the Hopi culture. It would appear that this patient is essentially narcissistically oriented. . . . Entirely from the point of view of the history there is the impression that when the impulses are those of anger, indeed rage, there is more or less paralysis or decompensation of the ego, in terms of lack of any filtration, leading to almost direct acting out of the impulses.

It is reasonably clear that it is hard for this girl to understand why she cannot do as she pleases without being interfered with by other people and although I feel that the superego cannot be well evaluated in a 16 year old, certainly the history and examination show there is very little evidence of a reasonably well functioning one. A review of the history in terms of episodes which appear to have been hallucinatory in nature indicates, it would be my feeling, that these represent, if indeed hallucinations at all, hysterical in contradistinction to psychotic hallucinations.

Impression: (1) Hysterical character with many evidences of poor ego filtration of impulses. Indeed, I would feel that the patient is essentially impulse ridden. (2) I do not feel that this represents psychosis. (3) Although I do not feel that the superego structure can be readily evaluated it occurs to me that this patient may well have a life-long superego deficit and that, therefore, much of her ability to conform in society may revolve around trial and punishment rather than anything related to internal self control.

Recommendations: (1) I do not feel that this case represents a good therapeutic risk, but on the other hand, the patient's ability to maintain herself in society will essentially revolve around her learning what she can get away with in terms of adjusting to the general cultural mores rather than internal control.

PSYCHOLOGICAL EXAMINATIONS

At the time of Lola's referral to the author, the personal and social history were not available and had to be obtained in later interviews. The immediate problem was to complete a diagnostic study as the basis for a possible rehabilitation, training, and/or therapy program. Accordingly, a battery of psychological examinations was administered.

The psychological test results obtained at the time of the second and third meetings with Lola should be viewed in relation to the attitude of the subject toward the test situation. Lola was ambivalent—she was grateful to the examiner for coming to see her and was apparently less hostile and suspicious than in the initial interview about his stated desire and interest in helping her. On the other hand, when she was pressed to take the tests, which meant working with difficult verbal materials and making decisions in structuring unstructured materials, she became angry, suspicious, and defensive.

The Rorschach examination, which was the last test given in the psychological examination battery, resulted in a definite shift in Lola's attitude to one of open hostility. She recalled taking the "ink-blot test" about a year previously. When she reached Card X she broke into tears, and it took several minutes before she became sufficiently composed for an abbreviated Rorschach inquiry to be attempted. She explained that she didn't like the ink blots, but would not or could not explain why the test distressed her so greatly. Following the Rorschach examination, her attitude was clearly one of pugnaciousness and hostility, an attitude which it took several interviews to overcome.

WECHSLER-BELLEVUE I.   On the Wechsler-Bellevue Scales (Form I) Lola obtained a Full Scale I.Q. of 91 (see Test Summary A). Obviously, the results of this examination must be interpreted cautiously because the Wechsler examination was standardized not on Hopi Indians but on other cultural groups. Nevertheless, the examination does serve to point out that she is not feeble-minded, as previously reported. As a matter of fact, her performance scale I.Q. of 102 is probably the most valid indication on the Wechsler Scales of her true intellectual level. Her relatively poor performance on the verbal scales (Verbal I.Q. 81) is not surprising in view of her cultural background and previous education. Examination of the content emphasizes her verbal impoverishment and lack of information in terms of the white man's culture. There is obviously educational retardation as measured by the ordinary scholastic standards for white adolescents.

On the performance scales of the Wechsler there is evidence of very good manipulative abilities, capacity to deal with abstract visual designs, as well as good problem-solving and learning ability. There were no indications in the Wechsler examination of any process of disorganization, or of organic brain pathology. On the Block Designs subtest, for example, Lola obtained a weighted score of 13. The performance scales, in general, suggest that she can perform adequately, efficiently, and intelligently when she is properly motivated.

FIGURE DRAWING. The Draw-A-Person Test further serves to confirm the findings of the Wechsler examination insofar as both contradict the reported feeble-mindedness. The drawing (Fig. 7–1) serves to point up a fairly well-organized, narcissistic, and egocentric individual who has difficulty in controlling her aggressiveness.

RORSCHACH. The Rorschach examination (Test Summary B) unfortunately produced a meager protocol and sheds little light on the underlying personality structure and functioning. There is a total of four responses, all of which were populars, clearly perceived: On Card I, "a butterfly"; Card II, "two people"; Card V, "a bat"; and Card VIII, "a dog or something." Her rejection of all the other cards is difficult to evaluate in view of her Indian background and her previous experience with the Rorschach. The inquiry period failed to elicit very much and no real effort was made to "test the limits" in view of her obvious emotional distress. The Rorschach examination does have value in this instance inasmuch as it points out that Lola is not confused and that she can perceive the world about her realistically.

TAT STORIES. In analyzing the TAT protocol (Test Summary C) it should be noted that this examination was administered approximately six months after Lola's placement at the training school. In the months since her initial examination, Lola has formed a positive relationship with the psychotherapist and, in the past month, with the new social worker. There have been no further trances or seizures, and although she still displays aggressive behavior intermittently, Lola's energies have been channeled into the school's manual arts program.

The TAT record will undoubtedly be of interest to the reader, particularly the response to Card 5. In this response, one is impressed by Lola's effort to avoid or deny seeing things which the white man's culture is likely to label as hallucinatory or hysterical phenomena. In Lola's words, "She tries to forget her because she is too frightened even imagining she sees her." That the person perceived is Lola's mother is clearly evident from the very next card, 7GF. Lola's perception of the situations depicted in these TAT cards is apparently influenced by her stay at the training school. It is likely that there was social pressure applied directly and indirectly by the other girls who tended to categorize Lola's earlier behavior (talking to the breath-spirits of her parents) as a sign of being "crazy."

Further evaluation of Lola's TAT record discloses that she generally perceives her environment as frustrating, punishing, and harmful. In general, she reacts with resentment. However, in spite of her feelings of frustration she tends to submit to the pressures of the environment after experiencing a significant degree of internal conflict and distress. In general, the heroine of her TAT stories is inadequate, maladjusted, or in conflict over her interpersonal relations.

Finally, a comment should be made about Card 14. Here Lola symbolically states her problem: "Going out in the world and doing things right and being a success so that he doesn't have to be locked up." Her final comment, "I really don't know what he can do" might be rephrased as a question: "What can *I* do?"

The over-all personality picture obtained is that of an emotionally unstable and highly aggressive Indian youngster. Her inability to adjust to either the Indian school or the home environment has resulted in her commitment. Within the limits of a carefully supervised and organized program of rehabilitation she may learn to control her aggressiveness and asocial behavior. There is apparently no other facility available for this Hopi Indian youngster in the state and unfortunately the academic and general program of the school is not geared to her special needs. Nevertheless, she is capable of learning more adequate patterns of behavior and deriving some benefit from the program of rehabilitation.

DISCUSSION

CULTURAL CRISIS AND THE INDIVIDUAL. The relations of the individual to his society and culture pose many interesting questions for the scientist interested in human behavior. Is there a connection between the mental illness or delinquency patterns characteristic of a given cultural group and the social norms that that group enforces? How much is the individual's life style influenced by the society's traditional culture? What complications arise for the individual in a period of cultural change or cultural breakdown?

The study of the relation of culture to personality can be carried on more rewardingly in the so-called "primitive" societies because of their relative simplicity. One such preliterate American Indian culture which has been studied extensively is that of the Hopi Indians. It is not the purpose of this study of one Hopi adolescent to make generalizations about other Hopi Indians, but rather, in presenting a developmental clinical study of this youngster, who was raised during a period of "cultural crisis," it is hoped that some light may be shed upon the diagnosis and treatment of individuals in similar conflict situations.

CONFLICTING IDENTIFICATIONS. In addition to a general economic and cultural crisis which faced most Hopi families in the 1940's when they lost most of their land to the Navajo, there were other specific factors which complicated Lola's family's existence. Lola's father observed "the Hopi Way" and was a respected member of the Bear Clan. Her mother, on the other hand, although a Hopi, was a "modern" (friendly) converted Christian. Typically, Hopi girls accept for the most part their mothers' standards, because the Hopi society is matrilineal and the bond between Hopi women and their daughters is usually very strong. Lola is somewhat atypical, for in her therapeutic interviews she revealed a stronger identification with her father.

Within Lola's family it appears that a great deal of conflict and friction were present. This undoubtedly added to the girl's ambivalence about being a real Hopi. In her interviews she indicated with pride her membership in the Bear Clan. Yet she revealed a reluctance to accept her responsibilities to the clan while she boarded at the Phoenix Indian School. With equal pride she recounted her achievement at the school as a pom pom girl, drum majorette, and cheerleader. These activities were frowned upon by the informally organized Hopi council there, and finally they did manage to bring pressure to bear that was great enough to result in Lola's disturbed behavior.

MEANING OF THE TRANCES. The seizures that Lola experienced and which were the initial reason for her referral to this author are very interesting from the standpoint of culture conflict. The interpretation of the dynamics might be attempted at this point in view of our present knowledge of the various conflicting factors. It should be noted that both the neuropsychiatric and psychological examinations, conducted before it was possible to obtain a social history, tend to rule out organic possibilities and suggest that the seizures were precipitated by psychogenic factors. The seizures always occurred in settings of heated argument wherein the predominant feeling was anger. One might speculate that Lola, conflicted by her intense outbursts of anger and her concept of being "a good Christian" and also a "good Hopi," was in an intolerable dilemma. "Passing out" or becoming unconscious was one way out of this dilemma. It is interesting to note that she withdrew from these situations and sought help in a fashion that is not unusual for Hopis, that is, she withdrew into a trance-like state wherein she consulted her parents' "breath-bodies" (spirits). This communication with her parents, when observed and evaluated by white men's standards, suggests a hallucinatory or hysterical type of experience. However, according to Hopi belief, the spirits of one's parents and ancestors are very much alive and available for consultation. Viewed in the perspective of Hopi culture and Lola's particular background, the symptom of "seizures" is not particularly pathological. The usual diagnostic labels of "hysteria," "psychotic type of behavior," or "delinquent adolescent," etc., do not appear to be appropriate and merely obscure our understanding of this adolescent's defenses. It is of further interest to note that since the beginning of therapeutic interviews which gave her an opportunity to verbalize her feelings there have been no seizures.

MEANING OF AGGRESSIVENESS. Lola's aggressiveness still remains the problem confronting the professional workers at the school. Her aggressiveness, both at the Indian school and in the home of her sister, was the basis for her commitment by the court to a school for female adolescent delinquents. Placement at this school, operated and administered by Catholic nuns, further complicated Lola's adjustment problems. The Hopi tribe is particularly distrustful of and negatively oriented toward the Catholic church and religion because of missionary attempts over four centuries to "civilize" them. As a result of the centuries of Hopi struggle against conquest and conversion by Spain, an intense enmity and suspicion of representatives of the Catholic faith was built up. In the light of this background it is rather apparent that Lola's placement in this Catholic school intensified her difficulties.

The importance of aggression as a factor in personality development has been stressed greatly in recent years. Aggression may be interpreted not only as a response to experienced frustration but also to the anticipation of further frustration. That is, the individual may strive to do something in an aggressive fashion when his physical or emotional comfort is threatened. Commitment by a court to a training school was interpreted as punishment by Lola, and her frustration was presumably intensified when she found that the school was administered by Catholic nuns.

In considering aggression among the Hopi, it should be explained that the young Hopi child is customarily indulged and literally the "lord of the manor" as far as his immediate surroundings are concerned. The adults in his environment cater to his needs and desires, so that the Hopi child discovers early in life that aggressive behavior brings prompt and effective results. Rather suddenly, however, at school age, this pleasant state is interrupted, and the child's relatively unrestrained personality is molded into its conceptually ideal pattern of a smooth, selfless, cooperative being. The egocentric, aggressive behavior which had been so pleasantly effective and easy during the first few years of life is the antithesis of that which is now expected of the young Hopi.

For the Hopi child in the 1940's the cultural, economic, and social crisis then in process created new sources of frustration. Unfortunately for Lola, her mother died when she was eight years old and so the "normal" pattern of Hopi socialization and learning did not occur. For example, the first initiation ceremonies usually take place when the child is between the ages of seven and ten. Lola, because of her mother's illness and subsequent death, had not gone through the initiation procedures, a fact of which she is acutely aware, and of which she was forcefully reminded by the Hopi girls at the Indian school. Lola did not have the typical Hopi learning experiences in socialization and one cannot help but speculate how effective her control of her aggressive impulses might have been in a more stable or typical period of Hopi society and in a more stable family constellation. That is, it is inferred that because of the general crisis and breakdown in Hopi cultural patterns, as well as in the family breakdown, it was not possible for Lola to acquire or learn adequate control of her aggressive impulses.

THE FUTURE? What does the future hold for Lola? Prognosis for adjustment is considered "poor" in either the Hopi or the "white man's" culture. Should the efforts of rehabilitation be directed toward Lola's return to the Hopi way of life? Or should efforts be made to integrate her into the "white man's" culture? Lola doesn't know what she wants. How can the various rehabilitation workers facilitate the adjustment of this so-called "maladjusted" or "delinquent" adolescent during this period of culture crisis or emergency, when there is a critical imbalance in one or more essential dimensions of the cultural structure? These are but a few of the practical questions raised by clinical study of this adolescent whose maladjustment may be viewed as the end product of a cumulative cultural stress.

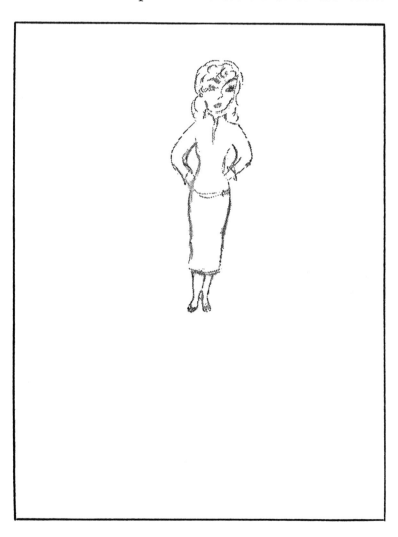

FIGURE 7-1. Draw-A-Person Test.

Test Summary

A. WECHSLER-BELLEVUE INTELLIGENCE SCALE (FORM I) FOR ADOLESCENTS AND ADULTS

Verbal Scale	Wtd. Score	*Performance Scale*	Wtd. Score
Information	5	Picture Arrangement . . .	10
Comprehension	6	Picture Completion	10
Digit Span	7	Block Design	13
Arithmetic	6	Object Assembly	12
Similarities	8	Digit Symbol	8
(Vocabulary)	–		
Verbal Score	32	Performance Score . . .	53
Verbal Scale IQ	81	Performance Scale IQ . .	102

Full Scale IQ . . . 91

Test Summary

B. RORSCHACH PROTOCOL

Response	*Inquiry*
CARD I.	
1. A butterfly. That's about all.	It's the whole blot. (Q) The wings.
CARD II.	
1. I don't know. (Rejects.)	
CARD III.	
1. Two people.	Over here (Q) Look like men (Q) By the head.
CARD IV.	
1. I don't know. (Rejects.)	
CARD V.	
1. A bat.	The whole thing. (Q) The wings are like flying.
CARD VI.	
1. I don't know. (Rejects.)	I can't see anything. (Breaks into tears again)
CARD VII.	
1. I don't know.	Don't know—nothing.
CARD VIII.	
1. A dog or something.	A dog. (Q) It just looks like a dog.
CARD IX.	
1. I can't see nothing.	Nothing

Response   *Inquiry*

CARD X.

1. I can't see nothing—I don't want   Nothing
to look at those cards. (She breaks
into tears—cries for a minute or
two.)

Test Summary

C. THEMATIC APPERCEPTION TEST

CARD 1.

I think that he thinks he has to take his violin lessons, and he doesn't
want to. He is thinking of how to get out of his lessons because he
doesn't want to. I think he doesn't know whether to ask to get out
of his lessons, so he'll take his lessons and maybe some day he will
become a musician.

CARD 2.

I think that this girl is glad that she can study and go to school
rather than stand out there and work. She is happy that she can get
an education, and not be there like her parents who are very poor
and work in the fields. She hopes to be a teacher or something and
make a success of her life.

CARD 3GF.

This girl has had a fight or something. She has been very hurt by
somebody. Somebody might have taken something she had and they
didn't want to give it up. She fought over it but she couldn't get
it back and now she feels hurt and she can't do anything more about
it. She tried talking and then argued about getting it back, and that
is about all she can do about it.

CARD 4.

This man he seems like he is hurt or something because this girl his
wife caught him going with another woman. His wife is pleading
with him not to feel bad because they can start things over. This
other girl looks like she wants to start trouble. They make up and
they get along and he forgets about this other girl.

CARD 5.

This woman is frightened because she saw something in the other
room. It was really just her imagination. (Q) One of her relatives,

a person. (Q) She often thinks of this person and misses her since she died. (Q) She has been dead for quite a long time. (Q) She tries to forget her because she is too frightened even imagining she sees her.

CARD 7GF.

This woman, this lady, is talking to this little girl. She is reading her a story but this little girl doesn't seem to be interested. This little girl is thinking about some other person that used to read to her and how she misses her. (Q) This other person that used to read to her was her own mother. (Q) The little girl feels unhappy right at the moment, she wishes it was her own mother, however she knows she has to forget and she tries.

CARD 8GF.

This woman looks like she doesn't know what to do and is thinking about what to do. (Q) She has so much to do and doesn't know what to do first, like housework or something. She feels she has to do as much of her work as possible and just doesn't know where to begin. She does her work and after a time she does manage to do all the things she has to.

CARD 10.

This woman looks like she is happy about something and she wants to cry with joy. (Q) Maybe she has had a child and she is happy and the man is happy as she is. (Q) They have a little boy, they just spoil him, but they live very happy.

CARD 12F.

This old woman looks like she is advising this woman to do something. This girl is not very happy about it, and the old woman is saying something will happen to her if she doesn't take her advice. (Q) She takes her advice and later she is happy that she took this old woman's advice. She wants to repay this old lady for her advice, but by then the old woman has died, and the only way she can repay her is by keeping on doing what this old lady told her to do.

CARD 14.

This boy looks as if he is locked up in a dark room. He is thinking about going out in the world and doing things right and being a success so that he doesn't have to be locked up. (Q) He might have disobeyed the law and they do let him out and he makes a success. He supports his family and they live happily. (Q) He joins the service and does all right, I really don't know what he can do.

8

A Stoic Faces Stress

George W. Hohmann

THE STRESS

John Yatsiti was hard at work on the railroad when the foreman of his section crew notified him that his father was seriously ill at their summer hogan high in the Arizona mountains. John left work, got his battered old jalopy, picked up a friend, and started up the main highway toward the high country pastures, where his family had taken their small flock of sheep.

About dusk that evening in 1953 John grew tired of driving so he let his friend take over and he went to sleep in the back seat. The next thing John remembered was his sudden awakening as the car lunged over a steep embankment. John was thrown from the car and landed on his head. When he regained consciousness he tried to get up to find his friend but he could not move, for John's neck had been broken, and he was completely paralyzed save for his head and neck. He called out to his friend, but he did not answer—for he was dead. And that is how this stoic young Navajo came to know his greatest stress.

THE BACKGROUND

CHILDHOOD AND EARLY TRAINING. Stress was no stranger to John for he had grown up under conditions of severe economic privation even for a Navajo. He was born thirty-two years ago in the mountain hogan of his father, where the family had gone for the summer months. John's parents were in their early twenties and had been married about a year. He was their first child and during the following twenty years, thirteen more children were born, two of whom died in infancy. Eleven of John's siblings are living and well. Four or five of the younger children are still at home with his parents, as well as an older sister who "is old maid, stay home with mother." Three other sisters are married to Navajo men who have left the reservation and work as miners. Another brother and sister are away in Indian Service schools.

During his early childhood, John recalls that his parents were always good to him and that the entire family "stick together." There were few arguments or signs of discord in the family. Although they were always poor, he recalls only a few occasions when "I cry because not enough to eat." They never had good clothes, jewelry, or other signs of wealth. He feels that his parents were not especially strict in disciplining him but, according to Navajo custom, as a son he was always spanked by his father. He believes he was a fairly well-behaved youngster and the main thing he got in trouble for was "teasing the girls."

There was little time for frivolity in John's life. By the time he was six years old, he was expected, as the oldest child, to do many chores. When he was old enough to go to school he had to work steadily helping his father tend their sheep, so that John has had no formal education. During most of his childhood and youth the struggle for more than a bare livelihood was interrupted only by occasional days spent visiting relatives, attendance at church on Sundays, where his uncle was the minister, and trips to the trading post where they bartered their wool, and the blankets his mother wove, for food and clothing. Sometimes they would attend tribal rituals or would gather with their relatives for a "sing" to benefit an afflicted kinsman.

MILITARY SERVICE. When John was eighteen, he was drafted into the army. He had some difficulty in getting along at first because he spoke only Navajo, but after a short period in a school where he was taught the rudiments of conversational English, he made a good adjustment in the service and enjoyed it. He was the only Navajo in his company and was occasionally annoyed when he was mistaken for a Mexican, for he is proud of the fact that he is an Indian. Throughout the four years he was in the service, he was assigned to a heavy construction unit, and his main duties were helping to lay temporary metal airstrips. He spent nearly two years in the South Pacific, where he contracted malaria, which finally became so severe that he was evacuated stateside. The malaria continued to bother him for about five years following his military discharge and was the only serious illness he had had before his accident.

ADULT LIFE. When he left the army he returned to his family on the reservation. Although he had liked the service and seemed to have looked on it as a great adventure, he felt no inclination permanently to leave his native culture. As he says, "The Navajo has his own way, and don't want to live no other way." When he came home, John found his family better off economically than they had ever been. He worked with his father and soon they had accumulated a flock of more than two hundred sheep. John found himself a girl-friend, and after nearly two years of courtship they had made plans to be married when an unexpected government regulation limited each family to sixty-one sheep. John feels they were exploited when they were paid only two dollars a head for those sheep they had over their quota. With this reversal, John postponed his marriage, left home, and found part-time and seasonal employment on the railroad. He continued his courtship when he was at home between jobs, and, at the time of his injury, once again had definite plans to marry.

THE ILLNESS

ONSET. It was the morning after the accident that someone finally noticed the wreckage and came to John's aid.

He was taken to an Indian Service hospital, and for several weeks it was doubtful that he would live. About two months later he was transferred to a Veterans Administration hospital where he could receive specialized treatment for his quadriplegia.

EARLY COMPLICATIONS. When he came to the veterans hospital, he had a complete paralysis and anesthesia below the shoulders. He had a few flickers of muscular control in the shoulders and upper arms. There was a complete loss of control of sphincters of bladder and bowel, and sexual functioning was destroyed. He had lost nearly a third of his body weight, had some pressure sores, and suffered from severe chills and fever due to urinary sepsis. He was completely dependent on others for all his physical needs and had difficulty in making these known, for he had forgotten most of the limited English vocabulary he had learned while he was in the Army.

PSYCHOLOGICAL REACTION. Despite all this, John always seemed to be in good spirits; he never complained about his predicament in general nor about any of his distressing symptoms. He never mentioned any pain, though this is usually a disturbing complication, especially during the first months after injury. Most of the time he either lay quietly in his bed, or, as he began to recall his English vocabulary, he was inclined to make jokes, tease nurses, and encourage his fellow patients. He soon became a favorite with both patients and personnel, and his subtle, clever sense of humor and his clowning antics cheered everyone.

"THE RECOVERY"

MEDICAL STATUS. John was a most cooperative and hardworking patient and he responded well to his complicated and tedious regimen of medical and physical rehabilitation, so that two years after he came to the hospital he had regained considerable independence. He is able to spend most of the day up in his wheel chair, and has regained enough movement in his arms to wheel himself almost anywhere in the hospital that he cares to go. He has very little use of his hands. His bladder function is regulated and his urinary sepsis fairly well controlled, though he must wear a urinal continuously. There has been no return of sexual function. His bowels are regulated by enemas though he sometimes may soil himself. His pressure sores are healed. He can feed himself with adaptive utensils and he can attend to most of his toilet but he must have help to get in and out of bed and to get dressed.

EDUCATION AND SOCIALIZATION. In addition, John has capitalized on opportunities for educational, recreational, and social activities. He has worked diligently with the educational therapists and has learned to read at about the fifth-grade level and to write on a typewriter with adaptive equipment. He also has studied arithmetic, geography, and history. A special interest in the history of the American Indians has been developed and he wants to "learn what happen to them since white man come to what call New World." He says, too, that he "want learn speak English real good, so I talk much like them college guys." Through recreational activities, he was drawn into a public-speaking group organized along the line of toastmasters. John enjoys making recordings and has done several Navajo chants and songs. He rarely misses a party in the recreation hall, and though initially he seems almost painfully shy and retiring in such situations, he says that Navajo men do not make small talk with strange women.

ADJUSTMENT TO DISABILITY. With all this, it is little wonder that John was considered so well adjusted that he was never referred for the customarily routine psychological evaluation. To be sure, he could sometimes be seen sitting alone in the sun in some remote area of the hospital grounds as though lost in troublesome thoughts, but he gave little overt evidence of the usual or "normal" turbulent reactions experienced by most patients during the first year or two following injury. Unlike most patients, he never seemed to cling, in an overdetermined way, to unrealistic hopes for a miraculous recovery or to deny the seriousness of his condition. He did not seem obsessed by a need to blame his predicament on himself with resultant withdrawal and depression. Nor did he blame others and become overtly hostile, negativistic, and aggressive. He rarely showed signs of irritation at the myriad frustrations he met daily, and he gave little indication of rebellion against his enforced dependency. Grief over his great loss was not shown by John. In short, he seemed to face stoically his troublesome life without letting himself or others really know his true feelings.

THE PROBLEM

PSYCHOLOGICAL TESTING. John first came to the attention of the psychologist when it was desired, for didactic purposes, to obtain test protocols on a patient from an Indian cultural group. Since John was known to be a cooperative person who might be intrigued by the testing, his help was enlisted. He quickly formed a comfortable relationship with the examiner and seemed interested in the testing. The first examination, completed in December, 1955, consisted of obtaining personal history data and administration of the Rorschach and those parts of the Wechsler Adult Intelligence Scale (WAIS) which he had the physical ability to complete.

WECHSLER ADULT INTELLIGENCE SCALE. On an abbreviated WAIS, he obtained an estimated I.Q. of about 88 (see Test Summary A). It is very difficult to get a measure of his actual level of intellectual functioning because on verbal tests he is handicapped by his language and cultural limitations, and on nonverbal performance items by his motor impairment. It is interesting to note that on Block Designs, a task which is not completely foreign to him, inasmuch as Navajo men sometimes draw designs for blankets, he obtains his best score. He achieved this success in spite of having to roll and push the blocks with the sides of his hands. It was evident that he perceived the organization of the designs quickly and constructed them systematically and correctly. On only one design did he fail to complete the task in the maximum time allotted, but in no case did he gain additional credits for speed, a limitation obviously due to his paralysis. This performance, combined with his ingenuity in working around his physical handicap and the rapidity with which he learns, suggests that he has at least average, if not superior, intellectual ability.

RORSCHACH. On Rorschach I (see Test Summary B), John gave a total of sixteen responses, with an average time of 47 seconds per response. His average reaction time to the achromatic cards was twenty-eight seconds and to the colored cards, ten seconds. Unlike the protocols of most Navajos, John's record consisted exclusively of "whole" responses with the exception of the popular large detail on Card VIII. The first Rorschach revealed dilation, an anxious use of shading (k), and a lack of formal intellectual controls (low F), which immediately suggest that all is not as well with John as his usual behavior and jovial façade would indicate. This impression was quickly corroborated by his response to the first card, where he expresses the dysphoric feeling of leaves eaten away by bugs. He goes on to give symbolically the apprehension and anxiety which he feels about his impaired bodily functioning in general, and more specifically about those functions located in the pelvic area. His feelings, which are readily given on a symbolic level, have been stoically denied in his daily behavior and verbalizations. These initial responses are quite typical of those given by most spinal cord injured patients about six months following injury, when they are at the depth of their depressive reaction brought about by the full impact of an awareness of the severity of their loss and the improbability of a complete recovery. Ordinarily such signs of depression will have largely disappeared by the twelfth to eighteenth month after injury, when the patients have had time to abreact the trauma of their loss and rediscover interests in their lives.

In the second card, John continues to be preoccupied with his physical functioning, especially with respect to sphincter control and sexual function. One cannot help but wonder why John, some thirty months after injury, is still so concerned about these disabilities when many patients, who clinically appear to have made much poorer adjustments, have long since lost these preoccupations.

The pervasiveness of the depression becomes increasingly evident on Card III, where its relation to anxiety and guilt about excretory functions and impotence is clear. Incidentally these complications of spinal cord injury are universally considered to be more severe than the orthopedic difficulties imposed by the paralysis. Under the impact of the same stimulus, however, John also gives, for the first time, a response (2) which is *not* laden with anxious, depressed affect, and some recoverability is shown.

Next, on Card IV, expression is given to the façade, the hard shell of stoicism, the defensiveness of maintaining that he is impermeable to the circumstances which have befallen him. But then he shows his inner sensitivity, an awareness of feeling which he is reluctant to admit and of which he is critical.

In the next two cards, John continues to show his basic sensitivity to interpersonal relationship but is also critical of it, perhaps because this basic sensitivity is one thing that constitutes a threat to maintaining his stoic façade. When confronted with the symbolism of female sexuality in Card VII, his response is one of great distance and coldness. We may well wonder whether John feels that any heterosexual relationship is quite as remote and unattainable as "Japan islands" and quite as cold as an iceberg. Following his distant, cold response to female sexuality, John turns to further concern about bodily function in the next card. This is interrupted briefly by the compelling "popular" animal response, which he apparently associates with warmer, happier days in the desert.

Through the remaining two cards, John continues his preoccupation with bodily functioning and expresses the depressive concern about wilting and decaying flowers. One cannot resist the idea that his first response, the bug-eaten leaf and the wilting flower are related to his self concept arising out of his agrarian background. He must feel that he too is eaten out, wilting, and decaying.

In testing the limits with him, John readily added to his human and animal movement responses, and gave nicely symbolized sexual responses (snake to the top of VI, and water coming through gates to bottom of VII). With but little encouragement he gave the usual sexual responses to these areas and admitted that he had thought of it when he first saw them. Thus it is suggested that he has control of his expression of feelings in this area, but without excessive repression or denial.

EVALUATION. In summary then we may say that John is a man who probably has at least average or better intellectual ability but who is prevented from fully demonstrating this by his language handicap, cultural difference, and motor paralysis. He gives clear evidence of a moderately severe depressive reaction, and his responses are typical of those given by other patients a few months following injury and are similar to those of anyone who is experiencing a grief reaction to a great loss. The question is raised as to why John's depressive reaction, as shown on the Rorschach, has continued at least a year longer than that of most patients, especially in the face of the fact that in his overt daily behavior he appears to have made a much better adjustment to his difficult circumstances than most. Could it be that John's culturally inculcated stoicism, which demands that he never show grief, sorrow, despair, or frustration, has prevented him from giving vent to such feelings and working them out with the support and understanding of his compatriots and the hospital personnel? With these thoughts in mind work was continued with John.

THE TREATMENT

CRACKING THE FAÇADE. By the time the testing was over, John obviously felt comfortable with the psychologist. He almost eagerly appeared before the trainee group for which the testing was originally undertaken and answered questions about his culture and his feelings about it. At the end of the testing sessions, he expressed some feelings of discontent with his lot for the first time known to anyone at the hospital. He began talking about his frustration in life on the ward. He told how, when he asked attendants to help him or do something for him, they are sometimes busy and irritable and tell John to "do it yourself." This hurts him very much and he recalled that "before I hurt, I big man, strong, work hard, do anything anyone do and many kinds of work before sundown. If I could, I do everything for myself, don't ask no one." When asked what he did when the attendants did this, he replied, "not pay attention, just do nothing or make like a cartoon talking, be funny and pay no attention." He then volunteered considerable information about his frustration and irritation over the implications of his disability and contrasted his present condition with his previous independence and vigor. When talking about how he was before his injury he came near to tears and said irritably, "I must be crazy in the head to tell this." He was offered support and reassurance that such reactions were quite understandable and that it might be well to share his real feelings with someone. There seemed some acceptance of this, but John did not reappear for a while.

EXPERIENCING THE DEPRESSION. When he did return, it was for a further "testing" of the psychologist. John's television, given to him by some philanthropic group, was broken, and since he is completely without funds, he had no way to get it repaired. This was arranged through the Special Services Division of the hospital, and it was learned from them that John previously had had them do this on his own initiative. With this testing of the psychologist successfully passed, the treatment continued in its informal way.

No definite schedule of appointments was made and no time limits were set, but John usually came two or three times a week to talk with the therapist for half an hour or an hour. Almost at once he began to unload his feelings. He spent a great deal of time recalling how he used to ride horses, herd sheep, work on the railroad. On a pleasant day he compared the weather to his desert home, on a foggy day he would yearn for the dry heat of Arizona. Often when he would talk about how he could have these things no more, he would be quietly tearful, or sit comfortably in long periods of silence. He seemed at last to be allowing himself to grieve. He rarely joked or ridiculed himself in the therapist's office, but when he was seen in the hall he always gave a greeting that grew out of a joke he once told the therapist.

John's behavior on the ward began to change. He became a bit more demanding and irritable, and there was less joking and clowning. Ward personnel were prepared for this change by the therapist and were most cooperative in accepting his expression of these feelings.

After a while he began to talk about his girl-friend, how he had hoped to marry for so long before his injury and how he felt he could never do so now. He spoke of his fondness for children and his frustration that he would never be able to have any. He verbalized his desire to return to the reservation, and faced the impossibility of his doing so since he has no way of supporting himself, nor are there facilities there for him to receive adequate care.

He grew much freer in expressing his sexual frustration and his desire for a close affectional relationship. He stopped by one day to say that what he really needed was "some suk-suk" and explained that this was a slang term for intercourse which he had learned from Japanese prisoners of war when he was overseas.

RECOVERY FROM THE DEPRESSION. About six months after the therapy began, John's mood began to take a turn for the better. By that time he could talk meaningfully about his problems without seeming overwhelmed by sadness. He said, "I been worry too much. What I gotta do is work hard, get strong, so I get out of here." He took a renewed interest in his work in the gym, enrolled in some new courses in educational therapy, and resumed his activity in a public-speaking group. He went to occupational therapy and it was suggested that he might do some weaving, to strengthen his hands, but he disdainfully informed the therapist that that was "woman's work."

As John progressed, it was noted that he was less reserved in social situations. One day some movie starlets were visiting on the ward and John was seen to be watching them intently. He was encouraged to talk with them, but he refused, saying, "They're for the white boys," but added that if a Navajo girl were there he would talk to her. Shortly thereafter he told the therapist he would like to "find nice girl and do some courting."

PLANS FOR THE FUTURE.   Some eight months after the therapy started, he began to show an active interest in an idea for employment which he had half-heartedly advanced at the time of the testing. Another Navajo, who was a patient here some years ago, has been employed as a "disc jockey" at a radio station in New Mexico. He does a record show and commercials in the Navajo language for the benefit of prospective Indian customers. John believes he might well be able to handle such a job, and has undertaken further speech training. Perhaps more importantly he has written to several radio station managers, and has received realistic encouragement along these lines. By this time he could talk freely about how he no longer felt he had to "make like the cartoon" and he was encouraged to utilize the energy he formerly had channeled into maintaining his façade, to cope with the very real problems he faces.

Ten months after John's psychotherapy began he spontaneously asked one day to "take them tests again; see how much I learn." At first the therapist thought he was referring to specific academic information, and educational achievement tests were suggested, but he quickly made it clear that he meant "I learn not worry so much. Feel better." And it was thus that the second evaluation was undertaken.

THE RESULTS

PSYCHOLOGICAL RETESTING. In the second testing, the WAIS, Rorschach, and certain cards of the Thematic Apperception Test were administered. His WAIS performance was essentially unchanged, except that he did considerably better on Digit Span, suggesting the possibility of less interference of anxiety in the performance of this task.

THE SECOND RORSCHACH. In this testing John gave twenty-five responses to the Rorschach, nine more than previously (see Test Summary C). He shows much less tendency to give poorly organized whole responses ($W\%$ is 44) and places greater emphasis on large detail responses ($D\%$ is 52). Thus his manner of approach is consistent with improved ability to meet practical day-to-day problems and, incidentally, with Navajo response tendencies. The dilation has largely disappeared; there is an increase in formal intellectual controls (marked increase in F), and considerable decrease in the anxious use of shading, k. Even at this level of interpretation, it is suggested that John's adjustment has improved.

As regards content, only three anatomy responses appear, in contrast to their great preponderance in the previous record. The occurrence of one of these on Card I reveals the patient's continuing concern with bodily functions. Relief from his depression, however, is suggested by the replacement of the dysphoric "bug-eaten leaf" by the more usual "crab."

On Card II, in place of the response indicating bodily preoccupation, he now gives the popular one of animal movement. He also demonstrates his freedom to give sexual responses in the presence of the examiner.

On Card III, he again relaxes his concern with anatomy and gives only the popular human response. There is a shift in sexual identity of the figures from male to female. In this connection it is interesting to note that as most spinal cord injured patients gain a realistic acceptance of their enforced dependency, such a shift in the sexual identity of these figures occurs. This does not appear to indicate any basic psychosexual confusion, but rather a realistic acceptance of an enforced passivity.

He drops his crustacean response on Card IV, which has been taken as symbolic of his "hard shell of stoicism," and gives only the response indicating his inner sensitivity, remaining critical, however, of such feeling.

On Card V, the shading response of which he previously (V,1) had been so critical, has been relinquished in favor of the well-conceptualized "fighting turkeys." This suggests that in his fantasy he is capable of returning more freely to his native environment.

Card VI first appears as a "tiger hide," later becoming a "sheep hide," which seems to have pleasant early associations for him. With his ability to recollect his past more comfortably he must feel that he is more of a whole man. At least he is now able to give a sexual response. Surely there is greater conscious awareness of his problems in this area and greater ability to handle his feelings.

Now on Card VII we have a clear change in John's feelings related to the female symbolism of this card. Not only does he give up his airplane view of a distant iceberg, replacing it with the more usual sexual response, but also in his unconscious symbolization he now perceives "Texas State," which is in his own Southwest, and for him much more attainable than the distant "Japan Islands." One might well feel that he is again capable and ready to live intimately with a woman.

After his improved response to the sexual symbolism of Card VII, John runs the gamut of responses to Card VIII, from a preoccupation with his bodily functions, through several responses related to his native background (tree, lizard, desert rocks), to a conscious sexual response. Perhaps the most interesting thing, however, is the way he suddenly reaches for his depression, which seems almost gone, and says, "I nearly miss it," then giving the only clearly dysphoric response in this protocol. While it seems evident that he has improved greatly, the residuals of his depression remain.

One may well raise the question whether, with the numerous sexual responses given, he is not now in the process of working through his feelings in this area. When this phase is accomplished he may again realize there are also other important areas of function.

On the last two cards, John is much freer than previously, and gives a total of six responses, all well seen and fairly benign, which primarily reflect associations to his home. By contrast, on the first examination he gave but three responses, two of which reflected his bodily concern and the other ("old leaves, turn brown") showed his depression. He still clings to his "Japan Island" response, but it is now given casually, to a more appropriate area, without the feeling of icy cold and distance.

THEMATIC APPERCEPTION TEST. John's TAT responses give some further understanding of his present feelings (see Test Summary D).

In these stories John tells us that he has sustained a great loss and is grieving over it. He is worried about himself and recognizes that he faces a difficult life. He feels his helplessness and realistically questions his ability to overcome his difficulties; yet withal, there is a general feeling of guarded optimism, suggesting that with perseverance, hard work, and time, he may return.

RE-EVALUATION. In summary, it may be said that in the ten months between evaluations John really has faced the stress with which he had been confronted for the previous two and one-half years, and which he had at first strictly denied. He has allowed himself to grieve over his loss, has received that support and encouragement which realistically could be offered him, has worked through some of his problems, and is beginning to face the future in a different way. The retesting leaves little doubt that he is less anxious and apprehensive, less concerned about his bodily dysfunction, and perhaps less guilty about eliminative accidents growing out of his loss of sphincter control. Most certainly he is less depressed. He still is concerned about his loss of sexual function, but sexuality no longer seems such a distant and cold thing to him, and he has gained the ability to share these problems. It is hoped that this is a step toward their optimal solution.

Much work remains to be done with John. He has faced many problems; others remain. His bodily concern has lessened but not gone. His depression has lifted but not disappeared. His sexual feelings are more accessible but unsatisfied. Perhaps most important, John is still in the hospital, and though he has a plan for leaving, it has not yet been implemented.

THE IMPLICATIONS

The striking thing about this case is not how much this Navajo, whose culture places great value on stoicism in the face of stress, differed from others in the reactions he had to experience when confronted with great loss. Rather it is of interest that his stoic refusal to indulge in the usual or "normal" grief seems simply to have prolonged his depressive reaction. It is a moot question as to how long he might have gone on with his inner depression and his façade of joviality had he not by chance been offered the opportunity to grieve over his losses and abreact the trauma of his injury and its sequelae.

It is suggested that the inner reaction to great personal loss is much the same for the stoic as for anyone else. Stoicism, a form of suppression, does not seem to offer a way of averting such reactions, but rather seems only to postpone them and interfere with the adjustive value of grief reactions in the face of loss.

Once a person has worked through his feelings about a loss, and has accepted it in a realistic way, stoicism may be an effective way of dealing with that over which one has no control. And so in the case of John, it is hoped that he may realistically face, with stoic resignation, those things in his life which he cannot change, and that he may channel his energies into salvaging his life and building for a constructive future.

Test Summary

A. WECHSLER ADULT INTELLIGENCE SCALE (WAIS)

Verbal Scale	Wtd. Score	Performance Scale	Wtd. Score
Information	6	Picture Completion . .	9
Comprehension	7	Block Design	11
Arithmetic	5		
Similarities	10		
Digit Span	7		
Vocabulary	5		
Verbal Score	40	Performance Score . .	20(50)*
Verbal Scale IQ	79	Performance IQ (Est.)	101

Full Scale IQ (Estimated) . . 88

* Prorated.

Test Summary

B. RORSCHACH PROTOCOL I

Response	*Inquiry*

CARD I. 5″

1. Looks like leaves from trees, something eat some of it.

   Just looks like leaves—hole here where bug eat part away. (Q) Nothing.

   W,S   F   P

2. Man right here where bladder is—like pictures they take—this be tail—this sides.

   (Q) Just looks like those pictures they take in G.U. room of man in this part (gestures to pelvis).

   W   Fk   At

CARD II. 6″

1. Looks like same thing but different—this is tail and this go on up.

   This part here (gestures to pelvis) the side here and this go up to back. (Q) Them same pictures.

   W   Fk   At

CARD III. 7″

1. Same thing but shows bones more, this is parts of body inside, the red spot.

   This is around the middle here and bones for sides here and this is tail part here—the red is the inside parts.

   W   Fk,C/F   At

Response	*Inquiry*
2. Looks like two guys holding something.	They hold this. (Q) Head, neck, arms, legs. (Guys?) (Patient smiles self-consciously) They just look like it.

W M   H   P

CARD IV. 35″

1. Just like some funny stuff in the ocean—hard animals that walk around.

W FM,Fc A

Like those things that bite with legs. (Q) Like have hard outsides—they got little stickers all over (gestures).

2. Like skin of a cow—see that, tail like.

W Fc   A obj

(Q) Head here, eyes, tail turned up here, legs. Not good job. (Q) Stretched out to dry. (Q) Fur side is showing.

CARD V. 14″

1. Something like you skin an animal. This is back here and you skin around. This be tail and side here.

W Fc   A obj

Skinned him—not good job—goes around here. (Gestures to abdomen.) Tail here and head up here. (Q) Looks like a fur.

2. Turn it looks like a bird. Going, fly up like you see them.

W FM   A   P

Mouth here, got wings out. Fly up here—tail out.

CARD VI. 55″

1. Don't know what kind is, but looks like skinned wild cat—don't look like they skinned it off right.

W Fc   A obj P

It's spotted like a wild cat and this looks like it was skinned off the head and face.

CARD VII. 32″

1. Sometimes ride airplane, see water around—break the ice like in Japan islands—other words, like some islands with gulf here.

W,S FK,C′F Geo

This ice broken away by water. (Q) It looks that color and is crooked (gestures) and stick up here. (Q) Yes, this looks closer.

Response	*Inquiry*

CARD VIII. 15″

1. Just about the chest in here—like maybe the heart here—hip would be down here and chest up here. This, outside body muscle.

I saw picture in book for Doctor show like that. (Q) Colored to show parts of the body.

W   F/C   At

2. This looks like two rocks, brown rocks, blue rocks, and something jumping across. Might be a small lizard, in desert, you know.

(Q) The lizard head, feet and tail here. He jump across rocks. Colored like in desert.

D   FM,CF   A   P

CARD IX. 13″

1. Looks like the same thing—inside the body. This looks like the heart and this is something.

Like those pictures colored to show inside parts of body.

W   F/C   At

2. This way it's the color, the leaves here, the stem and flower on top. This looks like the leaves are a little bit old.

Those old leaves turn brown. These leaves still green and this is a red flower.

W   FC   Pl

CARD X. 9″

1. This be right in here the body. This be—go to chest, breathe. Bladder is right here. That's all.

These others are different parts of the body—this where you breathe, down in here. (Gestures to lungs.) This is bladder. (Q) Like those colored pictures in a book.

W   F/C   At

Test Summary

C.   RORSCHACH PROTOCOL II

Response	*Inquiry*

CARD I. 4″

1. Like the bone right here (gestures to pelvis) what you call it.

(Q) Just looks like it, those pictures the doctor take, looks like the backbone here.

W   Fk   At

2. Or looks like a crab—that's all.

Legs out here, head, pinchers. (Q) That's all.

W   F   A

	Response	*Inquiry*

CARD II. 23″

1. Looks like a bear fight there. Heads here—or kiss each other.

    WᚷX   FM   A   P

Inquiry: Heads, ears, nose. (Q) Noses together.

2. Looks like a woman here (smiles). Don't want say nasty word.

    D   F   Sex

Inquiry: Just this bottom part looks like a woman—sex. (Patient explains in detail the differences between the Navajo polite and slang terms for female sexuality.)

CARD III. 6″

1. Looks like somebody, two—holding something.

    W   M   H,Sex   P

Inquiry: Head, body, legs, hand, and this something they hold, don't know what. (Q) Looks like women because this (indicates breast).

CARD IV. 3″

1. Looks like a cow hide, tail end, and head here.

    W   Fc   A obj

Inquiry: (Q) The color looks like it, and tail here has been cut off—skinned off here but not right, not good job. (Q) Like a fur, soft.

CARD V. 24″

1. Turn around this way, looks like two birds fighting, heads, feet, and feathers going back here.

    W   FM   A

Inquiry: Feet, wings, flying back together—turkeys fighting.

2. This way looks like a butterfly.

    W   FM   A   P

Inquiry: Butterfly, flying up. (Q) Just wings on each side, tail and head this way.

CARD VI. 2″

1. Looks like a tiger hide.

    W   Fc   A obj   P

Inquiry: (Q) Just the fur, like you touch.

2. An old sheep hide too, some old sheep hide.

    W   Fc   A obj

Inquiry: A sheep hide—an old one—fur just the same, is soft.

(a) This looks like a little snake.
    D   F   A
(b) But the peter too.
    D   F   Sex

Response	*Inquiry*

CARD VII. 18"

1. Looks like some kind of animal leg here.	Just this much, the foot and leg. (Q) Way shaped, leg here, hock up here.

D   F   Ad

2. This way looks like—don't want to say it—a woman again.	Just this way, with legs spread apart.

D   F   Sex

3. If a little more on this way, would be like Texas state.	Top part here, across here, ocean around here and up to Mexico.

D,S   F   Geo

CARD VIII. 10"

1. Looks like some kind of body, chest here, bladder here, ribs.	(Q) Looks like the bones. (Q) Like colored charts I've seen in doctors' books.

W   F/C   At

2. And here looks like some kind of lizard.	Hind legs, front paws and head. (Q) Just crossing over something.

D   FM   A   P

3. And here looks like a woman too.	Just the split down the middle.

D   F   Sex

4. Something a little bit like a tree.	Pointed top of a tree. (Q) Just the shape of it.

D   F   Pl

5. This right here looks like the rocks, you know those yellow stones—that's all (pushes card away, then takes it back).	Like yellow and red rocks in the desert in Arizona. (Q) No, just the colored rocks.

D   CF   N

6. One more, I nearly miss it. Looks like some kind of leaves which has been eaten up by an insect.	All of it, the holes are where insect eats. (Q) Like in fall, leaves turn all colors and still insects eaten some of them.

W,S   CF   P

Response   *Inquiry*

CARD IX. 42″

1. This way looks like some kind of tree to me.

 D FC   Pl

Just this tree in here, trunk and top. Some trees are flat this way—like red flowers on it.

2. And looks like some kind of elephant, ears too.

 D F   Ad

Ears big on each side, and nose here.

3. This way looks like an animal, some kind of coyote. See, ears go both ways.

 dr F   Ad

Ears here, head up to here, nose coming down to here. Long pointed face of a coyote.

CARD X. 12″

1. Jackrabbit sittin' way over here.

 D,S FM,FC′ A   P

(Q) Almost all of him, ears, nose, face, and white body down through here.

2. Grasshoppers here.

 D FC   A

The two horns and front feet. (Q) Green like a grasshopper.

3. Looks like some kind of island— Japan.

 D F   Geo

Just like it, looks like a map. Just the long shape of it.

Test Summary

D. THEMATIC APPERCEPTION TEST

CARD 1.

He thinking about how they make that and about how he will play it in his future life. He will be a cowboy like the movie star. (Happen?) He'll be able to play it, but now he's just a kid.

CARD 2.

This lady looks like she's tired. This lady looks like she is going home to make some chow for this man and this lady is sick or cross because it don't rain. Maybe she look this way and think about the rain. Looks like it's a little bit warm. (Happen?) Maybe it will rain. This ground looks like it's growing beans.

CARD 3BM.

Looks like this—is that a lady—looks like she's in jail, worry, thinking, crying. If she's in jail, is a wild woman in some kind of trouble. What's that on the floor, paper or gun? Looks like a little gun. (Q) Don't know, that's all.

CARD 4.

Looks like the man is going some place long way away and that lady looks like she worry. Some kind of loss. He gamble, looks like lost everything they were. He go away. (Return?) A long time, then he will.

CARD 8BM.

This guy looks like he's dreaming, walking, thinking about this thing going to happen. This gun—he go hunting, get shot, go to hospital and doctor operating. Maybe already happened. (Turn out?) Maybe he is still hurt and feel sorry for himself. Maybe think he never do it again.

CARD 13B.

This boy looks like he worry about that other boy that got shot. Maybe he's thinking about how he's going to get along in his future life in school. Maybe he lost something to play with, but he's worried. He try to find some way—maybe he find it.

CARD 13MF.

This man, looks like his wife died or is real sick and he start to cry. He can't do nothing about it. Maybe she's been dead and he came home to see it.

CARD 17BM.

This man looks like he's been in prison and is trying to escape. Maybe he'll make it.

Indian Postscript

Ella, whose father was Negro, provides a transition from Part I. Her mixed blood symbolizes her mixed-up identity. This young woman incorporated the culture conflict between her lower-class Negro father, who tried to seduce her, and her proud and dominant Iroquois mother, who rejected her. Although highly endowed herself, Ella felt that her physical resemblance to her father forced her into an alliance with him which isolated her from the rest of her family. Her harsh superego, the product of an unbending religious training, would not admit the intense hostility generated by her frustrating parents, and transformed it intropunitively into a masochistic character defense. As she decompensated, following her mother's violent death, she developed compulsive and depressive reactions with suicidal tendencies, which led her to seek the protection of the hospital.

Lola, the full-blooded Hopi girl, is not unlike Ella, insofar as she has experienced the impact of conflicting cultures. Although there was no ethnic discrepancy between her father and mother, they were in extreme religious discord as followers of the Hopi Bear Clan and the Mennonites, respectively. An added aspect of Lola's culture conflict was the breakdown of Hopi socialization patterns stemming from a major crisis at the tribal level. Under such circumstances the growing girl was offered no consistent pattern to follow. Without a strong superego to keep her in line, Lola was left to the mercy of her impulses and became so serious a behavior problem that she had to be committed to a correctional institution. Her culture conflict was further complicated by Catholicism, a faith avoided by the Hopi since the days of the early Spanish missions.

When Lola got into fights with her Indian schoolmates over tribal obligations, she experienced severe conflict between her parents' peaceful religious precepts and her stronger impulse to fight. In such crucial situations she escaped into hallucinatory trancelike seizures during which she "consulted" her dead parents. Viewed in the context of her culture, such behavior appeared less malignant than it would have in the rank and file of middle-class white patients. Nevertheless, lack of a stable frame of reference as a guide for personality growth makes the prognosis almost as guarded in Lola's case as in that of Ella, whose splitting ego finally shattered.

John presents a contrast to the other two cases. Firmly rooted in the native Navajo culture transmitted to him in a large, harmonious family, his identification pattern is highly congruent with the dominant culture. He early learned the highly valued suppressive technique of stoicism which served him well as a defense against anxiety and as a protection against social dependency. In the extreme emergency of his broken neck, however, this defense proved *too* "effective," prolonging his depression at the same time that it successfully concealed it from others. To dispel the grief and proceed with his plans to return to his reservation and work for "the people," John had to be encouraged to work through his mourning.

An overview of the small sampling of cases in this section contributes evidence of the role played by culture conflict in personal conflict and reveals more about the mechanisms of interaction between the culture and the individual.

PART IV

SPANISH LEGACY

Preview

Like the indigenous Indians, the Spanish groups [1] antedate the Anglo-Saxon colonists in the New World. The culture transmitted by the first Spanish settlers is a curious mixture of old Spain and the native folklore of the Indians whom they married. In spite of its many variants, this cultural mixture provides its members with a cohesive core of religion, language, custom, and values, which they can make their own, and from which they can reach out for identities in the larger society. If, however, the earliest contacts in the family circle are deviant, the individual is deprived of his birthright of solid ingrouping, and subsequently may have serious trouble in finding himself anywhere else.

The material in this section demonstrates some of the strengths and weaknesses to be found within different groups of Spanish derivation. We have brought together cases from a number of variants of this subculture. There is Manuel, a Mexican-American from Texas, whose psychological problems came not from identification with his ethnic minority but from his attempt to repudiate it. We have also included some Puerto Rican men and boys from New York whose lives reflect the disintegration of certain basic values prevailing on the Islands, with resulting personal disorganization. Finally, there is a Filipino youth from California who offers some interesting comparisons and contrasts with the other Spanish culture groups.

---

[1] For a compact picture of the various Spanish culture groups, the reader is referred to J. H. Burma, *Spanish speaking groups in the United States* (Durham: Duke University Press, 1954).

9

Search for Identity by a Young Mexican-American

Horace M. Peak

CULTURAL BACKGROUND

FROM RICHES TO RAGS. In spite of the romantic history and honored tradition of Spanish America, the attitude of the American population today toward the descendants from the early days unfortunately can be summed up as the "Mexican Problem."

The pattern of Mexican living varies somewhat throughout the Southwest, depending on whether it is Texas, New Mexico, or California; but the differences are not fundamental, and a description of living conditions in Southern California will not do any real violence to the facts of the Mexican way of life as it is found anywhere in the Southwestern states.

Most of the Mexican people in southern California live in *colonias*, somewhat separated in space from the Anglo-American parent communities. They vary in size from a few small homes or shacks to settlements of several thousand, invariably located on the "wrong" side of something. In large cities like Los Angeles, Mexicans live in "pockets" of settlement, similar in most respects to the *colonias* of the outlying districts.

It must be noted that Mexicans are not segregated so rigidly as Negroes. Their resistance to absorption is not necessarily a "sour grapes" reaction. While excluded from some restricted places and areas, they still may gain admittance to many locations that Negroes may not enter. If gifted by nature with physical attractiveness or social skill, they are at full liberty to "crash" the cultural barriers and obtain social and economic emancipation. But few ever do so. Most are unable to or, for that matter, do not even want to under the present circumstances. Resentful of the fenced-in nature of the existence forced upon their kind, many who could "pass" react by rejecting as unworthy the culture which has rejected them.

Mexicans are not foreigners in the American Southwest. Unlike most European minorities in America, Mexicans have had their roots in the country for centuries. They were here long before the Anglo-Saxons. Their ancestors settled here before the Anglo-Saxons had heard anything more than the merest rumor of the existence of the country. The Mexicans' relation to and feelings about the region in which they live are too important to be ignored in any adequate study of the problem.

SPANISH SUBGROUPS. The Mexican problem is further complicated by the subgroups within the Mexican minority. Aside from the Mexicans who are foreigners in the United States, we may recognize the Spanish-American descendants of colonists who moved into the country in the wake of early military and missionary expeditions. They married Indian wives, so that the Spanish-Americans of today are the descendants of the immigrants from Spain, New Spain, and the diverse tribes of Indians of the areas where they settled.

Mexican-Americans have many factors in common with Spanish-Americans. They have almost the same genetic background as the Spanish-Americans but with a larger proportion of physical characteristics from the Indian side of their ancestry. They are the descendants of immigrants from Mexico and as such lack many of the stabilizing influences which the ties to a common cultural past give to the Spanish-Americans.

The Mexican-Americans in particular are subjected in considerable degree to the forces of acculturation. The Mexicans have rapidly assimilated the utilitarian aspects of American culture, such as cars, household utilities, etc., but where cultural values have been involved the story is different. The Mexican has been much less inclined to give up the value ideals of his fathers.

Among those values which they are loath to relinquish may be named special foods, music, religion, and to a lesser extent, language. Even the young people who aspire to complete Americanization maintain their love of Mexican music. The Catholic Church remains as the strongest bond of unity and symbol of their communal needs and satisfactions. A Mexican who is no longer an active Catholic or who has embraced a Protestant faith, as in the case to be presented, has done almost as much as one can do to isolate himself from the main body of his people.

MEXICAN-AMERICAN FAMILY LIFE. Important differences involving values may often be observed between the Anglo- and Mexican-American family structure. The typical Mexican-American home of today is made up of the parents and dependent children. If grandparents or other relatives live in the home also, they very likely do so of necessity and by tolerance. But the extended household is still accepted in Mexican life and numerous homes may still be found in which married children, grandparents, aunts, and uncles, etc., have honored places. Adults in the family other than the parents may be parental in their attitude toward the small children of the household.

Older Mexican parents tend to cling to the ways of living associated with the Mexican culture. They believe in the family-centered life, in close family unity, in maintaining parental authority, and in unquestioning obedience from children. The father is the dominant figure, and the mother's role, overtly at least, is submissive. But the mother is respected and venerated and, covertly or subtly, may be a powerful factor in the home. The young children must accept and obey all older members of the family. If death or desertion has removed the father, mature male members of the family may assume authority and leadership.

SOURCES OF CONFLICT. From their contacts with Anglo children and other sources, including radio and TV, Mexican children learn of the Anglo way of life and the Anglo children's freedom from close home supervision and discipline. They discover the satisfactions to be had outside home life and the need for money to obtain these satisfactions. They become resistant to the institutional controls of the old culture.

Other important cultural differences are seen in basic personality traits and outlook on life. The average Mexican tends to be concerned with the present and the immediate past rather than the future. Security for him lies in the old and the stable and not in the new and unfamiliar. Mexican-Americans are not ego involved in their work as are Anglos. Work for them is not so apt to be an end in itself or even a means to an end; rather, it is the lot of man and they do only as much of it as is necessary. "Success" and "failure" do not have the same meanings for them as for the Anglo.

The Mexican is more likely to try to adjust to difficulties than he is to try to overcome them. This may be seen in his passive or docile reaction to authority or in his fateful inactivity in sickness. Nor does he see dependency in the same light as the Anglo. In his cultural background the unit of independence was the extended family or village, perhaps with its patron, and dependency on the part of any member was looked upon as normal. Dependency was subjectively defined and usually fully accepted, and any member's need became the unquestioned object of any or all who could contribute toward that need. The great differences in philosophy of acceptance and resignation, passivity, dependency, etc., between Mexicans and Anglos have been the cause of much misunderstanding of Mexicans by the Anglo population, who misinterpret Mexican philosophy and see these people as indifferent, lazy, or unambitious.

The expectations of the dominant American society confuse the Mexican people. In some circles the Mexican is expected to behave like a Mexican while in other places or at other times he is another "American." Many Mexicans can "pass" and, unlike the Negro, can do so without having to hide the facts of their birth and past life. But this passing subjects them to personal conflict. Shall they leave the ways and values of their own people and be assimilated into the aggressor culture? Certainly, the ambivalent, conflicted attitude which the Mexican has toward absorption can easily be understood.

The story of Manuel exemplifies the kinds of conflict that often complicate the lives of Mexican-Americans. In the present case, the only information available came from the subject himself. It follows, therefore, that many important data are missing, but it is believed that the biographical material obtained, supplemented by psychological testing, makes a valid description and analysis possible.

PERSONAL BACKGROUND

THE PICTURE OF ANXIETY. Manuel is a single, twenty-two-year-old Mexican-American who was referred to the psychologist by his college counselor following failure in his classes. He was tense and appeared unhappy when he came for the first interview, though he had been looking forward to the hour. He complained that he was failing in school and had been discharged from his job because of what he termed "attacks." When one of these attacks came on, he would begin to shake all over, feel dizzy, get pain like pin pricks in the back of his neck, feel panicky, have choking sensations, and perspire profusely. He was not able immediately to tell under what circumstances the attacks came on. He did emphasize, however, those attacks which occurred at work and talked at some length about the crude, vulgar, laboring Mexicans with whom he had to associate in his work. He said most of his friends were non-Mexicans or "Anglos" as he called them. They were refined, cultured people with whom he was proud to associate.

He had spent some time in his company hospital where he had a complete check-up. Here he was told that there was nothing physically wrong with him, that his trouble was emotional, and that he should seek psychological help. Not liking this diagnosis, he procrastinated and tried to struggle along in school. It was under these circumstances that he met the school counselor, who took time over a period of weeks to help him accept the idea that his troubles were of an emotional nature.

UPWARD MOBILITY. Manuel was born in a small city in Texas in what he called a slum area and under circumstances which he described as poverty. His father deserted before he was a year old and was never heard from again. His mother immediately moved with him and his older sister to New Mexico to live with her parents and brothers. Here Manuel spent his infancy and much of his childhood in continued poverty, the family being supported by the mother's father and brothers. When Manuel was nine, the family group managed to move into a better place; and the next few years saw a series of moves, each involving a step upward on the socioeconomic ladder.

Since they were likable people, the family managed to adjust fairly well wherever they went. However, they were Methodists, an affiliation that created some cultural distance between them and the Mexican population as a whole. Many of the Methodists were non-Mexicans or Anglos, and here Manuel had his first introduction to a bi-cultural conflict.

FAMILY AND FRIENDS. Manuel's mother did not remarry and at present makes a home for Manuel, whom she supports. She is an attractive woman, with very fair coloring and a vivacious personality. Her appearance was a source of considerable tension between her and her dark-complexioned in-laws who were more typically Mexican in appearance. She had only four or five years of schooling, a fact which worried her greatly and later entered into her relationship with Manuel. She managed to secure training and experience in simple clerical work, eventually attaining economic independence.

For many years she has had a close friendship with an American of Anglo-Saxon descent who has exerted a great influence over her and Manuel. His attitude is quite paternalistic, particularly toward Manuel who has come to resent him greatly because of his patronizing attitude. All the mother's friends are Anglos and have been for many years, a fact that has confused Manuel who did not have his mother's ability to "pass" in American society. She has always been over-protective of Manuel, and even now persists in treating him as if he were a small boy.

Manuel never knew his father, but was much influenced first by his maternal grandfather and later by an uncle who seems to have been the dominant male adult in his childhood. This surrogate father was in the home from Manuel's earliest childhood until his eleventh year. He took a lively interest in the boy, introducing him to various kinds of masculine activity including ball and other sports. He was also the disciplinarian, administering spankings when he deemed it necessary. In fact, he assumed the role of father and was accepted as such by Manuel.

Another early influence in his life was his sister. She seemed to have taken a motherly interest in Manuel, taught him to read Spanish, and encouraged other intellectual interests. Later she married an Anglo who is a member of a non-Mexican minority group.

When Manuel was nine years old the family moved to a better neighborhood where his mixed cultural associations began in earnest. There were only a few Mexican children in the local population; the remainder were Anglos, children of European descent, Jewish, Negro, etc. Some of them were children of well-to-do parents, and Manuel found association with them a source of particular satisfaction. Of this period he said, "My friends were little rich boys." His main techniques for securing their approval and companionship were usually those of compliance and subservience.

As a result of his older sister's help Manuel did fairly well in grade school. He ran into trouble in high school, failing in mathematics although he managed to get grades as high as B in some other classes. His verbal ability was good and he usually showed interest in and fair aptitude for anything involving reading and literature. His social life was also fair. His friends were mostly Anglos, although he always prided himself on being able to get along with the Mexican young people. He belonged to gangs of the non-delinquent type and never got into trouble, though there were occasional fights.

GIRLS. Manuel began dating when he was fifteen. His first girl friend was an Anglo but later he also dated Mexican girls. His interest in sex appears to have been normal. In spite of his passive, feminine-appearing ways he had sexual experiences involving intercourse, and there is nothing in his history to suggest homosexual tendencies. He describes his dreams as having been of intercourse with pretty girls.

At the age of nineteen he became engaged to a Catholic Mexican girl but his mother broke up the engagement ostensibly because of the girl's religious affiliations. He had his first anxiety attack at that time. This experience appears to have initiated a new chapter in his life in that it brought into focus his ambivalent dependency on his mother and his inability to break away from her control and enter adulthood on an independent basis.

Since this experience, and particularly since his illness, he has been very shy of girls. At the time he came for help he had begun to be interested in a fourteen-year-old blond Mexican girl who lived across the street from him. His behavior toward her was quite nonaggressive and nonmasculine.

SCHOOL AND WORK DIFFICULTIES. Manuel entered college with the idea in mind of becoming a teacher, but his grades were too low for him to continue. He tried a new college, but again failed. The second attempt was severely handicapped by disappointment over the refusal of the second school to accept a transcript from the first. His efforts to obtain an education were further obstructed by his mother's attitude. She severely criticized his school efforts, constantly demanded that he improve his performance, and upbraided his every failure regardless of how much he tried.

Employment became a very big problem in Manuel's life. While he succeeded in working quite steadily, he had to take ordinary laboring jobs which he detested. Aside from the operation of minority prejudice, his failure to secure the kind of work he wanted can be explained in terms of his passive, nonaggressive personality which in turn reflects his lack of self-confidence. He is constantly filled with resentment over his humiliation at having to do work, symbolizing all he has tried to leave behind and forget. His illness, while serving to relieve him of odious employment responsibility, has at the same time increased his dependency on his mother and exposed him to her continuous criticism.

CULTURE CONFLICT. Manuel's needs and conflicts are well illustrated in his interests and avocational activities. He prides himself on having high level interests, claiming to enjoy such books as *Crime and Punishment, Paradise Lost, Pilgrim's Progress, Modern Man in Search of a Soul.* Moreover, he says that he enjoys classical music and that he responds to the feeling tone. "I like anything that makes me think. . . . That is what keeps me apart from the Spanish people—my love of opera and deep books. The English Church accepts my ideas." The satisfaction he derives from these interests comes more from his self concept as a person who has them than from any intrinsic value they have for him. The interests do not win him friends, but tend rather to create social distance. In reality, Manuel is in no sense an intellectual; the discrepancy between his aspiration and reality levels is very great and indicates his confused ego identity.

More closely related to his "real self" is his enjoyment of bull fights, and the romance surrounding this tradition. It is significant that when he is angry with his mother, he likes to imagine that his pet dog is a bull and, pretending to be a matador, he plays out the preliminary teasing with a cloth for a cape.

Social activities and other associations further reflect the cultural and other personality conflicts of this individual. His closest friend is a non-Mexican-American married to a Mexican girl. Manuel teaches a Sunday School class in a mixed Mexican and Anglo church. Here he takes pride in displaying his learning, and the religious and philosophical ideas gained mostly from his reading. There is little doubt that he interprets smiles and other signs of patronizing interest from the Anglos as approval and acceptance while at the same time perceiving the disapproval of the Mexican members as reassurance that he has found a better way of life than the Mexican culture can offer him.

MOTHER AND GRANDMOTHER. Manuel found himself incapable of breaking away from the maternal bonds which, as he grew older, he resented more and more. He said, "I am dominated by my mother." He did not confide in her and kept away from her as much as possible. His usual practice was to give in to her. On the rare occasions when he rebelled openly he suffered great remorse afterwards. Of one such experience he said, "I stood up to her, and she gave in. I felt like a heel afterwards." He was away from her for about a year at college at one time and reported that he felt fine during that time although he was getting very poor grades.

One of Manuel's greatest sources of comfort as he grew up was his grandmother who shared the home with his mother and sister. She seemed to be all that his mother was not—comforting, encouraging, and accepting. She took his side against his mother, praised his school efforts, and in general gave him the emotional support he needed.

Shortly following his grandmother's death the most serious aspects of Manuel's illness began. He grieved greatly over her passing, experiencing repetitive dreams in which he was with her in the old relationship. In his simple, naïve, yet appealing way he said, "In my dreams I can have her again." After she was gone his hostility toward his mother rapidly fulminated. He had to face his mother alone, and her domination and goading stirred him to anger he dared not express. At home and at work he began to have the severe attacks that finally brought him to seek help.

FIRST ATTACK. The first incident occurred one evening when he was watching TV and his mother told him to turn it down. He went out of the house, slamming the door behind him. Immediately he began to shake all over. From then on attacks were frequent and some of them were very severe.

PSYCHOLOGICAL ASSESSMENT

Manuel presented himself as a neatly dressed young man of medium build and good posture. Although his complexion was quite fair, his features suggested a Mexican rather than an American background. He was friendly, smiling readily, and impressing one immediately with his gentleness and passivity, in striking contrast to the more usual Mexican masculinity picture. His behavior gave no indication of perceptual distortion or inappropriate affect.

For psychological assessment of his intellectual status and psychodynamics, an intelligence scale and several projective tests were administered.

I.Q. The Wechsler-Bellevue Intelligence Scale, Form I, was selected as the most appropriate measure of intellectual functioning. It will be observed from the test results (presented in Test Summary A) that the Verbal Scale I.Q. was 110 while the corresponding Performance score was only 87. The Full Scale I.Q. comes out 99. From this we can assume that the patient is functioning broadly within the "normal" range of intelligence, his verbal ability, however, reaching the Bright Normal level, with his performance ability dropping down into the Dull Normal distribution. The discrepancy between these two main parts of the scale suggests emotional instability. On the Verbal Scale, the only tests that measured below par, Arithmetic and Digit Span, are the most sensitive to temporary inefficiency due to fluctuations in attention. The patient's generally poor motor ability displayed in his performance test scores, may also be largely accounted for by his self-consciousness and distractibility. His failures on the Digit Symbol and Block Design tests, which involve learning and reasoning ability, are well compensated for by his high score on Similarities on the Verbal Scale. It seems reasonably safe, especially in view of the negative neurological findings, to attribute Manuel's wide inter-test scatter to emotional distractibility resulting from his extreme anxiety. It is these factors rather than inadequate capacity that undoubtedly explain his poor scholastic showing.

PROJECTIVE TECHNIQUES. The Thematic Apperception Test (TAT) and the Make-A-Picture-Story Test (MAPS) (see test summaries B and C) provided Manuel with a medium for projecting his goals, conflicts, identifications, and defenses. In these tests, Manuel's responses reveal his identifications with Americans of social and economic status higher than his own. His heroes are all middle-class non-Mexicans, as in the family scene described in response to MAPS, 1, "The Living Room." The villains in his stories, on the other hand, are non-white zoot-suiters, *pachucos*, colored B-girls, etc. A good example is afforded in his fantasy to MAPS, 2. In view of the sad lot of his people, Manuel's goal is clear: He will become a kind of Moses to lead his people out of the bondage of poverty. This sense of mission comes out repeatedly in his fantasies. Thus, in TAT, 2, he visualizes himself as a college-bred agricultural expert teaching the ignorant the latest methods of crop cultivation; in 13B, he returns home as a teacher, a lawyer, or a doctor to bring succor to his downtrodden people; and again, in 8BM, he appears as a doctor relieving their pain. The same theme is the basis of his fantasy on the MAPS, 7, "The Shanty," in which, after becoming educated and learning about minority people, he becomes a lawyer, a doctor, or a minister, in order to help his people rise up from the ground. Running through these altruistic aspirations is the more homely aim of his making his people proud of him through the personal glory he attains as a professional expert in the stories already recounted, as well as through other avenues to fame such as the fantasy on TAT, 1, of becoming a musician like Heifetz interpreting Mozart.

In the light of his low level of intellectual ability and achievement, the aspiration level in these fantasies is far out of line with reality. The unrealistic nature of his striving comes close to awareness in his story on TAT, 3, where he says: "It looks like a boy that's crying . . . weeping because maybe he's had some great disappointment. Either he didn't pass in school, or someone he loved very much has passed away." His need for his magic-helper grandmother is apparent, and comes out again in response to MAPS, 9, "Dream." In spite of the obvious risk of failure, he strives compulsively toward unrealistic goals, refusing to downgrade his unattainable ambitions.

PERSONALITY EVALUATION

CONFUSED IDENTITY. At the back of Manuel's losing struggle for status is his basic search for an identity which in a sense is a hand-me-down from his mother and his maternal grandparents. The grandparents' struggle for status had its roots in the early Texan-Mexican conflicts. Leaving the church of their father, they had identified with the American "aggressor" in religion. Whatever their motives for this defection from "the Faith," it served the purpose of obtaining for them some of the status they felt they could not find in old cultural ties. From his childhood Manuel remembers his grandfather's struggle to get his family "across the tracks," and the other side of the tracks meant, to them, becoming as Americanized as possible.

Becoming Americanized, however, did not mean ceasing to be Mexican. The mother's family lacked the ability really to pass the cultural barrier. Thus the family social and cultural pattern assumed a strange hodgepodge of mixed loyalties, identifications, and values. The mother was more seriously involved than other members of her family. What turn of fate or of unconscious dynamics caused her to marry into a Mexican family of the very type from which her family was trying to escape is not known. After her husband's desertion, she increased her social distance from her Mexican origin by entering into a relationship with an Anglo man. It is known that her husband's family was both jealous and ashamed of her. This can only mean that her attitude toward them revealed the inner conflicts that disturbed her relationships with her husband's people.

His mother's life, instead of giving Manuel security in cultural identification, intensified his conflicts in this respect. There had been a great deal in his Mexican background of emotional, if not material, gratification to give him warm feelings toward his own people. Close relatives, including the grandparents, uncle, and sister, had given him every support; and he recalls them all tenderly.

THE TIE THAT BINDS. Because of his Mexican appearance, his social contacts all tended to remind him that others saw him as Mexican. But instead of being permitted to make the simple and satisfying identification with his ethnic ingroup, he was forced out into the impersonal Anglo world of relentless struggle and strife. His mother's domination has resulted in a strong ambivalent tie that he is powerless to break. His passive dependency and identification with his mother and her Anglo values have spurred him on to more strenuous social climbing. The resulting failures have won only his mother's recriminations and more intensive goading, followed by ever more desperate attempts on his part to succeed.

The strangle hold his mother exerts came out in her disruption of his proposed marriage. His Mexican Catholic girl might have offered Manuel some security and stability of cultural identity. But he was powerless to resist his mother's interference. After breaking the engagement he even "leaned over backwards" in reaction formation against the danger of his inner rebellion, "identifying with the aggressor" by embracing evangelical Protestantism.

ROLE OF CULTURE CONFLICT. In evaluating the role of culture conflict in Manuel's case, we must ask ourselves whether he would be in his present emotional difficulties if he had *not* been a Mexican. Undoubtedly the ambivalent dependency on his mother and his passive aggressive personality with its repression of the slightest whisper of hostility might have occurred in any number of mother-son relationships regardless of culture. In this instance, however, cultural factors did give substance to Manuel's problems in several ways, one of which was the conflicting cultural models with which he was presented. At first there was the pervasive warmth of his original Mexican family, with his grandfather and uncle helping to mold his development. These early models were later replaced by his mother's Anglo friend who confused the picture for Manuel.

On the distaff side, the special person was his beloved Mexican grandmother whose values were to be reinforced by the girl of his choice. These gentle figures contrasted with the powerful and commanding mother who has played the "Devil's Advocate" in his life. His only means of coping with her indomitable will has been by passive compliance, coupled with strong reaction formations against any trace of hostility, which gives him his simple, bland façade. In his effort to avoid her displeasure he has tried to deny his deeply cherished identity with the people he resembles and knows best, and to set up the ego-alien ideal of intellectual and social strainer. His precarious defenses were sufficient to enable him to maintain adequate emotional balance as long as they were buttressed by his grandmother's support. With her death, however, and the inescapable demands and domination of his mother, he decompensated, developing disabling anxiety, loss of job, and school failure.

RECOMMENDATIONS

The outlook for Manuel is hopeful provided that he gets the help he needs to find himself again. This means helping him to drop the superimposed false identity and to accept himself for the loving, rather naïve person he is. His warm, early ties provide a firm foundation on which to build a sounder ego. His capacity for relating to people and for insight into himself have already been demonstrated in his responsiveness to the initial sessions of the individual therapy in progress.

It seems desirable to supplement individual interviews with therapy in a group of age peers, preferably Mexican in background, to strengthen his primary ingroup ties, as a first step toward a stronger identification and greater self-acceptance. In this emotional context, the more specific problems of overdependency on his mother, reduced intellectual efficiency, and vocational maladjustment have a better chance of being worked through to a favorable outcome.

Test Summary

A. Wechsler-Bellevue Form I

Verbal Scale	Wtd. Score	Performance Scale	Wtd. Score
Information	13	Picture Arrangement . . .	14
Comprehension	12	Picture Completion	8
Digit Span	6	Block Design	5
Arithmetic	7	Object Assembly	7
Similarities	14	Digit Symbol	7
Vocabulary	14		
Total	66(55)*	Total	41
Verbal I.Q.	110	Performance I.Q. . . .	87
	Full Scale I.Q. . . . 99		

* Prorated.

Test Summary

B. Make-A-Picture-Story Test

NOTE. The subject methodically placed all the figures in straight rows in front of him. He lost no time in making his stories and displayed a very good interest in what he was doing. Very little questioning was required.

1. Living Room.

The father is coming in with presents for the little boy. The boy is really supposed to be facing the other way but I can't find a picture that shows him that way. The dog is going to meet the father, the wife is going to meet him and also the girl is going to meet him. They are all going to meet the father. I guess it's the little boy's birthday. They are all very happy. Here is the grandmother also— she is sitting down. (No minority group figures were used in this story.)

2. Street.

I don't know. This is a B-girl going into the tavern. Two men are coming out. This man is standing on the corner looking at the girl as she is going in. He'll probably walk in after her. All four will finally go in and get a beer or something. This man (Negro figure) is a wino. This man (minority group figure) is a jitterbug. This man (Mexican figure) is a *pachucho—pachuchos* and jitterbugs —that's what they are. (Outcome?) This boy will try to pick the girl up and take her up to a hotel room. He's a rough, tough guy— just loafs around and don't do nothing or just a bum—or maybe just a man after a girl. (Q on girl.) She's a young girl gone wrong.

3. Schoolroom.

The man is giving a speech with all of the gestures. The teacher is explaining what is going on to the class—they are going to give a play. The man here is the scene director. He's got a magazine in his hand picking out the pictures so as to get an idea as to what the scene is going to be in back of the man. Could be putting on *Othello* or something. This man could be portraying Othello—this boy could be looking on—waiting his cue. He'll be coming on in a minute. The teacher is explaining to the rest of the class what is going on. (Asked to tell more about it.) This could be one of my classmates— this looks like my friend who is a very good drama student. This could be the dean of the school where I went—he was very good at creating scenery. This could be the public speaking teacher there.

4. Bedroom.

Just this one man—he is undressing and his wife is already in bed and he's undressing to go to bed—get a good night's sleep—got slippers on—getting his pajamas. The lady's asleep 'cause she's going to get up early in the morning to fix his lunch and get him ready to go to work.

5. Bathroom.

He's doing No. 1—man and wife. He's urinating—she's undressed because she's going to get into the tub and take a bath. He'll probably come over here and take a shave. She'll take her bath and probably go to bed. They'll probably go to bed together 'cause they are man and wife. That's the story.

6. Nursery.

A little baby is in here asleep in a crib—a little girl—she is the little sister of the little boy. They are brother and sister and they are looking at the baby brother in the crib. He has just started to cry and the little boy is going to pick him up and give him his baby bottle—the little dog comes in and looks. He will probably pick him up and take him to Mother who will change his diapers. He is probably wet—and give him his formula. That little dog could be my little dog—Duke. It shows the little boy and girl love the little baby enough to take care of him a lot. The little girl could be jealous because she's just standing there. Or it could be she is bashful and afraid to pick him up. The little dog just came along for the ride.

7. Shanty.

They live in a very poor neighborhood. The man don't have any food or anything to give to his children. (Figures in this story represent minority groups.) He must be a grandfather—the parents must be dead. The little boy wants to go to a movie—and he is crying and the man feels sad because he can't help. He is very old—can't work. Too poor—the house is falling to pieces. They belong to a minority group. The little boy must have been teased—called a nigger or some other bad word. Man is telling him not to worry—everything will come out right in the end—will tell him a little story—make him feel good. The grandfather and boy will probably go out and play together. The man is looking out and wondering where he is going to get the next meal from and his grandchildren and himself will go out and cut grass or beg—anything to get food—will tack up walls and windows to keep out the cold. They might beg—or the boy can go to school and learn how to better himself, or the man can become desperate and go out and steal or kill somebody—but they are good people so that is the last thing they will do. The boy will get a good education and learn about minority people. He will become a lawyer or doctor or minister so he can help his people to rise up from the ground. Now they will go out and play or get into a boxing game.

8. Camp.

There are no more soldiers so we imagine there is a whole platoon here. The captain is telling the lieutenant why he didn't get the men to shine their shoes better. He is bawling him out before the men—telling him if he doesn't get on the ball he'll take away his rank. He's strict—from West Point—a career man—wants everything just so. Shoes must have shine so he can see his face in them, etc.

9. Dream.

This could be my grandmother and me—I'm crying because I've lost her. The only way I can get her back is by dreaming about her. This is my little dog. I am telling her I fell down—or somebody called me a bad word, called me a "Mexican greaser." Later in my dream I grow up—she's telling me to be strong—not to be afraid of anything. It really happens a whole lot—I dream about my grandmother. I wake up and feel better. This way is the only way I can see my grandmother again.

Test Summary

C. Thematic Apperception Test

CARD 1. 5″

The boy thinks he wants to be a great musician. He's going to learn to play the violin. He is looking and thinking and making up his mind how a small boy wonders how he is going to put a big violin under his chin—the paper is the score—just a little simple exercise because he is just beginning to learn.

He wants to learn how because the expression on his face is serious. He doesn't want to go out and play. In the end he will learn how and be great probably as Mozart or Jascha Heifetz. (Where might the idea of being a violinist have come from?) He might have got it from listening to a record or from his teacher who told him about Mozart. Most little boys like a piano or a violin or guitar. Maybe his Dad plays a violin and he wants to learn or he might just have thought it up himself. He is very serious about this. His little eyes shine—he wants to learn.

CARD 2. 10″

The boy is working—and plowing the field. The lady is looking on and supervising. This is the boy's brother. The girl is going to school. She is thinking she doesn't want to be a farmer's wife. She wants to make a career in law or teaching other children. She looks like she might want to be a school teacher and come back and teach the farmers how to better themselves. The family is working and plowing the fields and planting potatoes or something, to enable her to go to school and finish her education. That is the story. (Tell more about the boy.) He likes the farm work. He wants to help his sister go through college. He's probably gone through college like A.&M.; learned how to rotate the crops. (Where might the father be?) The father is way over here working. He's with the other horse—they are not very advanced—must be poor farmers—they don't have tractors. The dress on the lady is old-fashioned dress. Maybe they are sacrificing themselves to put the girl through school. She has all the modern clothes. They are simple but I think this is the best they can do.

CARD 3BM. 4"

Is this a girl?—It looks like a boy that's crying—weeping because maybe he's had some great disappointment. Either he didn't pass in school or someone he loved very much has passed away. He's all by himself crying so that nobody will see him cry.—I think that is it. (What might the outcome be?) Somebody will come there and comfort him. It looks like he is a small boy wearing knee pants.

CARD 6BM. 2"

This is a boy telling his grandmother he didn't come out so good in a test. She is looking out of the window and listening to him. She is telling him that it is going to come out all right. Just do the best he can—she probably will give him something—the dish he likes best —sort of pamper him to get him out of the mood he is in—if he wants to cry she will let him cry on her shoulder. He will go out feeling very good. At least she will back him up.

CARD 13B. 3"

A little boy here. Don't look very secure. He's living in an old shack—staring out on nothing—thinking "how am I going to get out of this place—how am I going to better myself?" He wants to play with other little boys but they don't want to play with him. He must be by himself—he must be an only child. He's thinking that he wants to be somebody. He wants to go to school and better himself. He will wear shoes like the other children. Way it will end he will probably grow up and be a teacher to other poor children or a lawyer or a doctor and be a help to his own people and help raise their standards of living.

CARD 7BM. 6"

A boy is talking to his grandfather. He's telling him that he would like to learn how to play baseball and he knows his grandfather used to be a great baseball player and that he wonders if his grandfather will teach him now—if he feels up to teaching him how to play baseball. The grandfather says he will—he is up to it. Grandfather probably looking at him really fondly thinking how when he was young and he wants to help him. His grandfather will probably go out there and throw the ball—he is an old man—or will just catch the ball and let the boy throw it at him—he can't move around too fast like he could before. In the end the boy will be somebody the grandfather can be proud of. He'll be a good baseball player.

CARD 12M. 10"

The boy is sleeping—the man is going to grab at him. Like going to kill him or hurt him or do something to him—trying to harm him. The boy will get up and beat him off. The boy will probably end with winning over the man—and call the police to take him away.

CARD 4. 10"

It looks like the man was caught with this girl—this is the man's wife. She is asking why did he do this. He don't want to look at her—he is looking off to one side. He's ashamed to face her, and tell her—well she hasn't been a good wife or that he no longer cares for her or that he loves this other girl he's found with. She loves him—way her eyes are looking at him—but he don't like her. He's the sort of man who goes from girl to girl, marrying them off and getting tired of them. It looks as if he might run away with some other girl after he gets tired of this one and the same be repeated again. It looks as if he's found his match—she's just after his money. He's not going to get away too easy.

CARD 18BM. 12"

Somebody is putting their hands on the boy. He is drunk. His friend is helping him—pushing him up. He's going to help him—take him home and put him to bed—sober him up. He'll just have a hangover—he'll be grateful to his friend. (Is there maybe something else wrong that caused him to drink to excess?) Maybe he had a problem that he couldn't face up to—only way he could face it or get rid of it is to go out to some bar and drink—get so drunk that he will forget his troubles.

CARD 13MF. 8"

Looks as if he's gotten through having an affair with a girl. She's in bed. Somehow, he's very sensitive—so that when he gets done with a girl he feels sorry that he's used this girl in this way. He's crying because he's very sickened that he's done this. (What might have led up to this?) Some girl he's picked up in the street or a friend of the family. Some girl he knew. She's an innocent girl who didn't know anything about him. His urge overcame him so he's ashamed to face up to the girl's family and himself. He'll probably have to marry the girl in the end. This he feels is the only way he can make up to the girl. They'll both be very happy. He'll feel secure because he will know he had done the right thing. She loves him so she'll be happy. That's what's going on in his mind. He's thinking what he's going to do.

CARD 8BM. 10″

The boy is dreaming—he's a little boy—so he's dreaming. He wants to help other people. He wants to do this by becoming a doctor and relieving pain. This might be him after 20 or 30 years. He's very young—taking a bullet out of the man—he's just thinking this—maybe he wants to be an army soldier—represented by rifle in the picture. Just the thoughts that are going on in his little mind. He might end up growing up and being a doctor.

10

Dilemmas of Two Puerto Rican Men

Marvin K. Opler

SPANISH FAMILY VALUES AND ACCULTURATION PROBLEMS

Most Puerto Rican migrants come to New York to avoid the poverty and population pressure of the Island. They may carry with them the burdens of an original cultural heritage Spanish-American in spirit and tradition and quite different from the variegated pattern of beliefs in the metropolis. This cultural orientation will have stemmed from Spain and been modified in the rural districts of the Island or in the slums of San Juan. But if it is Puerto Rican at all, it will stress the dominance of males in most social activity, in paternal authority, and in patriarchal responsibilities, according to specific ideas of honor, respect, and shame. Families should be large as indicators of male potency. Providing adequately for them is a routine matter of honor and prestige. The lines of authority in the family go lineally from father to son, brooking no interference from subordinated female roles. The latter are to be protected within the family setting, with collateral male kin performing this function. Beyond this magic circle, all unprotected adult females are fair sexual game, and the young girls chafe at the perennial roles of baby-tender and sheltered homemaker.

This is the common warp of Latin cultures in the Island or

south of the Rio Grande. But everywhere, in cities and industrialized plantations, the weft of urban processes challenges such values. To the extent that women work for wages in some parts of Puerto Rico, man's role is less crucial. Besides this, countless women become dissatisfied with the role indoctrination of childhood and adolescence. They may become, in subtle ways, destructive in the intersexual and familial relationships that come within their control. The weakening of male role has meant higher rates of desertion in the lower class and of separation in middle-class population. Marriages are brittle, adding to the childhood deprivation and internal strains within the family. These strains, greater in lower classes, may be found either in San Juan or in New York City.

But besides these social and economic strains on family life, cultural conflict also takes its toll. There is the great gulf between ideal or original cultural expectations, already mentioned, and what the migrants find existing on the mainland. Their values—what they deem desirable, proper, or good—are rarely found. Male job downgrading and unemployment is more drastic here for males than for females. One street song begins, "I would not trade Puerto Rico for a hundred New Yorks!"

With such dislocations and the rapid pace of acculturation, the number of adjustment problems of Puerto Rican youth grows also. Here we describe two Puerto Rican young men caught in such culture conflicts. They are both second sons, in their early twenties, and both, not uncharacteristically, have fathers absent from the home scene.

The first was studied in a public hospital facility following hospitalization for a few months in the navy. His naval tour of duty had been short and his diagnosis was schizophrenic reaction, paranoid type. He was white and from the lower-middle-class stratum of San Juan. In the latter respect he contrasted with the second case, a colored ambulatory schizophrenic with paranoid traits who was from the lower class of San Juan's worst slum.

A LOWER-MIDDLE-CLASS VETERAN

Let us call the lower-middle-class veteran Alberto. He is twenty-one years of age. Both parents came from the lower-middle-class stratum of the city of San Juan. The father was twenty-three and the mother eighteen at the time of marriage, whereupon the father, after several lesser jobs and minor clerkships, secured the enviable post of policeman.

ALBERTO'S FATHER: GUAPO OR POLICEMAN? Alberto's father, from all accounts, was a much-spoiled eldest son of indulgent parents. The neighbors knew him by the Puerto Rican term, *guapo*, a lad who takes liberties—a headstrong adventurer. Alberto's uncle in New York described his elder sibling as having a swashbuckling exterior, but being really attached to an ambitious and manipulative mother. Alberto's paternal grandmother had prevailed upon her husband to sell his interest in the small family farm and join the general exodus of rural families from the district to the city. There her ambitions for an easier life ran counter to her husband's distaste for the new surroundings. The paternal grandfather felt his social and economic independence dwindle as his new responsibilities grew. With Alberto's father, he encouraged the *guapo* tendencies, vented sudden fits of anger and alternately allowed him every breach of discipline. Alberto's father, first as *guapo*, and later even as policeman, found it hard "to settle down." He was impulsive and volatile in temperament, the darling of his mother, and always in some scrape with authorities.

EARLY LIFE IN SAN JUAN. In San Juan, where Alberto's mother and the maternal grandparents lived, the household had consisted of the paternal grandparents, Alberto's parents, and the four children whom we shall call Roberto, Alberto, Melinda, and Elena. Alberto's mother had been subjected to the usual strict upbringing of Puerto Rican girls. She and her parents had lived in the rural countryside before they, too, settled in San Juan. Alberto's mother had viewed the marriage, arranged by her own father, as an escape from pressures of being an only daughter. She was married off at age eighteen.

Roberto, the elder son, was born in the second year of marriage, and Alberto, a year later. Neither pregnancy nor birth was unusual. The mother hoped to nurse both boys for well over a year, but in her rigid concern for this self-imposed schedule of nursing, she complained that Alberto's arrival had interrupted the suckling of the elder son. To compensate for this, "a better job" was done "for Alberto," who was nursed for two years. Both boys walked at about a year and a half, and were toilet trained, under constant urging, before two.

Both mother and paternal grandmother laid great stress upon learning language through constant repetition of words. In this, as in every aspect of child care, the manipulative older woman and rigidly strict mother vied and quarreled with each other. Disassociating himself from these female battles, Alberto's father would assume his most manly, decisive (and *guapo*) manner on the rare occasions when he was at home. Issuing orders in a deep, guttural voice, his decisions were peremptory and arbitrary. Often, he would side with his mother for no apparent reason or indulge in frequent fits of anger. In time, the sinecure on the police force led to illegal scrapes and shady deals, salted with a series of the extramarital liaisons sanctioned in this culture for males. The number of alcoholic sprees with boon companions increased. Alberto's mother salvaged her all-important marital status by rigid adherence to the routines of a meticulous housewife, becoming overly clean, orderly, and compulsive.

CLEANLINESS RITUALS. The boy's toilet training was one such instance. The mother exulted in claims that Alberto *wanted* to use a receptacle because Roberto used it. She argued with the grandmother that she was not forcing him —and the issue was drawn. Both boys were pitted against each other in the contest of cleanliness. Alberto, perhaps less accomplished than his older sibling in toilet training, had the advantage of occupying a hammock adjacent to his parents' bed. Besides the possible confusions of genital and anal functioning, he early began to cater to his mother's phobic fear of "city dirt and disease." In the daytime, he never liked to sit on the floor as did most children; he wished to be bathed by his mother frequently; and he delighted her by constantly washing his hands.

ANAL FEATURES: PSYCHOPHYSIOLOGIC REACTIONS. As the boy grew, these themes took other forms. The mother commented that Puerto Ricans often went barefoot whenever the occasion afforded itself, but Alberto preferred to wear shoes to be clean. With the central controversies over toilet training ringing in the household, he buttressed his claims to exemplary cleanliness by periodically developing severe constipation. As early as two and three years and on through latency, the mother gave a weekly, almost ceremonial dosage of castor oil or milk of magnesia. This was accompanied by considerable discussion of bowel movements. As the triumvirate of mother, boy, and grandmother dwelled on the bodily function, the father, in his sudden, brief appearances in the household, shouted his beliefs and decisions about these same matters. Alberto's confusion and desire to please everyone at all costs crystallized in the organ language of colitis, whereby constipation alternated with diarrhea throughout his life.

The matter did not even rest there. He and his siblings also had their share of worms, the childhood plague of Puerto Rico. In addition, two siblings, both girls, were born when the patient was, respectively, five and six years old. With all siblings, the castor oil was administered to counteract *Worms* and *Constipation,* the twin evils, but since Alberto's bowel involvement was the greater, he drew the greater attention on both scores. By age seven, when his female siblings required infancy care, his mother began to give him hot water enemas at least once a month. Later, at eighteen, during the acute onset of his schizophrenic illness, he tried to self-administer such an enema, but failed because he feared too much hot water, and complained, for the first time in his life, that his mother had given the children laxatives and enemas "when we didn't need them." To this was added, "it was done when father was away and he didn't care about the house anyway."

During the childhood diseases of whooping cough, measles, and chicken pox, further efforts were made to monopolize his mother's attention. Each siege was followed by a month-long period of being run down, requiring the mother's continuous care. By sixteen, a continual nasal discharge began. While his physical condition was excellent in all reports, the rhinitis and alternating bowel patterns were part of a larger series of vaguely shifting hypochondriachal complaints including claims of stomach trouble, dizziness, and poor sleep.

ANAL FEATURES AGAIN: SEXUAL BEHAVIOR. Sexual life is described as beginning in adolescence, coincidental with the father's separation and shortly after arrival in New York. Masturbation occurred frequently in showers and toilets, either before or after bowel movements. Heterosexual excitements are claimed in New York's crowded apartments, but despite more talk of divorce and desertion than in San Juan, he himself had neither dates nor girl friends and denies any homosexual experience. In late adolescence, masturbation began to evoke guilt. "It makes you dumb or dull and pimply." One should also know where to go for sex with women. His own busy life began to require his attendance at college in evening classes while working overtime as clerk. The patient added that there was too much preoccupation with homosexuality in Puerto Rican neighborhoods, but he was, at first, unaware of his selective attention to this matter.

Perhaps the most striking symptom on this score was the patient's compulsive need for having bowel movements in public toilets. At first, he was unaware of the homosexual motivations for this, but explained that he stopped several times at subway stations for this purpose. This pattern occurred about three times a week, with anxiety about going to work, and masturbation occasionally to lessen this anxiety. His notion of the homosexual had no shadings and was limited to one type not infrequent in Puerto Rican culture. In his definition, this was a man "who cannot make the grade, and doesn't want to be a man—instead he wants to think and be like a woman." Having studied biology in college evening session, he had come away with the notion that the adrenals stimulate either sex to its characteristic types of activity. To this he added that homosexuals are all passively oriented, masturbating and paying each other like prostitutes. Later, in the hospital, the projection of passive attitudes was indicated in his asking the psychiatrist, "Am I getting paid while I am kept here?"

FAMILY BURDENS. The patient entered public school at the usual age, skipped grades, and completed high school in less than the four years, at almost sixteen. He was graduated with honors and college was envisaged for the future. Since this was not economically feasible, he entered trade school and, at the same time, became a clerk. He contributed two-thirds of his small salary to his mother's household expenses. It was at this time that the rhinitis began and the fear and resentment toward his father turned to open hostility. The father, in turn, had succeeded in going from bad to worse, had lost his sinecure through shady deals and had moved the family to the mainland city of New York for economic reasons. A year later, the parents separated and Alberto's father deserted the family.

Alberto described how his father went from storekeeper to factory worker, how in New York he constantly used the phrase, "In Puerto Rico, even a dog can bark," alluding to thin walls in crowded New York apartments; and how he finally returned to the Island. Roberto, the older brother, regarded the father as "just no good." He himself entered the navy and completed a successful tour of duty. When Alberto's turn came to enter the armed forces, he too was at the peak of his resentment against the father for "running out on us," but by then he had added hatred of Roberto for "letting all the responsibilities fall on" himself as second eldest son. He had hoped to detach himself from the wholly feminine home scene, but with two dependent adolescent sisters now requiring supervision, he saw little prospect of doing so and blamed his father and Roberto for having defaulted in their tasks. At the same time, his ambivalence toward assuming an adult male role by Puerto Rican standards was no less marked.

A CARICATURE OF MASCULINITY. On first admission, Alberto was described as nervous, restless, hyperkinetic, and emotionally disturbed. Peculiarities of gait and posture included, most prominently, affecting the rolling gait of a seaman with legs swung in wide arcs and toes slightly inward. The upper body, in sitting or walking, was held stiffly, as if "at attention," chin well in and chest grotesquely expanded. This caricature, symbolizing ambivalence toward his brother, was mixed with imitation, equally bitter, of his father. For this, he dropped his voice constantly to the deepest register possible and expressed whatever he had to say in commanding and guttural tones, often repeating the words, "deep, deep." At times, the exaggerated hoarseness had the badly controlled lilt of a drunken man. All this was punctuated, as if in parody, by loudly clearing his throat, a barking cough, and pauses that merely emphasized the difficulty in speaking clearly and naturally. All this masculine symbolization for the two men in his family had been perfected within a few days of active service when homosexual panic was precipitated. In these few days with the armed forces, he had noted a tendency for his voice to become feminine in tone, controllable only by imitations of the father whom he loathed. He expressed himself as wanting to have something to hang on to, his voice sounding "queer" if he tried it out on himself, and his hips swaying unless he modified his gait to that of his brother. The usual panic at ideas of reference (being stared at, being called a homosexual) occurred largely because of his own preoccupation with "what" he was. The mannerisms he adopted embarrassed him as being not like himself, but they were self-perpetuating so long as the patient was unclear as to his sexual and personal identity. He was, indeed, Alberto, but a different Alberto. An acceptance of his caricatured male symbols gradually lessened his reliance upon them or his need for their expression.

RISE AND DECLINE OF SYMPTOMS. Hostile, anxious attitudes were expressed by restlessness. He kicked his feet spasmodically when seated and crossed or uncrossed his legs. Conversing could not contain his hostile and aggressive tendencies. Tension and excitation marked the hyperkinetic activity, sometimes seen in restless pacing. If seated, he smoked incessantly, gripped the arms of his chair, or flicked the ashes of his cigarette nervously. Orality, in the constant smoking, the "deep, deep" interjections, the drunken mouthing and exaggerated lip-play with words, seemed to be prominent.

Mannerisms of voice and gait disappeared as Alberto's life history was meaningfully discussed. At times, apparently distasteful allusions to ward or hospital activities brought back more pressure of speech, the rapid word flow containing some clanging. When tension disappeared, the high affective coloring did likewise. In the same way, the patient was at first disorderly, with wet hair, or soiled shirt worn outside his trousers. An early explanation of this was a defiant, "I like to feel loose." Later such symbols of hostility also disappeared.

In time, the background of his family in Puerto Rico emerged with clarity as the patient moved from a tense and anxious state, with hyperkinetic psychomotor behavior, to one of being more obviously depressed but, at the same time, less impulsive and aggressive. With the disappearance of manneristic controls over anxiety, Alberto also appeared more than normally placid, cooperative, or suggestible. Although ideas of persecution continued ("people" talking about him), he began to discuss with insight his hostilities aimed at father, mother, and brother. His restlessness persisted only in a desire to travel and join the merchant marine after full recovery.

DREAM ANALYSIS. Dream material was recounted. *Dream 1:* He dreamed he owned a horse; and stated, "You wake up and find it's no horse." *Dream 2* reflected similar

doubts of male potency, and concerned driving a car which
magically transformed into a broom or stick incapable of
motion. This dream was quickly associated, in frank Puerto
Rican terms, with others about sexual intercourse. Alberto
stated: "I think I need sex with a woman—dreaming of
intercourse and waking up with night losses or wet dreams;
the body must get rid of sperms because they accumulate."
Dream 3 concerned travel on a ship to Spain where he saw
the Pyrenees covered with snow; it all changed to clouds
as he awoke. In *Dream 4* an older nightmare was evoked;
he was dying, and all the persons around him were busy
nailing him into his coffin; he wished to tell them he was
really alive, but could not speak. In *Dream 5*, he was breaking windows and doing this fearfully, but he could not run
away like the friends with him. "I felt like I was nailed
down to the floor." *Dream 6* had him married and settled
down with a girl he knew back in New York; she was
described as being brunette and small, and was a person
occasionally seen in real life.

Still greater content was developed in a later series of
dreams, with undistorted and insightful interpretations.
In *Dream 1* a boat moving slowly out of harbor finds him
staring down at the eddying, green water which seems to
bubble with slimy dirt stirred up by the ship's wake; with
nausea, he wishes to vomit at its stench. The commentary
reminded him of his mother, and the bowel movements
with enemas. *Dream 2* concerned a tall priest and nun
to whom he explains his wish to marry; there is a figure
of a girl, covered with rags, but looking like Melinda in
age. The nun in white disappears while he is explaining,
and the priestly figure becomes a voice shouting farther
away. The associations indicated that the adult figures
may have been parents, and his father disappeared when
most needed. He liked his sister nearest in age, and felt
sorry for her, "although sometimes I think my sisters have
fewer troubles and worries growing up." *Dream 3* finds
him in possession of a small, pearl-handled knife which becomes a large switch-blade; he attempts to cut down clowns

painted white on a platform, but as he tries, the knife becomes "runt-sized" again with blood on it. His father
shouts that Puerto Ricans do not use knives, "People just
say that," and he takes it away. No free associations of
this seemingly obvious dream were elicited. In *Dream 4*,
he is a child dirtied by other children who try to burn him
with a stick-and-paper torch; he is afraid his family will
catch him in this state, but can neither move nor talk. Comments included that the fire warmed him through the mud,
and he really liked the way it felt. In *Dream 5* he wants
to drink at a public fountain, but the dirt and gum in the
bowl make him sick; when he drinks, it tastes like hard
liquor and turns his stomach. Here associations were made
to negative training of the mother and feelings of revulsion
toward the father.

MOTHER'S LACK OF INSIGHT INTO PATIENT'S PROBLEMS. The
mother, when visiting the patient in the hospital, proved to
be an extremely attractive, carefully groomed woman of
forty-one, with surface warmth and affability, who at the
same time gave the impression of underlying coldness. Her
icy manner developed in discussions of the family, particularly the father's role in family separation. There was distinct defensiveness about the patient's illness, of which she
had no real understanding. Her English was halting at
times only because of concern about the effect of her statements. What emerged most clearly was the strong-willed
and rigid drive to be accepted and admired.

While the patient was aware of the seriousness of his
illness, the mother denied any understanding of what had
happened to him, being more concerned with her expectations for him. In her eyes, the outlook was good if only one
realized he had been a good boy, clean in childhood, and
abstemious with women and alcohol in youth—in contrast
to the uncontrolled behavior of his father. She paraded his
successful school career and willingness to help her financially while working his way through college as almost
official reasons why nothing serious could be wrong. True,
the patient had complained of being tired from the combi-

nation of overtime work and college attendance, but he slept well and possessed a good appetite. Finally, to clinch it all, there was no history of mental illness in the family and she was overly vehement in denials of nervousness or tension in the patient's entering service. Like most Puerto Ricans, she preferred to describe mental illness as a simple matter of bodily malfunction (nerves), possibly brought on by overwork.

PATIENT'S GOOD INSIGHT AND PROGNOSIS. In Alberto's accounts of his two sisters, it is clear that they had become, for him, somewhat seductive figures representing, as did the mother, both a sexual threat and an unwelcome burden. The Melinda of the dream recounted above was ready for marriage. In one dream, he associated that he had seen his sisters naked and was obviously embarrassed. While the mother denied sibling rivalries and negative emotions in the home climate, Alberto's accounts indicate the daughters' resentment of their mother's authority, the sons' open rivalry, and the mother's nagging and planful means of getting her own way. Alberto never felt that happiness or accomplishment was for himself. His seemingly useless gifts to his mother, his castration fears and self-punishment patterns, his anal and homosexual preoccupations, and his passivity were not in accord with the appropriate pattern of masculinity in this culture. But neither was his home headed by an adequate father. It was fatherless and controlled by a manipulative, rigid, and demanding mother. As Alberto grew up, these reversals of role in his Puerto Rican family became increasingly untenable.

The patient's future, however, is not bleak. Disappearance of acute symptoms occurred rapidly with insight. The family has learned that he cannot continue to develop insight and alone carry the burdens of a problematic family in a setting far different from that of San Juan. His plans to travel are undoubtedly a means of removing himself further from the strong maternal control. Hostile and inwardly suspicious, he nevertheless is able to perceive the blocks to further self-realization. Alberto has learned to read the mapping of his own symptoms—the passivity in hypochondriacal complaints, the earlier lack of firm identification, and the long-buried resentments and hostilities. With good intelligence, verbal facility, and growing insight into a traumatic past, Albert is catching up with the half-lost years.

LOWER-CLASS COLORED PUERTO RICAN MAN

BRUTAL BACKGROUND.   The next case, an ambulatory male schizoid, we shall call Ramon. Like Alberto, he was in his early twenties when interviewed and also the second son in a family of four siblings. In contrast, however, Ramon was partly colored. His father, also partly colored, had abandoned the family. The mother and four children promptly moved to the worst slum of San Juan, and on the few occasions when the father visited the city, the parents fought violently. Ramon remembers his father beating the mother brutally and once trying to kill her with a gun. As a child, both parents punished him mercilessly, the father using his belt and the mother her broomstick. Ramon, whose lot fell with the mother ultimately, felt that she showed him no vestige of real affection. The slum was recalled as a place where "we were brought up among savages." Killings and beatings forced the young men to join gangs of hoodlums for survival. When baseball or swimming seemed boring, sadistic sports were substituted. One game involved being thumped on the back with a stick as long as one could bear the pain. Today, Ramon's brother is hospitalized and under treatment for mental disorder, following several aggressive and assaultative episodes.

BEHAVIORAL CONSEQUENCES.   Ramon's aggressive and excited behavior is indicated in an account of his trip to the hospital with an interviewer. With mirthless excitement, Ramon appeared on the street to walk to his medical appointment. To any young woman whom he met on the way, he yelled, "Hello, Beauty!" At every corner, he hesitated to cross, explaining that in New York City drivers run you over like dogs. Since he was going to the clinic for a knee injury, he complained of this, calling it arthritis. To the list was added neuralgia and other worries about his health. His account of endless physical disabilities was interlarded with his exploits with prostitutes. Ramon seemed to be saying, "I am ill and worried about my health, but on the other hand I am also a pre-eminent male."

In subsequent discussions, it appeared that his hypochondriacal complaints included ailments which caused him almost constant pain and discomfort. His joints were arthritic. He had a rhinitis reaching asthmatic proportions. A stomach "upset" was almost continual. Where organic ailments stopped, he complained of trouble with sleep, dizziness, tension, and frequent colds. Like Alberto, he smoked continually and stated he had succeeded in getting some maternal attention, if not affection, by protracting childhood health problems. He had also never dated, had girl friends, or married. Ramon impressed one immediately as a tense, overactive individual, looking younger than his given age and overly concerned about his health and sexual identity. Ramon's fears and emotional constriction were early developed. Hostility toward frankly rejecting parents could not be expressed. Far from becoming merely callous, Ramon was afraid to be alone and terrified of being ridiculed. He learned to avoid punishments, tried to escape parental tongue-lashings, but developed a lengthy covert set of fears including high places, strange people, drunkards, food poisons, and being cut. The stern expectations of his mother bred in him a feeling that things should be done perfectly, that one should not show emotions to others, and that one should always be guarded with people. The introjection of these rules, based on suspicion and hostility, he recognized as being far from Puerto Rican values. Yet Ramon preferred to keep such opinions to himself and to trust no one.

HEALTH PREOCCUPATIONS. For as long as Ramon can remember, his chief concerns were about his health and

unnamed or unspecified enemies. Discussions of his loneliness, though persistent, had a curious quality of being
diffuse and disjointed. It was as if Ramon, like Alberto,
hardly understood himself, while at the same time he described frankly his hostilities, his sense of inadequacy, and
his emotional isolation. While appearing cooperative on
the surface, he seemed blocked, disorderly in appearance,
and constantly nervous and agitated. His ailments and
imagined sexual exploits, such as nights spent with half a
dozen prostitutes, seemed hollow and unconvincing. His
suspiciousness and rigid compulsions were as frankly expressed in the same contexts and even more deeply rooted.

For example, Ramon's health rules were thought of as the
only road to precarious survival. Though restless and ener-
getic, he complained of being exhausted. This necessitated
going to bed early, often in the evening, and above all,
making sure of getting proper food. There was no use of
drugs or alcohol. As with Alberto, Ramon disdained his father's heavy drinking and became totally abstinent. While
his fantasy accounts of sexual exploits were many, he
thought of sexual activity as being debilitating or dangerous
to health.

ORAL FEATURES: SOMATIC AND MASOCHISTIC REACTIONS.
While not stereotyped into a system of defensive controls,
Ramon's behavior was at times most bizarre. Like Alberto's
enema to rid him of mounting dangers, Ramon too had
regulations centered less in the bowel than in the stomach.
The upset stomach required certain foods at certain times
and enough rest to digest that food properly. The arthritic
pains, in his private folklore, were connected with un-met
needs for just the right nourishment. While Alberto had
centered his concerns on anal levels, Ramon's aggressive
orality emphasized his nutritive needs. The arthritis he
attempted to cure by eating certain foods and avoiding certain food poisons. When this failed him, he poured boiling
water on his leg to ease the pain. The burns were extensive
enough to require hospitalization. A comment on the entire
masochistic episode was Ramon's cryptic remark, "A person

with an incurable disease should stick a bullet through his head and that's all."

Apparently, this sense of hopelessness was early in development. His mother described him as having no real friends as a child and reacting to problems by going off by himself. She described the time that he took iron rods and, in a fit of pique, went out in a violent thunderstorm to see if the lightning would strike him. Despite some contrasts in type of aggression, from Alberto's passivity and dependence to Ramon's oral aggressiveness, both men had lengthy histories of masochistic and self-destructive tendencies. Ramon's nervous stomach, lightning test, and burnt knee episode were not all. He would taunt his elder brother until he was cruelly beaten. While fearing pain, he was often hurt.

FATHER AS A NEGATIVE MODEL. Ramon's father deserted the family, as in Alberto's case, during the boy's adolescence. The father complained that family burdens were heavier than he could bear. The extramarital exploits, the periods of unemployment, and his drunken appearances made the decision a welcome one for his wife. But before this frankly pronounced desertion, Ramon's difficulty in identification with his father is well described. The father, a peddler, was a person only to be avoided. As for the mother—nagging, demanding, and punitive in his absence—Ramon resented her even more. Since the father was colored, and the mother lower-class white, Ramon was mulatto and open to her further rejection, especially after they had moved to New York. On the mainland, the ethnic discriminations led Ramon to feel doubly stigmatized, both as lower-class Puerto Rican and as mulatto. The mother reinforced the social rejection, taunting him with the knowledge that in their tenement he was at first not allowed into the building, ostensibly for racial reasons.

While many Puerto Rican males would not work in the women's garment industry, Ramon does. Excluded from certain aspects of community life, he visits no neighbors and has no friends. His entertainment is exclusively through mass media. On these grounds, too, the battles with the mother are constant and openly antagonistic. In Sentence Completion tests, the father is described as "anyone who wants to beat you." The definition of a mother is grounded in mutual exploitation. Ramon has firmly decided never to marry.

MOTHER AS SOURCE OF ORAL DEPRIVATION.   The mother's pathology is more overt than in the case of Alberto's family. Generally, in this group, the acting out of lower-class persons is franker or more overt than in the class above. Here the mother, obese and overeating, ostensibly because of Island food deprivations, states that she is "rotten inside" because of constant suffering. For the most part, she and her children had always been hungry and deprived. Her son reported hunger in Puerto Rico that had even robbed him of sleep, and he recalled feeling at such times the most unhappy person in the world. The boys begged food from neighbors and learned to steal. In this period of the lean years, Ramon's oral concerns and resentments grew. "My stomach was ruined then and it was there that I developed a big appetite." In field work, he asked a Puerto Rican interviewer for money repeatedly or begged him to buy coffee and snacks for him. The impression was that Ramon wished to use the interviewer as a "good provider" who bestowed gifts and thus compensated for the rejecting and punitive father.

RESISTANCE TO SCHOOL.   Schooling was likewise resented. One story concerned a teacher on the Island who, according to Ramon, pushed him and pinched him. He responded by running away. Ramon never liked school and had, at times, to be absent for want of clothes suitable for the classroom. The mother disagreed with the boy's attitude, stating, "Educate a person and you make him a man of worth rather than a *bandito*. Besides, here the only friend one has is the dollar in his pocket." At sixteen, completing third grade with the teacher incident recounted above, Ramon had obtained a bush knife from his father's cart and threatened to kill him with it.

IDEAS ABOUT SEX AND MARRIAGE. Ramon's persistent child-hood fears included the danger of being cut. On receiving a small scalp wound from a falling tree branch in a storm, the sight of blood had terrified him. Ever after, he was afraid of being cut. Possibly related psychodynamically was fear that he might "injure" a girl. An attempt at inter-course on the Island is described with tremendous anxiety. Because the girl cried, he felt he had injured her fatally, and he regrets the incident to this day. His rules for mar-riage include a drastic improvement in health, a steady job, and plenty of money. Yet he discounts the possibility of his health's ever improving. As for the wife, the criteria are equally rigid. She must be white, second-generation American, wealthy, fluent in English, and a hard worker. He despairs of ever finding such a person among the Puerto Ricans, and until there is, he must find solace in fantasies of prostitutes. His habit of complimenting all passing girls whom he does not know is, for Ramon, a persistent daily habit.

DREAMS AND FANTASIES. Ramon's dreams include several in which he plays a passive homosexual role. In one, he is slashed by a man with a knife, but emerges unscathed. Psychological tests [1] such as the Rorschach indicate that he maintains the tenuous balance of a bizarre schizophrenic. Paranoid ideation was consistently shown on all instruments, including TAT and Sentence Completion. There was con-fusion in distinguishing between genital behavior on the one hand, and oral or anal behavior on the other. On the Rorschach, for example, one of the cards is seen as an old man with a cat-face in which the "cat" is distinctly used as a feminine symbol. The story continues with the young man "somehow having intercourse," whereupon the old man of the story becomes angry because the younger has eaten everything. On Card III, following incoherent rambling about ostriches and a bow tie, the subject jumped up "to have coffee." After nervously gulping water, he complained

---

[1] Unfortunately the original protocols are not available.

that he saw eyes staring from the cards, and continued only with animal responses and poorly delineated entrails.

Interviews also evoked the same oral-sexual confusion. During them he begged for food, coffee, money, cigarettes, a particular pencil which caught his fancy, and a hot dog. Most symbolisms of this type were frankly phallic, and many of the supposed sexual exploits with prostitutes of his fancy were described seductively in terms of orgasm without intromission.

DIAGNOSTIC IMPRESSION. The leading diagnostic impression from the tests was that of a schizophrenic reaction, paranoid type, with sharp mood swings as well. Having heard from his mother throughout life constant devaluation of both femininity and of male potency, Ramon apparently adopted a pattern in his own symptomatology of his mother's hypochondriacal complaints, her concern for survival and her displacements to oral emphasis. He is certain that he once irreparably harmed a girl. His male identifications are largely guilty ones, and his rules against female companionship or seeking a marital partner are insurmountable except in fantasy. His personality integration and emotional balance have not progressed far beyond that of his starved childhood—of being the "unhappiest person in the world."

ALBERTO AND RAMON COMPARED

CHANGING FAMILY ROLES. In any culture, the intrapsychic status depends, in part, on family stability, on continuous structural settings for that stability, and upon cultural values capable of supporting, in realistic fashion, both family and structural setting. The family thus becomes an interdependent small group organization. It functions, for better or worse, as the major recognizable unit of a larger social system. It transmits, in more or less coherent patterns, those meanings and values of a culture which find support or meet rebuffs in the realities of a social world. In the family of Puerto Rican and Spanish-oriented cultures generally, extramarital and premarital liaisons for males in lower strata

are sanctioned as part of a pattern of total masculine control
or dominance. But these patterns are open to change and
have changed with the movements of rural population to
industrialized centers like San Juan and New York City.

While larger role expectations may consistently demand
a father's economic contributions to enhance his total cultural prestige and honor, the challenge of this general
pattern is hollow and meaningless if the economic position
of the male changes to the extent it has in Puerto Rican
families. Instead, the father, ideally representing the
weight of authority within the home, sees his economic
role diminish, and with it his importance and real authority. Thus, the economic pressures at the bottom of the
social scale in contemporary Puerto Rico are much like
those intensified in the New York scene itself. Males un-
dergo a general downgrading in jobs available and the
marriages become as evanescent as their dominance role.
There is no barrier in a weakened Catholic religious system
to formal separation or simple desertion. Both occur increasingly. As families bear the ultimate of poverty, migration, and cultural dislocation, so their component members
may break under the strain of rapidly changing or burdensome family organization.

FATHER. Alberto's and Ramon's fathers, reflecting separation and desertion norms of their respective classes, emerge
from two backgrounds. The middle-class father stems from
a background of maternal overprotection, and Ramon's still
weaker and less effectual father, from his own background
of neglect. Both are weak paternal figures. Caught in the
transition to urbanism, which, for Puerto Rican culture
means increased status for women, the masculine roles of
each are further challenged and undermined.

MOTHER. Alberto's mother, beyond the uniqueness of
her particular struggle for independence, represents a
psychological compromise between the cultural ideals and
the expanded role of the Puerto Rican woman. By sustaining the family through a compulsively organized manipulation of her egocentrically conceived status of matron, she

exploitatively uses what the culture designates as her best weapons in life—her sons. Through techniques of seductiveness, increasing narcissism, and competitions between siblings, she produces a passively oriented, masochistic, compulsive, and ultimately confused second male child. Ramon's mother, fighting a more stark battle of survival with fewer means, develops in her child the aggressive forms of hostility which are closer to the surface, out of a welter of neglect. Both children fail to make a masculine identification and both avoid any real interests in female companionship.

EFFECTS ON BOYS.   In each case, the cultural expectations for male role performance are channeled for a time into male sibling rivalry which serves to reinforce hostility toward the fathers. Alberto experienced his repulsion from any actual role a few days after enlistment, and thereupon played his grotesque satire of the male world as he knew it. Ramon built his rules against marriage and the female world slowly and carefully over the years. Outside of parental and sexual relations, Alberto felt a hopeless lack of confidence and self-esteem, social and sexual inadequacy, and a poverty of positive emotions. Ramon's concerns about each of these areas was long in developing, but the combination of Puerto Rican and colored status finally crystallized his negative self feelings. Perhaps because of stricter lower-middle-class standards, Alberto's insecurities received less ventilation, leaving him for long behind a façade of successful accomplishment in school and work. His passive dependent and anal orientations were slowly and relentlessly imposed from without, held in rigid control, and finally transmuted into manneristic and carefully fashioned symbols. With Ramon, the acting out of aggressive and sexual impulse was more constant and gradual, consistent with his cruder slum background. The oral deprivations and affect hunger are mirrored in symptoms which center around eating.

Alberto's formalized and rigid defenses have as frantic a quality as Ramon's fantasies and rules. For both young men, the lack of a positive father figure finds no compensation in the culture beyond what a male "should be." Social norms do not exist as personally experienced reality, and acculturation has robbed each, through social and economic processes, of any stable context for behavior. To father desertion, more violent in Ramon's case, and male job downgrading, more obvious in Alberto's, one may add the brittle marriages and parental instabilities on the distaff side as centrifugal forces disruptive of binding home influences.

For Alberto the imagined solution was to flee from the family scene, while for Ramon, always more lonely, it was to lose himself in urban anonymity. Therefore, despite his colored status, Ramon was unwilling to leave New York while Alberto pinned his hopes on extensive travel. In both men pent-up affect was siphoned into somatic symptoms in accord with their psychodynamic needs. In their psychoses they show much sudden discharge of affect. Alberto, with better education and advantages, has settled down into the passive role of patient and must measure, with his own insight, the steps to maturity. Ramon, with fewer such assets, vacillates between a long-ingrained will to survive and his depressive reactions and suicidal trends.

CULTURAL FACTORS IN TREATMENT. Treatment in each case requires not only seeing defenses in balance but noting the cultural conflicts, the social experiences, and the role expectations of both men. Lacking the devious disguises of presumably more sophisticated people, such patients describe or act out their real problems with less evasion. Where they block, as in Alberto's occasional repetitions and symbolizations, or Ramon's interruptions of Rorschach, the signs are usually frank and direct as to what the individual can, and cannot bear, in amnestic material. Ramon remembers his childhood hungers with severe intensity, but his emotional hunger, like Alberto's, must be measured before one can proceed. Beyond the class-differentiations, seen largely in the greater tendency to act out in the lower and to control in the middle classes, these cases appear to be "typical" among Puerto Ricans.

11

Two Puerto Rican Boys in New York

Lauretta Bender and *Sol Nichtern*

CULTURE AND MATURATION

Growth and development in the young are characterized by progressive differentiation of function and behavior. As this maturational process unfolds, the interrelationships between developing life and environment become an integral part of the emerging personality structure of the child. These relationships are projected in the behavior patterns of the individual which may be accentuated by the stresses of culture conflicts. The process is particularly evident in the emotionally disturbed child who frequently demonstrates poorly integrated biological, psychological, and social maturation. The effect of a language and cultural barrier seems to enhance this lack of integration. In some instances in our experiences, this conflict and resulting behavior have led even to the clinical impression of an acute psychosis. However, careful observation of these cases has resulted in the final opinion that the severe distortions in behavior were more likely the product of culture conflict superimposed on specific aspects of personality development.

The role of nature and nurture continues to stand as a challenge to every worker studying human development. The historical attitudes have fluctuated in their emphasis from geneto-hereditary and constitutional to environmental and interpersonal factors. Our experiences with children would serve to minimize any attempt at such a specific

245

delineation. We emphasize the need for recognizing that personality is based on an orderly process of maturation involving biological, psychological, and social growth. Any factor interfering with this orderly process introduces a pathology of sequence which may then significantly alter the course of human development. Thus, when viewing normal or deviant behavior, all elements involved must be properly evaluated as to their contributing role. Many of the observed psychopathological processes of childhood have been described elsewhere. The following two cases are presented as examples of deviant behavior and sequential pathology arising from culture conflict superimposed on specific aspects of personality development. They represent examples of an acute and a chronic process. Contained within them are a number of major features seen in children of Puerto Rican origin observed on the Children's Ward of Bellevue Psychiatric Hospital.

JOSÉ

PROBLEM. José was an attractive, small, white, Puerto Rican boy of ten years, who came to New York City from Puerto Rico seven months prior to hospitalization. He was referred to us by the Bureau of Adjustment of the Domestic Relations Court. This child was brought to the attention of this service by the complaints of a maternal cousin who was currently caring for the child. José was described as "incorrigible and ungovernable." He was staying out late at night, truanting from school, and disturbing classroom routine when he did attend. He was described as having mood swings and unpredictable behavior. He would become aggressive and violent to his young cousins and other children without provocation, both at home and at school.

FAMILY BACKGROUND. Review of his family history revealed that José's mother and father were both born in Puerto Rico. They were married in a religious ceremony. José was the only child born of this union. The father deserted the family prior to the boy's birth. The mother died of tuberculosis two years later. José was cared for from birth by the maternal grandparents, who recently gave up this role because of illness and senility. A maternal second cousin assumed responsibility for the child and brought him to New York City. The foster mother was a warm, pleasant woman who had three children of her own, aged eleven, five, and four, respectively.

She knew little concerning his early development. She had merely heard that he had been a good infant and child and knew of no outstanding illnesses or accidents. In her own experiences with him he had eaten and slept well. José's foster family lived in a crowded working-class area of the city. Their housing was poor but adequate. The family was self-supporting and described by a social agency as stable.

NEUROPSYCHIATRIC STATUS. In the hospital, physical and neurological examination showed a normal healthy ten-year-old child, who was small for his chronological age. Psychiatric observation involving several examiners showed the same pattern of behavior. Initially he was unwilling to talk. He was tense and impulsive, cooperated poorly, and withdrew at times. After several interviews he began to cooperate and relate in a more normal manner. He appeared confused and without real comprehension of where he was and why. This appeared to be real and unrelated to his ability to understand. He demonstrated mood swings which were quite marked during the initial period of hospitalization. At times, he would sit by himself, obviously anxious and sad. Then suddenly, with only the slightest provocation, he would explode into a frenzy of impulsive aggression. As he adjusted to the ward activities, the hospital school, and the personnel, his behavior became progressively better and showed fewer fluctuations.

During interviews, José demonstrated poorly defined concepts of himself. His comprehension of his own body structure, differences between sexes, and family constellation showed confusion and a degree of integration ordinarily seen in a much younger child. He was not sure what struc-

tures were inside the body. He talked of the several women
who had cared for him as his mother and had difficulty
separating them in his mind. His fantasies reflected his
picture of a threatening environment. In his dreams, people
were always attacking him. He wanted to be a policeman
when he grew up in order to make people good. No bizarre
thinking, delusions, or hallucinations were ever demonstrated.

PSYCHOLOGICAL EXAMINATION. Psychological examination was reported to reveal interesting variations in performance. His reactions appeared unpredictable. At times
he was alert and caught on very quickly to the tests. At
other times he seemed confused and dull. He obtained an
I.Q. of 80 on the performance scale of the Wechsler Intelligence Scale for Children, classifying him as dull normal (see
Test Summary A). He functioned at about the same level
on the Grace Arthur Performance Scale. His basic endowment, however, seemed to the psychologist to be somewhat
higher than the obtained score. The impression was reinforced by the knowledge that José had only been in New
York for seven months and was obviously still going through
an acute adjustment reaction. On both tests there was a
great deal of variability, with scores ranging from defective
to average. On certain tasks he became extremely rigid.
However, he showed adequate learning and reasoning
ability as indicated by the Block Designs. His poorest
performance occurred on tests which were weighted with
meaning appropriate to American culture. His perception
of everyday features of his environment was very inadequate
and he was unable to structure simple picture sequences
as noted in his poor performance on the WISC Picture
Arrangement and Picture Completion tests.

On the Bender Gestalt Test (Fig. 11–1), a more purely
maturational test, he showed fairly good visuo-motor organization, although he had some difficulty in drawing angles.
His figure drawings (Fig. 11–2) were poorly integrated
and defined. When viewed as a body image test, these
drawings revealed confusion with reference to body bound-

aries and the attachment of limbs to the body. There was some elaboration of the face, but the body was empty and amorphous. The opinion of the examining psychologist included the following statement: "While the data are necessarily incomplete because of the language barrier, there would seem to be evidence of serious emotional disturbance in his variability and peculiar pattern of abilities . . . leading to the impression of childhood schizophrenia." It should be noted that this pattern of test performance has been seen in the nonschizophrenic child.

RESPONSE TO TREATMENT.   José did well in the hospital. His stay was deliberately prolonged beyond the ordinary period of observation in order to expose him to structured routine, the protected school situation of the hospital, and the milieu of his peers under close adult supervision. This treatment method, which provides a substitute for a lost, primary ingroup, is often effective with Puerto Rican boys. His adjustment was excellent, and after two and a half months he was discharged to his maternal cousin and returned to public school. Currently he is apparently making a good adjustment.

PABLO

REASON FOR REFERRAL.   Pablo was a ten-year-old, white, Puerto Rican Catholic boy, who came to New York some five years prior to his admission to the Children's Ward at Bellevue Psychiatric Hospital. He was admitted as a result of a neglect petition from the Children's Court. He had previously been known to the Bureau of Child Guidance of the Board of Education of New York City. Pablo was referred for observation because of outbursts of aggressive and disruptive behavior in school and running away, for which he was reported to have received severe beatings from his father.

PARENTAL ROLE REVERSAL.   Review of his family history revealed that the entire family migrated from Puerto Rico when he was five years old. There were two older sisters.

The father had been the wage earner for the family in Puerto Rico. However, prior to the move to New York, he had experienced some kind of illness with loss of consciousness accompanied by temporary loss of the use of his extremities. He was hospitalized at that time and never quite fully recovered. At the time of his son's hospitalization he was described as suffering from high blood pressure, severe diabetes, and other physical ills associated with "an emotional disturbance." These disabilities have posed financial hardship, resulting in the family's requiring public welfare assistance from time to time. The mother had assumed the role of the principal wage earner since coming to this country and worked full time in a factory, while the father cared for the home.

HOME AND SCHOOL ADJUSTMENT. The information obtained from the mother concerning Pablo's early development indicated normal development, the usual childhood illnesses, and no real problem until the current behavior difficulties. There was a history of a recent allergic rash, nail biting, and thumb sucking. The father described recent sleep walking and running away at night. His school adjustment in New York had been consistently poor. He had received unsatisfactory ratings in all grades. His behavior was characterized as eruptive. Change of any kind seemed to disturb him. He was first suspended from school at the age of eight, and although he received special remedial reading help at nine, he made no apparent progress. His asocial, aggressive behavior continued in school and led to his admission to the hospital for observation. His parents were not cooperative with various community agencies which were trying to help resolve some of these difficulties.

MEDICAL EXAMINATION. In the hospital, physical and neurological examination showed a white Puerto Rican boy of small structure and no physical abnormalities. He was right-handed, right-footed, and right-eyed. There was good muscle tone, normal ocular convergence, poor right-left discrimination, and fluid whirling responses to postural testing. Psychiatric observation resulted in the impression of an impulsive, anxious child who used withdrawal as his main defense. He had frequent uncontrolled outbursts followed by sullen, quiet periods. During his "rages" he would attack other children without obvious reason.

This boy seemed to use difficulty with the English language as a defense against communication in interview situations. In spite of expressed confusion with the language, he was frequently observed to speak English spontaneously in his contact with other children on the ward. In repeated interviews he responded with a persistent negativism and frequent withdrawals. He expressed real anxiety about difficulties with his school work and problems at home. At no time were any bizarre productions elicited. His ward adjustment was poor. He frequently started fights and quarrels with other children and then complained that they were picking on him.

PSYCHOLOGICAL TEST FINDINGS.   A psychological examination performed when the patient was eight years old by the Bureau of Child Guidance resulted in an I.Q. of 93. This was considered minimal. Another examination performed during his period of hospital observation resulted in an I.Q. of 86 on the performance portion of the Wechsler Intelligence Scale for Children. His use of English was too limited to evaluate accurately the verbal items of this test. He was a complete nonreader and had virtually no other academic skills. The subtest scores on the performance test were only moderately scattered with some failures on easy items and successes on considerably more difficult ones (see Test Summary B). He tended to give up rather easily when faced with an initial difficulty and kept seeking approval from the examiner. He showed perseveration not only on the WISC but also in response to the Rorschach cards.

Pablo's performance on the Bender Gestalt figures was relatively good. Figure 11–3 shows that six of the figures are crowded into a little over one-third of the available space, while the last two are disproportionately large and overlap. In the recall of the Gestalt the patient "contaminated" by combining into one the parts of two different figures. He tried to avoid drawing the human figure and had to be cajoled into making the attempt. His three preliminary attempts all lacked legs and hugged the margin of the paper. There seems to be an avoidance of the sexual area, although the emphasis on a beard and pipe in his final construction (Fig. 11–4) would indicate strivings toward a virile masculinity.

The language limitations made a thorough Rorschach impossible, but even his limited responses showed a tendency to stick to a response he initially found satisfactory despite its later unsuitability. When he departed from this "safe" percept his answers became increasingly impulsive with little regard for the form of the blots.

Throughout the entire testing he appeared anxious and withdrawn, consistently evading difficult situations by either giving up easily or acting in an impulsive and unplanned manner. In spite of previous testing, he showed no recognition of the materials, and neither enthusiasm nor distaste for the task. However, no psychotic content was revealed.

OUTLOOK FOR THE FUTURE. Pablo showed little improvement or change during his period of observation in the hospital. He was returned to the Children's Court with recommendation for placement in a residential school for boys and for special attention to his educational disabilities. While awaiting such placement he was returned home on probation. As last reported, he has continued to make a poor adjustment and was continuing to pose many problems in management.

JOSÉ AND PABLO IN CULTURAL CONTEXT

FATHER AND MOTHER. The social histories of both sets of parents were quite typical of the Puerto Ricans migrating to New York. The prime motivation of both individual and family migration could always be found in socioeconomic factors. There were a number of interesting features in these case studies which occurred with great frequency among Puerto Rican children. José, the product of a broken home, was consistently reared by members of the maternal family, since the natural father, although living in New York, refused to accept responsibility for the care of his child. This was the prevalent pattern of child rearing. The Spanish Catholic social customs, centering in a strong patriarchal household, exerted strong influence in Puerto Rico. In such a setting, the mother was completely submissive to the father's authority, and her dominant role in child rearing was clearly established. This exact definition of responsibility and social role resulted in a number of well-defined practices and attitudes which often failed in New York. In the disrupted family, the maternal side always assumed the care of the children. This practice was so deeply rooted that we frequently found children of broken homes bearing the name of the maternal family.

The mother was invariably considered the focal center of the family and was particularly so in the eyes of the children —both male and female. Girls in Puerto Rico from earliest childhood were more protected and cloistered. Close identification with the mother and the maternal role were firmly established. On the other hand, from the time of a boy's birth, efforts were made to make him display his masculinity. He was endowed very early in life with a sense of importance of his sex. He was encouraged to be virile and tough. He was frequently given special privileges and was not required to stay at home but allowed to roam the streets. This ultimately served as the base for assuming the authoritarian role of the father in the family. In this setting the father's major responsibility emerged as the provider of the material necessities of life for the family. He handled the more severe punishment. Corporal punishment was approved, accepted, and commonly practiced. The father's personal life and recreation was separate from the children and frequently outside the milieu of the family.

IDENTIFICATION PROBLEMS.   In this structuring, the girls seemed more easily able to establish an identity.   The boys appeared to be at a distinct disadvantage in that they were not permitted to develop close identification with either the mother or the father at any stage of formative development. It is interesting to note that both José and Pablo had difficulties with human figure drawings. If these drawings are viewed as projections of body image formation, both children clearly reflect through them the structure and stresses of their family setting. José's figure drawings (Fig. 11–2) were poorly integrated and defined. They showed confusion over boundaries. They represented a very immature attempt and were considerably below his mental age as scored on the Wechsler Intelligence Scale for Children. Pablo showed many of the same features with the additional emphasis on a beard and a pipe, indicating some of the strivings for a virile masculinity (Fig. 11–4).

When the family role of Pablo's father is examined within this cultural setting, a significant dichotomy appears. Because of a physical disability and economic factors in New York which make it easier for the Puerto Rican woman to find employment, a reversal in family role was forced on this man. He became the homemaker and had to assume responsibilities for child rearing. By culture and social indoctrination he was ill prepared for this role. His subsequent rigid, authoritarian, and punitive attitude and behavior appeared to take a heavy toll of Pablo's development. It frustrated several attempts by social agencies to help this family. He could not be dissuaded from his use of severe physical beatings. Unwittingly he became a persistent cause of his son's delinquency. It is interesting to note that Pablo ran away from home and roamed the streets in his attempt to defend himself from the threats of his family and hostile environment. These were the very same practices in which all Puerto Rican boys were encouraged.

FRIGHT, FIGHT, FLIGHT. For both José and Pablo marked aggressive behavior was a principal presenting complaint. Examined within the structure of the aggressive, masculine indoctrination of Puerto Rican family culture, it was no wonder that their reaction to certain threatening and frustrating situations nearly always resulted in direct physical counteraggression. Both of them had serious learning difficulties in school, where they demonstrated aggressive and disruptive behavior. The same was true of José in his new home and in his initial period on our ward. In the relatively protected environment of the hospital situation, however, José's behavior underwent rapid improvement. Pablo's conflicts of much longer duration, however, showed little alteration. These responses were common for many of the children observed in our setting.

Other consistent reactions present in the two children were negativism, withdrawal, and denial, which were in operation repeatedly during their period of hospital observation. These mechanisms were used only with authority figures and were repeatedly encountered in interview situations. Simultaneously, behavior with peers on the ward was consistently aggressive. This pattern seemed to reflect the cultural practices. These children, coming from a society where strict obedience was demanded by the authoritarian role of the father, were able to respond to the threatening aspects of the interview situation only with negativism and withdrawal. There was little room or conditioning for any other kind of response. On the other hand, with their peers, they were motivated to establish active, aggressive relationship.

This behavior was rather uniform for many of the Puerto Rican children observed. Fright, fight, and flight appeared to be the dominant pattern of response. It is interesting to speculate that this type of primitive phylogenetic and ontogenetic reaction pattern goes with the immature, plastic, and sometimes poorly defined psychological structuring so frequently seen in the emotionally disturbed Puerto Rican child. It is as if the combination of biological, psychological, and social events in the child's life served to prolong the gelling process of personality formation. As a result, performances and responses reflected younger and more primitive patterns. We have repeatedly observed primitive responses among Puerto Rican children in their visuo-motor organization, body-image concepts, and fantasy life, as well as in their social responses. This amorphous quality in some respects makes them more vulnerable to social stress. However, it also seems to give them a greater resiliency and their recovery and progress can sometimes be amazingly rapid. José's improvement during a very short period of hospitalization serves as an example.

PROBLEMS OF LANGUAGE. The special problem of difficulties with the English language was of major importance. José had been in New York for seven months prior to hospitalization and had not acquired even a rudimentary grasp of the language. Pablo had been in New York for five years and still demonstrated severe confusion with English. In interview situations his confusion became so great that he refused to speak English at all. Part of this may have been defensive withdrawal, but his difficulties in school indicated a real confusion in the area of language.

Our observations of Puerto Rican children as exemplified by José and Pablo raised a number of interesting points for consideration. Are we dealing with a specific language disability stemming from the Spanish-speaking bilingual environment? This appears unlikely in that a number of other languages have the same root origin as Spanish and have not presented a similar problem. Neither can it be a disability stemming totally from culture conflict. If it were so, other ethnic groups exposed to the same circumstances would produce similar problems. It would therefore seem most plausible to seek the explanation in a combination of the stresses of culture conflict with the internal maturation of the Puerto Rican child.

LANGUAGE AND MATURATION. Speech is a symbolic expression of feelings, thoughts, and ideas. It is the verbal means of communication and may be regarded as both a tool and a manifestation of language development. Children have an incomplete system of symbols and try to work them out in a continuous process of experimentation in which the aims and the drives of the total personality play the leading part. The free process of experimentation may be hindered either by the difficulty of the subject matter or by the threats which originate from the situation or from the attitude of adults. The actual process of symbolism lags behind the general state of development in the perceptive and emotional spheres. The child comes to reality and proper symbol formation as a result of his own biological and psychological maturation and his own experimentation. If these processes are themselves immature and poorly constructed, the lag in adequate symbol formation is even greater.

In the more obvious disorders of language development, such as speech defects, reading disabilities, and developmental aphasias, there is already considerable evidence that these conditions are developmental lags in specific brain function. Also, many types of brain disorders are frequently associated with language disturbances. From a phylogenetic point of view, language is a recently acquired function of the mammalian brain. As such, there are more likely to be lags in development.

LANGUAGE AND CULTURE CONFLICT. When one examines the case histories of José and Pablo, an impressive number of hindering events in their lives can be demonstrated. Their dislocation from one culture to another must certainly have posed a whole series of difficulties in subject matter, situation, and attitudes. These problems, in addition to the boys' immature and poorly constructed psychological maturation, could only serve to increase the lag in adequate symbol formation. Their language disability thus would appear to be a specific product of their total situation. As Spanish-speaking children with both incomplete symbol formation and language, they were exposed to a second language. Added to this was the conflict of culture and minority group status, exerting their known detrimental forces on personality development. As a result, there was created an ideal situation for abnormal symbol formation and language disability. Thus we seem to have an ethnic group in which personality deviation may be both the cause and effect of a lag in general language development. The child who does not have the normal understanding or use of language may become seriously handicapped in his personality development. Language exists, but within a distorted framework of psychological maturation and social adjustment. This kind of personality deviation can almost be considered as a special problem of culture conflict. Children should have the opportunity of approaching the reality of their level of maturation and experimentation untrammeled by fear that distorts the total process.

SOCIAL PROBLEMS. Both children presented serious behavior and learning problems in school. Certainly the language difficulties contributed extensively to this situation. Other social factors, however, were also at work. Many Puerto Rican children experienced a real lack of continuity in their schooling. Formal education began later than that of most of their age peers in New York. They frequently by-passed one or more of the earlier grades in regular sequence. In transferring from Puerto Rican schools, they may have been up-graded in order to be placed with their age peers. In Puerto Rico, grade placement was based upon achievement and not upon age as in New York. For various reasons there was a higher percentage of school transfers in New York of Island-born Puerto Rican children. This appeared to be an important disruptive factor, and aggravated an already unstable situation. Instability also characterized the domestic scene, expressed in broken homes, overcrowding, and working mothers.

This combination of school and home circumstances could only serve as a further disintegrating force to children who already demonstrated poorly defined and unstructured personality development. Examination of both José's and Pablo's social patterns revealed many of these factors.

RESPONSES TO TESTING. The responses of both children to psychological testing took on greater depth and proportion when re-examined within this maturational and social prospectus. José's reactions were described as unpredictable. At times he was alert and demonstrated excellent comprehension. At other times he appeared confused and dull. His performance showed a great deal of variability ranging from defective to average. In spite of some extreme rigidity, he had good learning and reasoning ability. In spite of satisfactory perceptual performance, social comprehension was inadequate. Body-image concepts were poorly defined. All these distortions and variabilities led the examining psychologist to the impression of childhood schizophrenia. Yet when the various aspects of testing were viewed against the background of the social forces which had influenced José's development, they assumed different significance. Each of the psychological distortions appeared to reflect the social patterns to which the child had been subjected. It was as if the child, through his psychological testing, mirrored the distortions of his experiences. These results could be better viewed as products of the environment than as an indication of the internal personality disorganization as seen in childhood schizophrenia. José's subsequent behavior on the ward and rapid adjustment to community living strongly favored this interpretation.

Many of the same features were present in the psychological performance of Pablo. However, the disruptive element of his living experiences were of much longer duration. As such, they appeared to have become more fixed within the psychological maturation of the child and resulted in a much more rigid pattern of behavior.

This clinical survey of José and Pablo clearly defines the close interrelationships among maturational processes, social experiences, and cultural patterns in a child's growth. The importance of the proper and complete sequence of various phases of development becomes apparent when their behavior, reactions, language, learning, and productions are examined. In several areas of their performance, a pathology of sequence introduces deviations which affect every phase of personality. In others, the culture conflict finds a fertile field for the rapid stimulation of personality distortions. Early recognition and correction of these disruptive forces become the therapeutic goal, if we are to help children like José and Pablo achieve their full potential as human beings in our increasingly complex society.

Test Summary

A. WISC RECORD FORM: JOSÉ

	Raw Score	Wtd. Score
Picture Completion	5	4
Picture Arrangement	6	5
Block Design	10	9
Object Assembly	19	10
Coding	28	8
(Mazes)		

Sum of Performance Tests . . 36　　　　I.Q. . . 80

Test Summary

B. WISC RECORD FORM: PABLO

	Raw Score	Wtd. Score
Picture Completion	11	10
Picture Arrangement	16	6
Block Design	14	9
Object Assembly	16	7
Coding	27	8
(Mazes)		

Sum of Performance Tests . . 40　　　　I.Q. . . 86

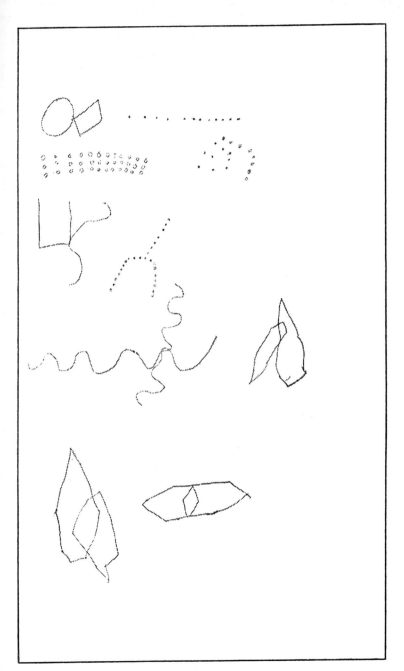

FIGURE 11–1. Bender Gestalt Test (José).

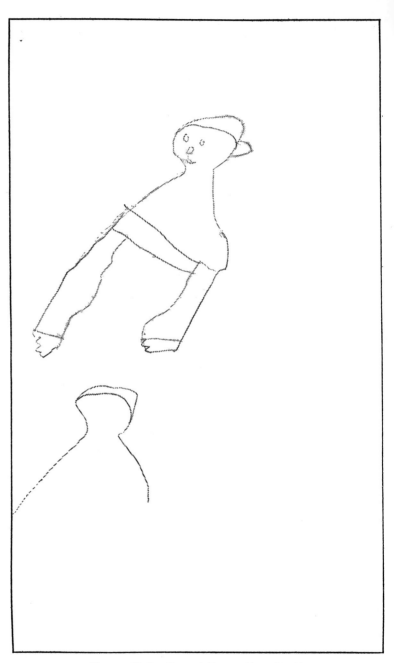

FIGURE 11–2. Draw-A-Person Test (José).

262

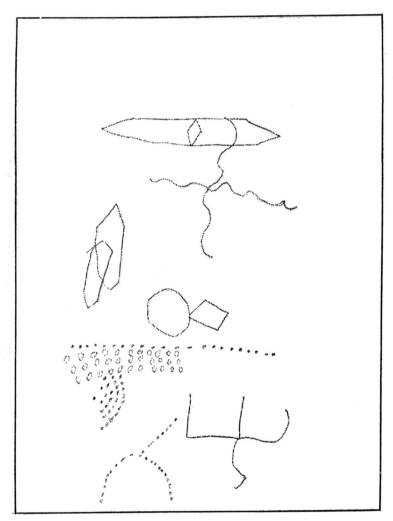

FIGURE 11-3. Bender Gestalt Test (Pablo).

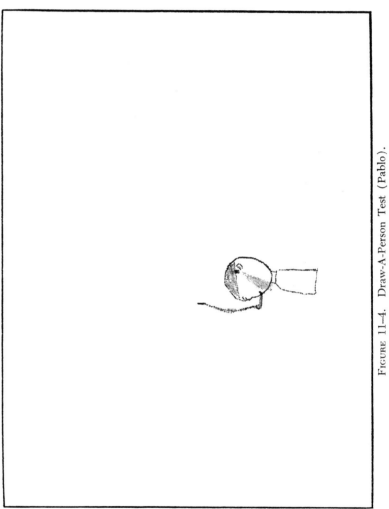

FIGURE 11–4.   Draw-A-Person Test (Pablo).

12

A Filipino in California Copes
with Anxiety

H. Elston Hooper

UNDERSTANDING THE FILIPINO

Psychological evaluation of the Filipino may fail to present some of the more obvious problems often encountered in the interpretation of cultural differences. The examiner will not ordinarily find grossly deviant responses to tests that have been standardized on subjects in the United States. The differences which are manifested, however, are generally of a more subtle nature and as such may more easily allow for errors in interpretation and may have important bearing on the evaluation and treatment of these people.

EDUCATION. The absence of gross cultural deviation in the responses of this Malayan group may be directly attributed to the fact that their country was occupied and governed by the United States from the time of the Spanish-American war until very recently when they were granted independence. Perhaps the most important of the American influences in the Philippine Islands was the development of an advanced system of public education. Schooling had been instituted by the Spanish as part of the Roman Catholic missionary movement, but it remained for the Americans to extend schools to even the most remote village. English

is taught in the schools and often the textbooks used in
elementary education are American. It has been stated that
the Filipino child may know more about George Washington than about the Filipino leaders. This has given the
Filipinos an understanding and belief in democracy. They
have been taught that "all men are created equal." When
they come to the United States, unlike certain other minority groups they often refuse to accept their assigned places
as inferiors in our culture. Many of the unfortunate incidents
which have marred relations between Filipinos and other
groups in the United States have been attributed to this
discrepancy between their expectations and the reality.

FEUDAL LIFE. In any study of the Filipino people it is
important to note that the economic structure of life in the
Philippines retains many elements of a feudal system.
Capitalistic development of industry and manufacturing
has been retarded, and the economy remains highly centered around farming and very small business ventures.
Some of the farmers own a few acres of land from which
they are able marginally to support a family. Many others
work the land of wealthy landowners and must yield the
greater part of their harvest to the landlord. This has made
for a class structure with marked differences between the
peasant, who lives in conditions close to poverty, and the
small but powerful wealthy class. It has also resulted in the
restriction of opportunities for the lower classes to achieve
any betterment of their condition. This frustration of opportunity for advancement is in direct opposition to the
efforts of the progressive educational system and creates
within the people strong but usually unfulfilled strivings
to surmount their obstacles. There are few avenues for
advancement available to the lower-class person. If he
can achieve a higher education he may be able to enter
the teaching profession. Government service, including the
United States armed forces, provides another source of
opportunity but is also dependent upon education. Emi-
gration to Hawaii or the United States has provided a

further chance for the Filipino to better himself and this has been the objective of many thousands of Filipino youths.[1]

STRIVING FOR SUCCESS. The vast majority of the Filipinos that come to the United States are in search of education. A degree from any college here will almost automatically insure success and prestige in the Philippines. Unfortunately they generally come poorly prepared, both scholastically and financially, to achieve their goals and have to resort to picking farm crops or work as house boys or cooks in order to maintain themselves. Their families in the Philippines have such high hopes for them that they are ashamed to return in failure and continue, therefore, in the meager living that is available to them here. Almost all eventually plan to return to their homeland. Their stay in the United States is made additionally difficult by the fact that the social life of the Filipino is extremely restricted as a result of a ratio between the sexes of about twenty males to every female. Interracial contacts and marriages have been frequent, resulting in considerable discord between groups and rather extreme discriminatory attitudes and actions on the part of white Americans.

In this chapter the history and psychological evaluation of a Filipino [2] patient will be presented, and we shall discuss

---

[1] Most of the nearly forty thousand persons who make up our Filipino population live on the West Coast and are especially concentrated in Los Angeles, Stockton, and Seattle. The greatest influx of immigration to this country occurred prior to 1935. At this time the Philippines were promised their independence from the United States and a formal quota of fifty per year was established. This was raised to a hundred in 1945, when full independence was granted.

[2] It should be noted that the Filipino is but one of several Malayan peoples that dwell in the Philippine Islands. The earliest inhabitants were the Negritos, a pygmy race who live in a rather primitive state. Later an invading force from Malay, the Igorots, drove the Negritos into the forests and jungles and settled along the coast of Luzon, the most northerly and largest of the islands. Centuries later they were, in turn, driven back by invaders from Malay who settled the lowlands of Luzon and spread to other islands. This group has become known as "Filipinos." A fourth wave of invaders from Malay, the Moros, had been converted to Islam by the Arabs and continue to be almost fanatic in this belief. They occupy parts

the psychological significance of the test protocols in the light of his cultural background. We have selected a patient who demonstrates many of the typical characteristics of the Filipino groups in the United States as they have been seen in a Veterans Administration hospital where they have undergone treatment for tuberculosis.

A SHORT HISTORY OF THE PATIENT

POOR PARENTS.   Our patient, Juan, was born on the island of Luzon. His was a typical farming family. On a few acres of land they managed to grow enough rice to provide their supply of food. Juan was the youngest of the three sons. Even before school age, he can recall working hard in the fields. His mother had a small business selling material and other supplies from a pushcart and was able in this manner to meet the various needs of the family. Although the family is generally a very close-knit unit in the Philippines, Juan can recall little closeness with his parents. He states that his mother "talked very little" and describes his father as "always very busy with the farm."

Under the educational system of the Philippines each *barrio* (a village unit consisting of up to one hundred families) had an elementary school. Juan started at the *barrio* school at the age of five. After one year, it was decided that he should go to live with his grandparents so that he might attend school in the *poblacion* (town). During the next six years he saw his parents for a period of only two months a year.

RICH UNCLE.   After completing the seventh grade, Juan wanted to continue his education by attending high school. As the nearest high school was fifteen miles away over poor roads, it seemed impossible to arrange more schooling until

---

of the most southerly islands, principally Mindanao. The Filipinos are the most important group in the Philippines. They control the governmental functions and make up the majority of the educators and professional people. It is from this group that the emigrants to Hawaii and the United States have chiefly come.

an uncle offered to take him into his household. At the age of twelve, he traveled by bus and boat to his uncle's home which was on a smaller island to the south. It took him twenty days to complete the four-hundred-mile trip. The uncle was a wealthy landowner, who in addition to his country estate maintained a home in a city of about fifteen thousand population. It was here that Juan lived during school semesters. There were two servants to maintain the house. On vacations and special days he would go to his uncle's estate which was "a good six hours' ride by horse."

Thus Juan became part of a new family—one vastly different from that in which he had spent his earlier years. The family consisted of five boys and two girls, all about his own age. Being well-to-do the family was well educated; all but the youngest child entered college and all are currently pursuing professional careers. Two of the sons have college degrees in agriculture, two are engineers, one is attending medical school, and one of the daughters has a master's degree in education. This family must certainly have reinforced Juan's already strong drive for education and success.

The uncle owned extensive land and had many tenant farmers from whom he collected 60 per cent of the crops. In the summers Juan worked for him supervising the harvest and collecting his uncle's portion. Juan found the contrast between the wealth of his uncle and the poverty of the tenants difficult to accept and occasionally reacted strongly against his uncle.

AUNT'S INFLUENCE. It is significant that he calls his aunt and uncle by the names "father" and "mother." The aunt was an understanding person to whom he could turn for advice. It was she who advised that he plan to utilize his intellectual abilities and not attempt to work for a living with his hands. As a maternal figure, she was undoubtedly the dominant person in the family in accordance with Island custom. Her influence was especially felt in regard to religion. Since the time of the Spanish missionary efforts, the vast majority of Filipinos have been Roman Catholic, and Juan's family were quite devout in this religion. His aunt always insisted that the entire family meet together for daily prayers.

WAR. The war with the Japanese started while Juan was in his last few months of high school. During the initial period he stayed in the city to protect and maintain his uncle's home. After the occupation, he was employed by the Japanese as a house boy. Because of his contacts with the enemy, he was induced by the Philippine guerrillas to pass information to them regarding Japanese military installations. When the guerrilla artillery showed amazing accuracy, Juan, along with other Filipinos, was forced to leave the town and went to join the forces in the interior of the island.

With the arrival of American troops in 1945, Juan decided to enlist in the United States Navy. He recalls that "the whole family had to be called in to make the decision, and they all approved. They viewed it as a great thing to have a representative of their family in a United States military unit." He was disappointed to find that his assignment in the navy was that of a valet to officers (at one time he served an admiral) but managed to accept this for several years. He began to demand that he be allowed to do something better. It was finally decided that he might go to a technical school to become a weatherman.

While in the service, Juan was married to the daughter of a well-to-do businessman. She was a devoutly religious girl and had been in a Catholic cloister. They have had two sons. His navy pay enabled his wife and children to live in Manila at a high standard of living.

TUBERCULOSIS. Juan had been in the navy about four years when he was hospitalized for tuberculosis. The disease at that time was mild and after seven months he was returned to duty. The following year X-rays revealed further progression, and he was again hospitalized in a naval hospital, from which he was transferred to the VA hospital after his discharge from the service eight months later.

Prior to leaving the navy, he had obtained his United States citizenship and decided to remain in this country and continue his schooling. He immediately began making arrangements for his wife and family to join him. There were many complications involved in this, and it was several months before his wife arrived and almost a year and a half before the children joined them.

RISE OF ANXIETY. Soon after his admission to the hospital he was routinely interviewed by a clinical psychologist. No significant problems were seen at that time and the comment was made that "the patient is intelligent, alert, and a very likable person." After sixteen months, however, his tuberculosis did not seem to be responding to treatment, and ward personnel noted that he seemed depressed and worried, complained of headaches and insomnia, and was concerned because others were beginning to notice his distress. It was at this juncture that he was first referred for extensive psychological study which was followed by supportive psychotherapy.

PSYCHODIAGNOSTIC STUDY

STRATEGY. In the three years of Juan's hospitalization he has had many contacts with the clinical psychologists. On two occasions extensive test batteries have been administered, including the Wechsler-Bellevue Intelligence Scale or the Wechsler Adult Intelligence Scale, the Rorschach, and the Minnesota Multiphasic Personality Inventory. In addition to the usual considerations in the study of psychological test materials, we have been interested in making some determination of the extent to which the difference in cultural background of the patient may have affected the interpretation of the protocols. Equally important has been an effort to obtain an understanding of the influence of acculturation during the five years in which he has been living in the United States. We might also anticipate finding evidence of Juan's reaction to situations involving discrimination against the Filipino.

Of special importance in understanding Juan is an appreciation of his reaction to his illness. Much of his test material reflects marked anxiety over the disease and the prolonged treatment with its occasional exacerbations. Tuberculosis is a highly feared disease among the Filipinos. The poverty of their living standards and inadequate hygiene have made for low resistance, and the course has most frequently been a fatal one until recent years brought improved methods of treatment. Under these circumstances it is readily understandable that the discovery of tuberculosis usually precipitates marked fear of death, of exclusion from the close family ties, or of being handicapped in making a success of life.

The tests should be interpreted, therefore, with an awareness of the influences of the cultural handicap, the effect of acculturation, and the fear of tuberculosis on the intellectual and emotional functioning of the patient.

TEST-INTELLIGENCE, 1953 AND 1956

GENERAL COMPARISON. Juan was given the Wechsler-Bellevue Intelligence Scale (W-B) in 1953 and the Wechsler Adult Intelligence Scale (WAIS) in 1956.[3] A study of the results should not only reveal cultural influences but may provide evidence of the effect of the patient's continuing contact with American culture. A profile of weighted scores for the two tests is presented in Fig. 12–1. The Verbal Scale I.Q. for the W-B is 104 with a Performance I.Q. of 92 and Full Scale I.Q. of 98. His best scores are obtained in the Information and Similarities subtests. Digit Span, Picture Arrangement, and to a lesser degree Picture Completion lie below the average subtest level. Inspection of the profile suggests that Juan has the capacity for above average intellectual functioning in verbal tasks as evidenced by a good store of knowledge and the development of superior

---

[3] The author is aware that comparison of the W-B with the WAIS must be made with considerable caution because of differences in content and standardization.

abstract thought processes. Digit Span may indicate the presence of anxiety which was described in the clinical history. Picture Arrangement is known to be highly specific in culture content and would be especially worthy of analysis. A more detailed consideration of certain of the subtests will be found later.

The WAIS, which was administered in 1956, resulted in a Full Scale I.Q. of 94. The difference of four points between this and the W-B I.Q. of 98 obtained in 1953 is too small to be of significance. What difference there is was contributed by the verbal tests, the Verbal Scale I.Q. dropping six points. The change suggests the disrupting effect of increased anxiety on the patient's newly acquired and presumably not well-assimilated language. Certain of the subtests of the W-B and WAIS have been selected for detailed consideration. Special attention will be given to items that appear in both tests.

INFORMATION. This was one of the most stable tests, yielding scores among the highest on both scales. This seems to demonstrate that in regard to his store of knowledge, such as might be gained through schooling, Juan shows familiarity with many aspects of our culture. Correct answers to items such as the height of the average American woman, Washington's birthday, and habeas corpus illustrate this. Some of the items, on the other hand, might be said to lie well within the scope of his "native" instruction. Such items include knowing the source of rubber, the capital of Japan, and what the Vatican and the Koran are.

The WAIS answers illustrate the new fluency that he has acquired and indicate that he has amassed a considerable technical vocabulary. Many of the answers are over-specified. This is illustrated in his reply to the question, "What does rubber come from?" On the WAIS he says "from a tree, from Ceylon, Dutch East Indies. Grows mostly in tropical areas where there is an abundant supply of rain. How would you like this answer—geographical, economical, or what?" Juan seems to be doing more than answering, he is parading his knowledge. For the most part his answers are accurate but in neither test does he know the number of weeks in a year.

COMPREHENSION. As with Information, this subtest remained at about the same level in both testings. The use of over-intellectualization is even more evident and proves to be more inefficient. This is best illustrated by the answer to the question why people who are born deaf are usually unable to talk. In 1953, Juan stated, "I don't know. Must be relations between the voice part of the body and bone perhaps." In 1956 he says, "There is an impairment in the main organs that connect the main nerve of the olfactory nerve and the nerve connecting the eye to the brain." He shows acquaintance with the general concept of nerves and their transmission of impulses to the brain. His use of this concept, however, is inaccurate, and the introduction of "olfactory" and "eye" into the answer indicates very loose thought processes. On the "taxes" item he gives an irrelevant extension: "Economically if people weren't taxed, one group of people would own the nation's wealth." This elaboration was perhaps determined by Juan's reaction against the economic inequality of classes which is so prevalent in the Filipino culture.

SIMILARITIES. This is probably the most significant of the subtests. It had the highest weighted score in the W-B but was lowered to third position in the WAIS. Examination of the answers reveals that in the WAIS his attempt to be more erudite prevents him from giving the generalized abstraction which is required for highest score in the items. This is especially true of the early items. For the similarity between an orange and a banana he had said "both fruits" in 1953 but says "both plants, biology" in 1956. For coat and dress he replaces "both wearing apparel" for "Have utility purpose. Both give protection, are warm. You can say help appearance." Instead of "animals" for dog and lion he incorrectly refers to both as "canines." At the same time, he shows marked improvement on certain of the more difficult items which require more abstract concepts such as poem, statue, praise, and punishment, suggesting that his capacity for abstract thinking is actually improved.

VOCABULARY. This test must be evaluated in the light of the fact that English is a secondary language for the Filipino. The people of the Islands generally are bilingual or trilingual. Their primary language is one of the dialects of the Malayan group.[4] In addition, a large number of the population also speaks the languages of the two principal occupying nations, Spanish and English. Juan studied English in his school years and had developed fair proficiency by the time he entered the hospital. Undoubtedly some of his errors in Vocabulary on the W-B can be accounted for by limited familiarity with the language. His definition of "cedar" as "a kind of drink," for example, might suggest that cedar is not a species of tree that he has had an opportunity to become acquainted with. The Vocabulary test of the WAIS shows fewer evidences of this type of handicap. His definitions are, on the whole, precise and accurate. The results on Vocabulary, along with those on Information and others of the Verbal tests, suggest that Juan's true verbal intelligence would be within Bright Normal or Superior limits were it not for the cultural handicap and emotional disturbance with its compensatory over-intellectualization.

PICTURE ARRANGEMENT. On both W-B and WAIS, the Picture Arrangement weighted scores are among the lowest. The story material of the tests is in general specific to our culture and may pose special problems for subjects from other cultures. Lowering of scores in this test may also indicate difficulties in interpersonal relationships. It would be anticipated that the minority group member, such as Juan, who is attempting to adjust himself to a foreign and partially unaccepting environment, would face problems in interpersonal dealings and that these might interfere with his perception and handling of situations in the test.

---

[4] The principal dialects found in the Philippines are Ilocana, Tagalog, and Visayan.

RORSCHACH ANALYSIS. The Rorschach was administered as part of the test batteries of 1953 and 1956. The test results provide information in regard to crucial considerations in the understanding of this patient. It will be recalled that in 1953 Juan was undergoing a state of emotional disturbance with depression and some agitation. It was important to know whether this represented an actual or potential disintegration into a psychotic reaction. Treatment considerations included a choice of psychotherapy or the physical therapies of psychiatry. Some estimation of the danger of suicide or explosive hostile outbursts was needed in order to determine the feasibility of maintaining the patient on an open ward setting. Decisions regarding these matters are normally difficult enough; in considering a person from a different culture they become even more hazardous.

The 1953 Rorschach had but eleven responses. All but two used the whole card. The content may be briefly described as follows: I, a flying bat out for a fight; II, the bleeding mouth of a person; III, a red plus mark and a person trying to attack someone; IV, black clouds; V, animal hide; VI, chest X-ray; VII, clouds; VIII, climbing animals; IX, TB sputum; X, germs under microscope. (See complete protocol in Test Summary A.)

There were three prominent features of this first Rorschach. Most striking was the expression of crude and explosive hostile concepts associated with physical attack and injury. Second, there were evidences of extreme fear and concern about tuberculosis. The third feature was the rather ineffectual attempt to use defenses against the manifestations of anxiety. This was seen in the use of concepts of X-rays, clouds, and views under a microscope.

Consideration was made of the role of culture in these factors. Interpretation of the significance of the expression of overtly hostile responses is an example of the problems imposed by the difference in culture. Juan's response to Card II was "Looks like a mouth of a person that's been hit —could have been hit and he's bleeding." This rather crude response was probably induced by "shock" reaction to the color of the card and represents hostile impulses that are close to behavioral expression. The minus form-level is an indication of the true extent of the disturbance. In a patient from our culture this response would suggest a very severe personality disintegration, probably of psychotic proportions, and the danger of overt hostile behavior. The hostility seen in Juan's record may, however, represent a more adjustive reaction to severe frustration than would be true for subjects of our culture. The Filipinos are permitted more overt expression of hostility and are expected to "fight" for their rights. In Juan's case, we must also remember that for several years he was engaged in rather bloody guerrilla warfare in the Islands. The problem of the interpretation of hostility expression awaits a group study of the psychological makeup of the Filipino. Our present state of knowledge can only suggest caution in our deductions.

We must be equally cautious in regard to Juan's disturbance over his tuberculosis. As was previously indicated, this is a disease that is greatly feared by the Filipino. Undoubtedly an exacerbation in his progress, following several years of treatment, might easily have brought these fears to the surface and resulted in the intense emotional upset that occurred in 1953.

Consideration of these cultural variables led to interpretation of the Rorschach as indicating a rather severe anxiety reaction rather than a psychosis. There were elements of personality disintegration in evidence, and it was felt that unless the stresses were lessened and more effective defenses instituted there was a possibility of development of a schizophrenic reaction. It was this danger that made the immediate start of a supportive form of psychotherapy so imperative.

The 1956 Rorschach results are of great interest. We wished to know whether our interpretations of the patient's personality organization were accurate, i.e., was a psychosis averted? The record was also examined to determine what the effect of continued contact with our culture might have had on the personality structure of the patient as revealed through comparison with his previous Rorschach.

The quantitative summary of the Rorschach immediately suggests that changes have occurred. The number of responses has doubled. This increase, however, is seen to result from increased elaboration of responses in an attempt to integrate all parts of the blot into the concept. It was frequently necessary to score each element of the response with a D and include them in an over-all W. The locations were as follows: $W = 5$; $D = 16$; $Dd = 1$; and $S = 1$. In comparison with the 1953 results, there has been a marked increase in the number and percentage of M responses. F responses are more frequently seen; one Fc is given. In the color area, he is now able to give responses in which the shape is predominant, although CF responses are still more frequently seen.

The nature but not the number of content areas has changed. Instead of clouds, blood, and X-rays we now have objects, nature, and fire. The patient seems to have replaced a rather constricted responsiveness with greater elaboration and increased use of his intellectual potential. The predominant emphasis has changed from outgoing color-dominated concepts to a more introspective preoccupation with the self. Form-level is superior to that of 1953 and the patient seems to have better intellectual controls. Concern with tuberculosis as a threat has lessened, and he now appears to be preoccupied with more abstract and philosophical matters such as the eventual outcome of the struggle of life.

The essential content of the responses is as follows: I, a black bird swooping down on its prey; II, animals in a duel with punishment by fire for the loser; III, female dancers; IV, a black gorilla ready to jump; V, stretched out animal hide; VI, long-necked animal about to attack; VII, squirrels in an argument; VIII, animals in contest to get to top of tree; IX, devils fencing with loser to burn; X, animals trying to escape from walls of hell and some who have gotten out. (The complete record will be found in Test Summary B.) Comparison between his two Rorschach performances shows that hostility continues to play a very important role in the concepts. Whereas, in 1953, the hostility had been primitive and poorly controlled, it has now become channeled into competitive strivings and controlled through use of intellectual and compulsive defense mechanisms. The response to Card II is a good example and contrasts with the 1953 "bloody mouth" response:

These two things here are more or less animals I would say. They are, more or less, in a duel. By the time they reach this point they will have combat. I believe the loser will fall down here through this space. There's a leg of one animal here and these are the wings. This is a cave and the loser will fall through here in cave—or the fire will eventually burn the loser. This looks like a furnace—the moment one falls it will burn the loser.

This theme is repeated in responses to several subsequent cards and appears to indicate that he has formalized and to some extent intellectualized his hostile impulses. In this manner he is not only defending himself from the threat of being overwhelmed by the hostility but is also rendering the impulses far more acceptable to a culture in which their repression is necessary to social acceptability.

Anxiety over feelings of inadequacy in competitive situations is the most important theme of this Rorschach. This anxiety probably relates primarily to his school life where competition for grades continually faces him. It also appears that his breakdown with active tuberculosis has symbolized failure in his struggle with life.

His present conception of his environment indicates that his already strong strivings for success may have been reinforced by an acceptance of our middle-class value placed on upward social mobility through the competitive process. To fail is for him to be condemned and the punishment is symbolized in hell-fire. The intrusion of this "religious" conception of punishment suggests that elements of his early religious training have taken on very significant proportions in his obsessive concern about success in our culture.

The 1956 Rorschach seems to confirm the previous impression that a schizophrenic reaction could be averted by the development of adequate defense mechanisms. The test shows that Juan has utilized an obsessive-compulsive defense system with emphasis on intellectualization. As was true in the WAIS, these defenses are not fully effective in controlling his anxiety. There has also been a marked increase in doubts about his adequacy, not only in the general sense discussed, but also as regards interpersonal and sexual relationships. It seems, therefore, that the present adjustment is a transitional one in response to intense stresses represented by the tuberculosis and by the threat of failure in our culture. It has served as protection against complete disorganization of personality but does not represent an efficient use of the potentiality of that personality. The need for the reconstructive efforts of psychotherapy remains as vital as in the past.

MMPI. The MMPI was given to Juan on three occasions. In addition to being part of the 1953 and 1956 batteries, it had been administered as part of an experimental battery in 1951, just five days following his first admission. A profile of T scores from the three administrations is found in Fig. 2. It will be noted that the majority of scores fall above the 70 T score line. This is evidence that at all stages of his hospitalization we were dealing with considerable personality disturbance.

Certain of the scales in which there has been a consistent progressive change throughout the years are worthy of note. The *Hs* scale profiles show a drop in T score for each of the three testings. This probably represents a lessening of concern over his general health, consistent with treatment for tuberculosis and increasing understanding of the disease. The short term fluctuations in his condition do not seem to have counteracted the generally lessened hypochondriacal preoccupation. *Hy,* on the other hand, has progressively increased. This may be the result of the general development of more systematic defenses to combat the continuing state of anxiety and depression. *Pd* may be interpreted as conformity to the social demands of our culture, with the progressively less deviant scores on this scale reflecting his increasing acculturation. A similar interpretation might be made for the *Sc* scale which also decreased with each testing. The MMPI results seem to confirm the interpretations of the other tests. It appears that the patient underwent a very disruptive period in 1953 but that the general trend has been in the direction of a more stable state with neurotic defenses.

SUMMARY

SOURCES OF CULTURE CONFLICT. In our study of a Filipino patient we have found evidence, both in the history and in the psychological evaluation, that his life has been filled with severe struggle and conflict. His early childhood witnessed his participation in the struggle for existence which is the life of the lower-class farm family. In order to continue his education he left his home to live with grandparents and, later, with his wealthy uncle. Here he vividly experienced the vast contrast between wealth and poverty which is characteristic of the feudal-like class structure on the Islands. As a member of the lower class he could not help but rebel against the injustices of the system but, at the same time, he sought to identify himself with what his uncle represented. This period of conflict seems to have resulted in the intensification of already strong strivings for self-betterment. He realized that the avenue for social and economic achievement could only lie in education and this became his primary objective. This goal was frustrated, however, by the Japanese occupation of the Philippines in the early years of World War II and Juan was drawn into active participation in the guerrilla warfare which the Filipinos conducted against their enemy.

When the war ended, Juan was financially unable to return to school and, after a family conference, decided to enter the United States Navy, intending to make this his career. The navy provided good income, by Philippine standards, and he was able to marry and establish a home. He was immediately confronted, however, with the prejudice within the service which limited him to duty as an officer's valet. For several years he fought to be allowed to demonstrate that a Filipino could perform other duties. His requests were finally granted only to have the onset of tuberculosis result in his discharge from the navy.

RISK OF DEFEAT. An often discouraging struggle with tuberculosis followed. His disease proved to be very unstable and periods of good progress were interrupted by exacerbation. It has been necessary for him to be hospitalized during four of the six years since his discharge. This has been a period of almost complete frustration of his status strivings. Caught in this impasse, Juan has reacted with panic-like states of anxiety and severe depression.

The patient's veteran status has proved an advantage in permitting him to obtain schooling in the United States. He selected accounting as a vocation and has already completed several years of study in that direction. He has established a home here and is now undecided as to whether he will return to the Philippines.

In reviewing Juan's case, we note that the achievement drive which he brought with him to this country was congruent with the middle-class competitive values he found here. In fact, they added fuel to the fire of his ambition and led to a losing battle to better himself. He has been unwilling to yield to the pressures that would restrict him to a place in the social order which would be viewed as undesirable even by other ethnic minorities. The added struggle this proud attitude has entailed sometimes proved too much for him, and has precipitated relapses in his tubercular condition. With supportive psychotherapy, however, the patient's adjustment has stabilized and the prognosis for getting along in civilian life has improved.

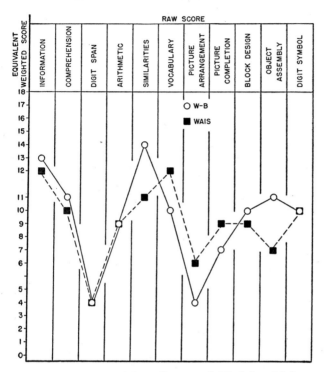

FIGURE 12–1. Wechsler-Bellevue and Wechsler Adult
Intelligence Scale Weighted Profile.

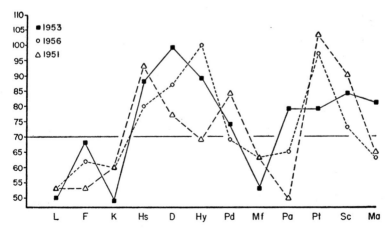

FIGURE 12–2. Minnesota Multiphasic Personality Inventory Profile.

Test Summary

A. Rorschach Protocol Comparisons

<u>1953</u>

<u>1956</u>

CARD I. 20″

1. ∧ The way I look at it—a bat wings spread out in flying motion. He'd be out for a fight—you can see his claws. That's all.

W   FM   A   P

Inquiry: (body?) Patient points to middle area. (out for a fight?) The position of the claws in either defensive or offensive fight.

CARD I. 5″

1. ∧ My impression more or less is that it's a bird—a big black bird ready for fight. It has its claws out for swooping down on its prey. The feathers here seem as though they're falling down from the bird itself. That's about all.

W   FM C′,Fm   A   P

Inquiry: (how much of the blot?) The whole thing. The claws are here, the wings here, and here are the feathers dropping off. (black?) The color of the card is black and so is the bird. (ready for fight?) It just looked like it's ready to strike with its claws out like this (gestures). (middle?) That's the body of the bird.

CARD II. 20″

1. Looks like a mouth of a person that's been hit—could have been hit and he's bleeding.

W, S   F, CF, mF   Hd

Inquiry: (black?) That's the face. (bottom D?) Dripping blood. (face or just mouth?) Mouth first then figured out it was a face. (bleeding?) Because of the color. Reminds me of with cultures—used red pencil instead of blue or black. (man or woman?) Just my personal imagination—fight between two men.

CARD II. 5″

1. These two things here—more or less animals I would say. They are, more or less, in a duel. By the time they reach this point they will have combat. I believe the loser will fall down here—through this space. There's a leg of one animal here and these are the wings. This is a cave and the loser will fall through here in cave—or the fire will eventually burn the loser. This looks like a furnace—the moment one falls it will burn the loser.

$$
W \left\{ \begin{array}{lll} D & FM & A \\ S & F & N \\ D & CF & Fire \end{array} \right.
$$

1953

1956

Inquiry: (how much?) Top here (red) is the animals more or less in a duel. The opening here into the cave with this down here being the fire. (animals?) The shape—not the color. The color was important here, though for the fire. This here makes it look like they're arguing or dueling—looks like when a person talking and there is some spray. Here is the head and the wings more or less obscuring the body. Here's the leg. (cave?) The opening here—open spot in blot. Loser will fall into fire down here. (fire?) The coloring underneath here—to burn the loser.

CARD III. 15"

1. V   Red marks remind me of the pluses doctor puts in your chart. Uses red pencil.

   D   FC   Abst

   Inquiry: Just the color.

2. V   A person with his hands like this (raises hands over head) trying to attack somebody.

   W,M   CF   H   Blood

   Inquiry: Big eyes here—just like Frankenstein. (feet?) Didn't see them. Could be blood of man he was attacking. (head, face?) No could be big goggles. (how see?) Just from waist up. (middle red?) Blood stain from injured part.

CARD III. 7"

1. Looks like two dancers here—this could be a table here—and they come together from time to time while dancing—and these could be ornaments hanging around. Here are their shoes, arms, legs. Could be females because of their big chests here and the hair—more or less, tied up.

   W, M   FK, Fc   H   P

   Inquiry: (how much?) The whole thing—the dancers here, table here, ornaments here. (dancers?) the shape—look female because of chest and hair. Hair is short style. (hair?) Yes, here—lighter in color. (table?) This is table here—shape of a round table with glass. (glass?) Yes can look through it to under part of the table. (ornaments?) Just the shape—just hung for attraction. (dancing?) The shape of the shoes and their position—could be a dancing contest.

CARD IV. 14"

1. Looks like ordinary cumulus clouds—clouds which are forerun-

CARD IV. 5"

1. This one is a—could be a black bear with legs here and arms

1953

ners of thunder—storms—black ones—eventually big rains come with lightning.

W   KF, C'F, mF   Cloud

Inquiry: Clouds are black (clouds?) Bulky. (describe?) Looks like cloud developing—this protruding part will eventually engulf this portion and build up to a big one.

CARD V. 12"

1. V The hide of an animal—a goat hanged and spread out to dry.

W   F   A obj

Inquiry: Outer covering of an animal being dried—spread out. (outer covering?) The shape (anything other than shape?) The end of other sides.

CARD VI. 11"

1. If there were ribs here this would be an X-ray. Just like an X-ray.

1956

(gestures) seems to be so mad to me though—as if it were about to frighten someone. It's sitting down on a certain—stool and it's just about ready to jump on its particular objective.

W   FM, Fc,FC'   A

Inquiry: (how much?) The whole thing—it's sitting down waiting for his enemy to come. Its shape (gestures) like a black gorilla—its whole body is expanded. (black?) Color of the card. (gorilla?) The shape and things up here like muscles—this lighter part on the neck—stands out like when the animal is mad. There are the legs here and its fur is standing up. (fur?) These fine things here are like fur (rub card). (stool?) This here—like a stool on which it would be sitting waiting to pounce on its enemy.

CARD V. 8"

1. Looks more or less like a hide of an animal stretched out—a hide exposed to the sun, on the outside, to be drying. This would be the legs of the animal, this the neck and tail.

W   Fc, m   A obj

Inquiry: (how much?) The whole thing, legs here, tail, head and neck. The head is cut into two parts here and it's stretched out to be dried. (stretched?) Just looks tight like when drying skin in sun. (skin?) It's smooth (rubs blot) like hair is flattened out—pressed flat while drying.

CARD VI. 7"

1. Another animal here. A long necked animal just like the pre-

1953

There look like some cavities there too.

W   kF   X-ray

Inquiry: Shape, neck—this is chest cavity. (anything other than shape?) No. (top D?) Didn't use that. (outer D's?) As this is developed film they can be extra portion.

CARD VII. 10″

1. Looks like clouds—cirrus type— high altitude. That's all.

W   KF, mF, Fc   Clouds

Inquiry: Decreasing from this portion spread out—will fade and be gone. (cloud?) Shape and some of the lighter coloring here.

1956

vious ones—I would say—this— well, he's just about to attack something—the ears are protruding out and so are the arms and legs—it's just about to attack too.

W   FM, Fc   A

Inquiry: (how much?) Whole thing. A long necked animal—something like the gorilla, but in a different posture—ready to engulf its enemy. It's got a spread neck, extended like a snake about to strike. (what kind of animal?) I don't know. Just a long necked animal. Doesn't have a tail; the tail could be forward. (rubs card) It has skin with spear-like fur—something like that animal—porcupine—on neck too, so if enemy comes it could snap its neck and stick it. (ears protruding?) This here, just the shape here.

CARD VII. 10″

1. This is some—like two squirrels here discussing something. Might not have come to a point yet— coming to a bad argument and looks like are ready to fight— and whoever will fall down here is the loser. Their ears are up, and ready to devour each other— I can almost hear what they're saying too.

$$W \begin{cases} D & M & (H) \\ D & F & obj \end{cases}$$

Inquiry: This part here are squirrels—like two persons yelling at each other. Their ears are up and their tails out—mad at each other. This down here looks like a platform and the loser will fall through here. The platform is locked now but will open here (gestures) and the loser will fall down from great height into

<u>1953</u>

CARD VIII. 9"

1. These two here seem to be small animals trying to climb up this stem.

    D→W   FM   A   P

I don't like the color. Red always keeps reminding me of some tragedy that could happen to me.

Inquiry: Animals climbing up a tree stem. Maybe trying to race up the tree. (animal?) Perhaps a mouse.

CARD IX. 18" (laughs)

1. Looks like spit of a tubercular person. Blood in his sputum.

    W   CF   Blood

Inquiry: Spit—blood spread out. (Rest of it?) Some cases have green sputum like this color. (Impression?) Just the color.

<u>1956</u>

nothing. (squirrels?) Only animal I could make out of it—could be rabbits though without ears up here —just seemed shape of squirrels.

CARD VIII. 12"

1. These are two animals walking over stone—colored stone; and this is, more or less, a tree that grew up through here. It looks like a contest—whoever reaches the top of the tree is the winner. They seem to be awful mad— this one wants to get the other.

$$W \begin{cases} D & FM & A & P \\ D & CF, cF & Rock \end{cases}$$

    DR   F   N

Inquiry: Whole thing. These are animals here and this is rock. This is spread of tree and this is top of tree with branches going out. (animals?) Look like animals, identical animals with legs, tail and head here. The expressions in face— mouth here where lighter color makes them look mad. It's a duel or contest to climb up tree. (kind of animal?) Those—like a mouse— rats. (tree?) Shape—top of tree here with this being spread out. (rock?) Just the way it looked. Red-colored rock with rough look in here—these light and dark spots.

CARD IX. 7"

1. These are—look like devils to me with swords here. They're fencing and there is fire here, down here. Whoever falls on side here will fall down and get burnt. The swords are closing together. This is the head of one devil here and here is the other. This looks like a big fire—or it could be blood

<u>1953</u>   <u>1956</u>

too, from one of the devils, which has flowed down into the fire.

$$W \begin{cases} D & M & (H) \\ D & F & obj \\ D & CF & Fire \end{cases}$$

Inquiry: (How much?) The whole thing—devils up here fencing—standing on this platform and the fire is down here. Looks like a big duel with the swords crossing. (devils?) They have heads like devils—terrible, confusing, terrifying—their heads are, more or less, like a mask. Here are arms and these are swords —body here and that is the platform where they're standing on and fighting. (fire?) This red—fire—and this can be blood which dripped out here on fire. The drips there make look like blood. It's running down through here, where it's lighter, and drips down here (points out drips) where it's burnt by the fire. Whoever loses will fall down through here into fire.

CARD X. 10″

1. Reminds me of a picture I've seen—under a microscope. Some germs shaped like this. (points to green)

W, D   CF, FM   Sputum

Inquiry: Picture I've seen. Showed magnified under a microscope. Sputum of TB person. This looks like germs crawling. (rest?) Just the specimen placed on the slide. Could be other germs.

CARD X. 9″

1. This is just the reaction of everyone on this ward here—nothing but confusion—animals trying to get out. Some creature confined here trying to move out, but there's an obstacle here which has to be surmounted. I don't believe this one will ever make it. (laughs) Could be me.

$$W \begin{cases} D & F & obj \\ D & M & (H) \\ D & F & (H) \\ D & F & obj \\ D & M & (H) \\ D & M & (H) \\ D & FC & obj \end{cases}$$

1953   1956

Inquiry: (How much?) Whole
thing—animals here by these red
walls. This is obstacle here. (blue)
Look at this one looking up (yellow)
and this one down here is worst of
all (green). This is like a lid on top
(grey). Here's one who made it
out (side blues)—looks real happy
with arms in all directions waving
and this one here who made it over
the wall looks happy running away
(side grey-brown). These red areas
looks like the walls—like the walls
of hell. Just one big mass of confusion—everyone wanting to get out
—but this one doesn't looks like he'll
ever make it.

Spanish Postscript

Although typically the Spanish legacy consists in a snug family and *barrio* life, supported by an intimate Church with many colorful fiestas, Manuel, a Mexican-American from Texas, enjoyed few of these treasured values. Instead of a protector-provider father, his was a deserter; instead of a warm, permissive mother, his was a social climber who "passed" for Anglo, and tried to force her son up the social ladder with her, adopting evangelical Protestantism on the way. Out of this deviant background, Manuel emerged with a confused identity and a false self concept, in which he substituted ego-alien intellectual ambitions for his deeper needs to share the values of his ingroup. After the loss of his grandmother, who served as buffer between him and his mother, the façade finally collapsed. The therapeutic problem is to help Manuel find the way back to his real self.

The Puerto Ricans, Alberto and Ramon, share with Manuel the fundamental disgrace of deserting fathers and hard, unloving mothers so uncharacteristic of the typical Spanish family. As in the case of Manuel, Alberto's status-conscious mother stimulated in him competitive striving that led to bitter disappointment when he found himself socially downgraded in New York. What was even worse for him, however, was his weak masculinity which broke down completely in homosexual panic on his entrance into the armed forces.

In Ramon's case, which paralleled Alberto's in many ways, the impoverished father image was further devalued by virtue of his being a Negro. A violent upbringing with no compensatory cultural supports developed in the boy para-noid trends with strongly masochistic features. Impulses were more directly acted out in accord with this patient's lower-class background, in contrast to the bizarre symbol-ism in which the middle-class Alberto expressed himself.

The Puerto Rican children, José and Pablo, provide an obbligato to the themes of Alberto and Ramon. Again we

find an atypical family, the father role removed by desertion in José's case, and weakened by invalidism in that of
Pablo. The subcultural pressure on these boys to exhibit a
masculinity for which they lacked training generated great
anxiety expressed in fighting with age peers and schizo-
phrenic-like withdrawal from the stronger and more fear-
some authority figures. While the prognosis is poor for the
adults who lacked the ego strength to cope with the serious
social disintegration around them, in the case of the children, the hospital seems to have gone far toward replacing
their lost ingroup so that good identities may be developed.

Filipino culture, although sharing with others of Spanish
tradition close family ingrouping, differs from them in its
greater congruence with American upward social mobility,
encouraged by the American educational system on the
Islands. Direct contact with the mainland, however, often
reveals a wide discrepancy between the *official* "equality"
ideology and *actual* minority discrimination. For Juan, this
was the major source of strain. The high socioeconomic
status he enjoyed in civilian life on his rich uncle's estate
made a shocking contrast to his naval assignment as officer's
valet. The obsessive intellectualizing defense he adopted
to control his anxiety, although more appropriate to his ego-
syntonic social strivings than the similar defense attempted
by Manuel, could not hold down the anxiety which eventually broke through in somatic illness. With good response
to counselling, the prognosis for Juan's making a realistic
adjustment is favorable.

Beneath all the diversity presented by the various forms
through which the Spanish legacy has been transmitted,
there is a common bond: the close ethnic ingrouping which
provides the member with a fundamentally sound ego that
is strong enough to integrate whatever experiences may result from contact with the main cultural stream. In cases
where the background has deviated from the typical
"Spanish" picture, the basic identity is lacking and, as a
result, the individual flounders in his attempt to find his
place in either the minority or the dominant culture.

PART V

EAST MEETS WEST

Preview

The vast differences between occidental and oriental ways of life are a source of serious culture conflict to members of those minorities trying to integrate them. The aim of Part V is to demonstrate some of the problems in which this cultural difference has played a part. In the interest of clarity it seemed advisable to remain within a single frame of reference by restricting our comparisons to only one of the oriental cultures. Because of the special problems created by World War II, the Japanese subculture was selected.

Within the Japanese-American group distinctions are made among the three generations in the United States today: *Issei, Nisei,* and *Sansei,* derived from the terms *ichi, ni,* and *san,* which, respectively, mean one, two, and three. A fourth group, the *Kibei,* or "returned," are unique. Usually eldest children of Issei rural families, they are sent to relatives in Japan for rearing and education, and are later returned to America. Differences in training and family status result in differences from both their Nisei siblings and their Issei parents.

Each of these groups of Japanese-Americans has had its own peculiar problems of acculturation. The Issei, with their Japanese upbringing, have some cultural identifications with their native land. Their conflict may be thought of as largely *external* inasmuch as they attempt to protect themselves from the inevitable inroads of the alien culture around them. This situation has resulted in much prejudice and counterprejudice.

The problems of the Nisei may be seen in general terms as involving more *inner* conflict. Like various European immigrant groups they are caught on the horns of an identification dilemma.

Of all the groups of Japanese ancestry the Kibei have the hardest time. Although they often become persons of broad cultivation and sensitivity, the identification problem is always crucial and may result in extreme social discomfort and feelings of rejection by both cultures.

In the present section we shall try to illustrate some of the salient problems faced by these groups. The first chapter presents Jiro, a young Kibei in collision with his native land on his return from Japan at the opening of international hostilities. Then there is Aki, an aging Issei struggling with an identification conflict paralleling many of the features of Jiro's problem. The third patient is a Nisei woman, whose problems in certain ways are closer to those of the first two cases than of the remaining two Nisei men. An interesting aspect of her dilemma results from sex differences in cultural pressure.

The final two chapters are clinical studies of two young Nisei men with strikingly similar problems and equally favorable outcomes. In Ichiro's case the progress of psychotherapy is mapped by the application of psychological tests at intervals throughout treatment. The other provides an opportunity to follow a detailed account of the course of psychoanalysis, in which cultural and individual factors are carefully integrated as it proceeds.

13

Cultural Dilemma of a Kibei Youth

Marvin K. Opler [1]

THE PROBLEM.   The patient, Jiro, was a Kibei male youth detained at one of the War Relocation Centers, California. In keeping with Japanese attitudes toward mental illness, he was brought after dark to the hospital by his father. For some time, Jiro had avoided his family and lived in another barracks apartment with Kibei boys who reported that his conduct had become strange. He was mute and withdrawn. While under observation in a bare hospital room, containing only a cot and chair, Jiro had attempted suicide by hanging. When helped to the cot, he rose and sat stiffly on the straight-backed chair. He remained there, with an alert and frightened look, eyes staring intently at any intruder. He refused most nourishment and ate only if left alone.

The last interview with Jiro before commitment showed him to be catatonic and rigidly controlled, but not entirely out of contact. Initial attempts at the usual handshake or bow elicited no response. When patted on the shoulder, the immobile facial muscles relaxed for a fleeting instant into the merest smile of recognition. He began to mouth the word, "Sensei," and succeeded only after difficulty to

[1] For detailed information concerning the project from which this case was taken, see E. H. Spicer, M. K. Opler, *et al., Impounded people* (Washington, D.C.: U.S. Government Printing Office, 1946).

manage the first syllable.[2] Minutes passed during which
Jiro shifted uncomfortably and stiffly in his chair. Slowly
and quietly the examiner addressed him as follows: "Jiro,
you don't have to speak now if you don't want to. What is
bothering you will pass away soon, I hope. Better feelings
will take their place. I will shake your hand, and either
write or come to see you." His face changed almost im-
perceptibly to the former look of alertness and fright and
there were no further signs of recognition. When he shook
hands, his arm seemed weak and his hands were cold and
clammy. But years later he repeated these four sentences
perfectly and added, with enthusiasm, that they had helped.

CULTURAL BACKGROUND

THE "NOTHINGEST." Jiro was twenty years old at the
time of acute onset. He had been living in a center bar-
racks-apartment with four Kibei boys for about a year.
As the center enlarged, following government policies of
segregation affecting Kibei as a class, his group moved to
the newly built ward or district known as "Manzanar." At
the time, Jiro, who seemed to evidence prodromal symptoms, explained, though not too convincingly, that he was
glad to move because he disliked being near his family in
the old ward.

In appearance, Jiro was smaller than most California
Nisei age mates. He seemed, at twenty, younger than his
years. Shy and withdrawn, he was also more self-deprecat-
ing than is demanded by good Japanese etiquette. He had
no outlets or interests and, in comparison to his four roommates, he described himself as the *nothingest.*

Jiro had returned to the United States in 1940 at the age
of fifteen, having gone through Japanese middle school.
The year following, as an adolescent still trying to get his
bearings in a strange new world, he was perplexed by the
prejudices unleashed in wartime and the social rejection

---

[2] "Sensei" for professor, any teacher or physician, in Japanese, was his
common term of address for the author.

implied by forced relocation to the centers. Living in centers from age sixteen to twenty, he confided that his horizons had shrunk to the one square mile of barracks and that his various interests had gradually diminished accordingly. His favorite phrase, complementing his own feeling of nothingness, was that here, or in the future, there was nothing. Since his feelings of hopelessness were not duplicated in hundreds of other Kibei in similar circumstances, it seemed important to pursue Jiro's story further.

FAMILY SETUP IN AMERICA.   His family was not atypical in composition. It consisted of an elderly Issei father of sixty-one years, bent on retiring as his sons came of age. His mother was a conservative Nisei woman of forty-five, obedient and compliant. Much rivalry was felt toward a brother, two years his junior, but who towered more than a head above him in height. In view of Jiro's conflict with and distaste for his family, there was allusion to this brother's becoming the future family head. A sister, three years younger than Jiro, had nothing in common with him. At the point of commitment, all family members were concerned about the blot on the family reputation since mental disturbance, like venereal disease, tuberculosis, or outcaste status, could prevent good marriages. Both Jiro's trip to the hospital at night and the general family embarrassment could be interpreted partly in this light.

At Jiro's birth, his father was forty, but his paternal grandfather had reached the official Japanese age of retirement, sixty-one. Birth was attended by the customary registry of his name in family records abroad, along with solemn agreement, after the letter of announcement, to send him abroad for education to the grandparental home following his weaning. This custom was viewed as an act of filial duty of sons who could not themselves return to lighten parental burdens or hasten their actual retirement. Accordingly, two years later in the company of a paternal aunt, Jiro traveled abroad. His mother, to impress her father-in-law's ménage, saw to it that he was toilet trained after a fashion and weaned by the end of the first year. She reported that he walked before a year and a half. As to her own feelings in the matter, they were expressed as follows: "After marriage, a wife no longer belongs to any family but her husband's; when I was married, the white wedding dress was our color of mourning—of leaving our family behind."

Jiro's father had come to Sacramento Valley at thirty years of age. His pioneering history was a typical one. He hired out as a farm laborer after failing to get steady work in San Francisco. Farming was his métier, but he found the methods quite unlike those of the family farm outside of Hiroshima. In both instances the land seemed poor, but the rocky, tree-stump hillsides of the valley were more untamed. A first assignment—to plow a contoured hillside—found him coaching the horse the night before to familiarize both man and beast with the task. The story of the tired horse, sweaty and spuming foam, was exchanged good-humoredly with other exiled farm hands, but his father was dedicated to sobriety and hard work. Lacking a citizen's right to own land, he had worked his way tirelessly as tenant, removing the stumps and boulders in the pioneer days of this fruit orchard country. He married soberly at forty, after nine years of sweat and toil, picking a daughter of the small Japanese-American community duly selected by the *baishakunin,* or go-betweens, of his own and a neighboring family.

The couple, quite disparate in age, hardly knew each other. Jiro's mother was a hard-working and dutiful daughter whose elder sister had yielded a son to her parents by *yoshi*-marriage [3] two years before. This son-in-law's adoption led to his taking the in-laws' surname, and made this second nubile daughter somewhat superfluous. She had done a man's work on the farm, consistently being eclipsed by her sister. Gaunt and appearing older than her age, anyone would have taken her to be the Issei wife of an Issei husband. In the center, freed for once of her daily labors,

---

[3] Yoshi-marriages among Japanese occur where a couple without male offspring adopt a husband for their daughter, calling him "son," bestowing their family name on him, and making him legal inheritor.

she spoke Japanese almost exclusively, visited her available relatives, and attended classes in flower arrangement, tea ceremony, dressmaking, and the functions of the Buddhist Church. Her Nisei children, quite the opposite, were versed in California slang and before segregation wore the saddle shoes, bobby socks, *yogore* (slang for *pachuco* or zoot-suit) costumes of typical West Coast Nisei. Somewhere in this intergeneration conflict and in the confusion of relocation and its aftermath, Jiro's homecoming was lost.

Both parents agreed that the artificialities of center life estranged the generations. Their conservatism, however, increased as their former tenancy holdings were wiped out, along with other tangible property, by relocation and enforced segregation from the mainstream of American life. They learned the small farm had gone to other tenants and deteriorated beyond repair. As economic, political, and social securities slipped away, they clung to their last vestige of respect—a cultural identity. An enlargement of the father's photograph had gone into one of the five suitcases brought to the center. This was bowed to before and after school and, now, upon leaving the barracks or on return. The mother referred to her husband as *anata*, spouse or lord, and never by name. The father's generally sober nature turned dour and tyrannical with his fears of the future. In the rifts between Issei and Kibei occurring generally in the center, his anger exploded on Jiro. Despite a life of unremitting labor, he had now reached the age of retirement only to see his efforts brought to nothing. The *nothing* was repeated, even if the thin barracks' walls and limited privacy allowed little else to be said. With Jiro he would insist on the ultimate respect demanded by filial piety, even as he had insisted before in sending the boy to his own father in Japan.

For this family, there was no way out of the segregation center. Although Jiro had, in fact, returned to this country at age fifteen because dual citizenship made him eligible for future Japanese military draft, American policy labeled him Kibei and, hence, suspect. Were he older at the time of relocation, better versed in American ways and language, or eligible for service, he might have found his way out. In his own conception, the decade and a half from 1925 to 1940 had made Japan itself brutally harsh and military, but here in the United States he was just as much a citizen without a country. To political insecurities were added pervasive psychological insecurities.

FAMILY SETUP IN JAPAN. Jiro's Hiroshima-ken grandparents were delighted, in principle, to receive a two-year-old grandson, but the grandfather was by this time sixty-three and had suffered financial reverses. The grandmother was sickly. To add to the inauspiciousness of the moment, anti-American feeling ran high, particularly in Hiroshima, due to our Japanese Exclusion Laws. To cap it all, Jiro himself was violently ill on the voyage and remained so for two months afterwards. The family reports "stomach trouble" with violent retching and vomiting. According to the aunt's account, her trip also was made difficult and it was difficult to welcome Jiro to his new home.

EARLY EVENTS IN JAPAN. Both Jiro and the family were able to piece together subsequent events. The grandmother's illness went from bad to worse, and she died when Jiro was in his fourth year. Hushed rumors in the household mentioned tuberculosis. In Japan, venereal, tubercular, or mental illnesses, are, like former outcaste or *eta* family origins, topics not to be discussed in polite society. Any one of these dread diseases is enough to prevent a good marriage and is searched for by the diligent *baishakunin.* Jiro long remembered the rumors and the threat they aroused. He recalled the lowered voices and polite circumlocutions used. Years later, when his grandfather spoke bitterly of Jiro's adding more than the grandmother could bear, he felt the whole weight of impossible obligations heaped upon himself and merged with terrifying scenes of his grandmother's coughing and grasping her sides. The sense of feeling worthless and lonely, of having done wrong, again took root, and he experienced a helpless sense of embarrassment and the wish to be sent away. He reported memories from before school age of a widowed aunt helping with his care and of his being carried astride her back to and from work. In the early school period, the austere image of the grandfather again intervenes, along with the harsh stiffness of the teachers. There were shameful episodes of enuresis, rare in Japanese schools. Three years before Jiro's return to the United States the grandfather died, and he recalls his sense of relief as he went to live with the widowed aunt while completing his education.

EARLY SYMPTOMS

SEXUAL FEARS.   Sexual interest was recalled as beginning and ending abruptly during this period of flight from patriarchal authority. Masturbation was denied throughout. Intersex bathing in the large wooden tubs of hot water, used for soaking in the evening, is described for more than one farmhouse. At one, contiguous to his aunt's, there were fantasies and daydreams concerning a female cousin. Besides the semipublic bathing, household nudity was common. Much of this evolved into private sexual guilt if not shame. Because of the circumlocutions in his grandfather's household concerning tuberculosis, venereal disease, and kindred matters, he was fearful of prostitutes.

At one gathering, the more elderly ladies became drunk and ribald. One of them, the most boisterous, spirited Jiro outside. She weighed more than he and, in her state of agility, she threw him on the ground calling him little boy, a term reminiscent of his grandmother's call. She attempted to have intercourse, but he was overwhelmed with shame and disgust. Having visited dubious restaurants in Hiroshima City with his grandfather, he recalled the raw, direct, and gaudy pornography at which he had stolen furtive glances, the scenes on cups and dishes and wall drawings. The net result was to increase his revulsion and distaste, whereupon the last raucous laugh of the elderly lady was left ringing in his ears. Comparing notes with others of his age, he imagined he had become impotent. Refusal to visit the city for the purpose of going to a house of prostitution lost him his best friend soon after.

INFERIORITY FEELING. Accounts of early memories concerning symptomatic items are sketchy in the extreme. Much of this Jiro later helped to assemble. He recalled a stomach disorder, with violent retching, for several days following the incident with the elderly lady. Earlier fantasies and daydreams concerning the female cousin do not appear to be significant symptomatological clues. Throughout his most commonplace accounts of events, however, his sense of inferiority, in households, sports, or school, is a consistent thread. He felt weak and insecure, small and insignificant or, at times, helpless and afraid. In school, the parading of the amazing deeds of patriots and historical figures convinced him, "I shall never be a man like these." Revenge stories of the Forty-Seven *Ronin* or Masterless Retainers, who after years of waiting conspired to wipe out shame visited upon their Lord, inspired him with terror. Japanese movies with the same themes of vendetta or revenge, which form an equivalent of American westerns, upset him. The more fantastic ones of marvelous magicians and transformers left him soothed and satisfied.

RETURN TO THE UNITED STATES

FACT AND FANCY ABOUT HOMECOMING. Strangely enough, Jiro's social and personal history took a turn for the worse as he re-entered the land of his birth. On the surface, homecoming should be auspicious for the eldest son of an Issei father and a conservative Nisei mother, particularly where he is conversant and moderately well educated in things Japanese. But just as Jiro had been *persona non grata* in the decade of the Twenties in Japan, following our Exclusion Laws, so in the wartime Forties in America he found himself an unwelcome citizen. While he arrived on these shores in a time of uneasy peace, his family, especially his siblings, had changed during the dozen years of his absence to the point where they no longer resembled the Japan that he knew.

From the viewpoint of his own insecurities, Jiro could hardly make the accommodation quickly. He had always been jealous of friends abroad who enjoyed the pleasant pampering of their own families, and he had been almost distrustful of their tolerance for his awkward, shy manners. Homecoming had long been viewed with intangible yearnings, with fancies that Japanese education would count for much among the Japanese-Americans of the United States, both young and old. He hoped that his status as first-born son would insure him immediate prestige in his own home. A sister of the same age as the erstwhile female cousin would have her circle of schoolgirl friends. And in this Japanese-American oasis, far from the "White" gangster males and loosely disciplined, immodest females who peopled the America of prewar Japanese propaganda, Jiro felt he could regain his human dignity.

The *dramatis personae* of these homecoming fantasies had been built up for some time in the haze of social distance. His father was well along in years and, like his dead grandfather, figured vaguely. His mother, much younger, was cast in the role of the vivacious paternal aunt. Instead, he was greeted by a sombre and exacting father, by a mother who seemed as worn and exhausted as his grandmother had been, and by other relatives who seemed distant and meant nothing. A brother of thirteen and his highly Americanized friends towered above Jiro. His sister's clique of sophisticated schoolgirls, obviously critical of his speech and manners, unnerved him. In general, the Nisei, with their smattering of Japanese and their even more incomprehensible Japanese-American slang, were different from all expectations. Both his English and his parents' Japanese, with archaic terms and curious additions, seemed untranslatable.

HOSTILITY TOWARD FATHER AND BROTHER. At first, the Nisei, within and outside his family, were the target of his well-controlled hostility. Their preferences in clothes and food were different. They danced, the sexes together, in athletic gyrations which seemed to him undignified or immodest. While his mother adopted the shuffling female gait of Issei women (toes inward and hunched-over shoulders), he himself seemed to walk more stiffly, in his rapid, mincing step, than either brother or father. Already shy and self-conscious, all speech, gait, and gesture seemed awkward or inappropriate. In Japan, where fixity of etiquette and polite consideration for the feelings of others constantly sanctioned even the most commonplace behavior, here such reassurances were strangely wanting. So fully occupied were his own siblings in their adolescent groups, that the first day home he walked three miles to speak with another Kibei and, as he put it, felt all alone.

In time, however, his father proved the greatest disappointment. Reared to respect age and paternity, it was hard to discover in himself the true nature of these feelings. Many Issei who came to this country in the early waves of immigration, before Exclusion, were disgruntled second sons who could never inherit in impoverished Japanese families. So it was with Jiro's father. Arriving in this country long past youth, penniless, unmarried, and with no trade but farming, he had toiled and sacrificed to attain marital status and patriarchal dignity. Jiro regarded his mother's lack of information about modern Japan as pitiable, but his gruff father also struck him as being hopelessly behind the times. He felt that his own status as first-born son was not honored by a father who had himself been "a second son." He resented his brother, Ichiro, for his very name since that name meant *eldest son*. It was as if he, Jiro, was written off as dead and sent to Japan at his brother's birth. In Japan, there is a phrase, "A brother is a beginning of a stranger." Jiro felt this rivalry in every way possible, and it was linked with even greater dislike for a remote and distant father who, in poor times, had hoped his eldest son would somehow make his way in Japan. That it was not customary to name a second son "Ichiro" was part and parcel of the many barbarisms of the household, for which he secretly blamed his father. He felt that his father had awakened too late to the thought that the future of his united family lay in America. Now this father, like the grandfather before, viewed him as a burden.

Since the age of fifteen is less confused and more focused than four, all hostilities toward the irritable grandfather that had been dissipated in infantile helplessness were mobilized in new form. He was estranged from brother and father. Later, in the center, as the Issei-Kibei rifts widened, the father was blamed in a variety of ways. When the family future in remote Northern California seemed a thing of the past, Jiro would ask, "Why did you bring me back? To rot in a concentration camp?" Or taunt, "Now I suppose your Ichiro will grow up to hold land in America!" The theme was disillusionment, insecurity, and hopelessness.

Because Ichiro knew American ways, because he could hold land when of age or help in dealings with the surrounding community, the father looked to him as a mainstay. On countless occasions, Jiro would be called almost absent-mindedly to do some task and then dismissed with reminders that he could not accomplish that particular job. In the primogeniture system, sibling rivalries are bound to ensue; but where every family decision and most tasks hinge upon the abandonment of this rule, the normal tensions are exacerbated. A father of retirement age increases this potential. Where he is indecisive or confused about his own family's future, there is no mitigating set of sanctions anywhere in Japanese culture. Here, indeed, the father insisted on sole and continuing authority with sons who had not yet come of age. But in this family, uprooted and at bay in wartime relocation, the father clung to authority at the risk of reducing Jiro to helpless ineffectuality. And so the clock was turned back to the same helpless fears that marked childhood in Japan. Jiro described this quite well. Before the center period, there were recurrences of childish nightmares, night sweats, sleeplessness, and terrified awakenings.

ESTRANGEMENT FROM SISTER AND PEERS. During the same period, "A brother is the beginning of a stranger" applied to his relations with his sister. In Japanese custom, an elder

brother, of age, may regulate a sister's conduct to unusual
lengths. He may sanction or prevent her marriage, and,
until she moves to her husband's household, he is, like his
father before him, the custodian of her morals and protector
of a family's good name. With his sister of the soda-drink-
ing, bobby-sox set, Jiro was at once the stranger in quite
another sense. Ichiro's friends were greatly preferred. In
the sister's presence or with such groups, Jiro found himself more than usually inarticulate. Between being tongue-
tied in public, and issuing peremptory commands to her in
the household, Jiro felt more and more that their relationship was untenable. The sister, in turn, like others of her
group, was either amused or frightened by the gruff manners and curt address of the Kibei. He avoided the school
or country church dances in part because dancing was
strange to him, but even more so because Nisei added to
his feelings of fright and estrangement.

Some of these feelings, in the peer group, were not due
to empty fear and embarrassment. Like other Kibei, Jiro
overheard discussions of himself and others of the Kibei
class. He was doubly resentful that these young people, so
sure of themselves, did not even know the many rules for
preventing face-to-face embarrassment, minimizing shame
in others. These girls, who knew other rules, who rose as
if at a signal to dance with boys, and whose sense of pro-
priety was fixed less by family than by gossip and rumor,
succeeded in adding to his anger and resentment. In the
same context, he disliked the lordly Issei all the more for
prattling about old-fashioned ways while they controlled
none of these changes. It seemed that the upstart Nisei escaped family surveillance even more than his kind who
were expected, in passive solidarity, to differ from the majority of the younger generation.

These girls and women of his mother's generation, Issei
picture brides or Nisei, were separated by a deep gulf. The
older generation was passively the property of their husbands. Dressed in shapeless calico, dutiful daughter types
were not like the younger generation. He missed the type,

well-known in Japan, who through intelligence or connivance almost ran the home from behind the scenes. Or else the family solidarity, down through generations, seemed lacking. Whatever it was, few older women seemed capable of the dignity or even of the ribaldry and abandon he remembered from earlier years. His mother, sickly and worn, he saw only as a pale and helpless reflection of paternal authority. She appeared colorless, imitative, and, like himself, passively dutiful. He even felt that, in these qualities, he took after her. At any rate, going full circle in his family group, Jiro found no solid attachment. He was thrown back upon his own sense of loneliness and ineffectuality.

During the year before relocation, these attitudes crystallized rapidly. Morose at home, he found companionship only with a few scattered Kibei acquaintances. He avoided sports, like the ubiquitous baseball (*basu-boru*). Intersexual contacts were absent. Speech and manner became, if anything, more awkward and constricted. Energy went into suppressing anger and controlling the tongue. Private rages found him tearing away handfuls of leaves and grass or biting his fingers. He became restless and, he thought, quite different from other Japanese, always trained for poise and patience. The Nisei California slang contained a characteristic phrase, "waste-time," for anything useless. He thought of the phrase constantly as he deliberately wasted time on lonely, aimless walks. Angrily he thought, "Where are the Nisei, with their bad manners, hurrying to? Where are *they* going?"

THE UPROOTING OF RELOCATION

MOUNTING TENSION. The answer came abruptly after Pearl Harbor. With the first events, he was momentarily glad of American citizenship, of avoidance of further training abroad. For once he understood briefly the Americanized Nisei who were flocking toward enlistment. However, they were rejected on obvious grounds of prejudice. As this happened repeatedly, his sarcasm grew, along with a sardonic sense of their being, after all, somewhat like himself—with no roots anywhere.

Soon, however, he realized what was really happening. Families, by Western Defense Command dogma and decree, were uprooted and herded en masse into such Assembly Centers as the converted stables at Santa Anita and Tanforan race tracks. From there, the trek to hastily constructed and half-finished centers seemed like a bad dream. Faced with bare barracks and a few army cots and potbellied stoves, with pine knotholes gaping into neighbors' rooms, anger and helplessness became endemic and diffused. In some families, fathers were interned elsewhere. In any case, families were literally thrown together. Privacy was minimal. Mass feeding at twenty cents a day per capita began. The Nisei took over center work at $12, $16, and $19 per month, the last restricted to technical or professional services. At first, there was not enough resurgence of things Japanese for most Kibei to function. As a group, their common resentments grew. Many insisted, as Jiro also felt, that Issei blind compliance and the Nisei knuckling-under was the wrong way, and that, first and foremost, citizenship rights should be restored.

MOTHER'S ILLNESS. In the general and hasty exodus from the valley the mother became ill, and only months later, in the center, did she recover. Jiro felt in his mother's illness and long convalescence the same pangs of shame and undercurrents of rejection and helplessness that attended his grandmother's death earlier. From the coughing, he was afraid that tuberculosis was involved, and here in center conditions, this was not something which would remain a private family affair. Even without a hospital diagnosis of tuberculosis in the family, the fear continued. With no privacy, the merest dispute with his father now declined into a silently endured paternal lecture in a barracks room apartment where the neighbors on each side could hear all. The custom grew in the center, particularly during loyalty registration, for Kibei boys to room together for self-protection. At first, he and the four Kibei friends took up their separate living quarters in the same ward as his parents—known as "Sacramento" district. It was later, during the transformation of the center into a segregation camp, that the group moved to the "Manzanar" ward of the project.

BREAK WITH FAMILY.   Many center events are interwoven with Jiro's final break with his father and family. Loyalty registration was incorrectly presented to the center residents as an army draft of the loyal. With some families still disunited, and all resentful of the sudden forced relocation of all men, women, and children, rumor and confusion beset the center. An Issei committee, sensing this, requested time for the program to be presented accurately in both Japanese and English to all the population. They even offered to conduct the governmental education plan. This suggestion the project director refused. Kibei were categorically blamed for the confusions which further ensued, since some Kibei had requested careful elucidation of the program. Their bachelor quarters were searched in the center. Not until Issei and Nisei leaders were browbeaten and beaten literally did the program of a few days get underway. Even then, it dragged on amid confusions for several months. A modicum of real peace was never fully restored at the center.

Community analysis was instituted shortly after the height of difficulties, and it was then that we met Jiro and his roommates. If not Jiro himself, then his circle, had made attempts to control hotheads in the center. His family felt hopeless about the center as well as the future; and they were in that part of resident population which had adopted a *shikatiganai* (a hopeless and fateful "it-can't-be-helped") attitude. They had, at first, recoiled from the center turbulence, hoping to register loyalty when the confusion died down. It never did, whereupon they hoped to hold together as a family—the last remaining security. In this interim, not only were Japanese-American Citizens League leaders beaten, but Kibei bachelor quarters became storm centers of the general turbulence.

One event stands out in Jiro's mind as a measure of his inadequacy during this period. His small group, like many of the "Sacramento" ward, was rumored to have registered loyalty already. Another Kibei group of *judo* and *sumo* (wrestling) experts decided to pay a serious call. Jiro's judoist friend was absent at the time or matters might have gone differently. Instead, Jiro was alone when he saw the visitors approach, and he quickly hid himself under a cot and barricaded himself with blankets. He was, of course, found and, being unable to talk from fright, he was beaten for no good reason at all. The quarters were ransacked. Since word passes quickly in a center, his friends soon reappeared and saw the chaos. In subsequent weeks, his group circulated throughout the ward, explaining intricacies of registration to confused rural people. Jiro did not. By the time the center had cooled down, the joking sobriquet his friends had given him was widespread. The words implied "at home, but at the same time not there." When able, he registered affirmatively to loyalty, but with the popular Kibei qualification, "if my citizenship rights are restored." His brother, Ichiro, registered a simple "Yes." In the further confusions of segregation time, his brother and sister were eligible to move to another center. But Jiro and his friends were blocked by Kibei status, and his own case was doubly confused by the qualified answer.

SEGREGATION AND EMOTIONAL ISOLATION. Before segregation and the second family separation, Jiro and his friends moved to the "Manzanar" ward of the project. His resentment of his father's inability to carry him through relocation outside center confines grew apace. Segregation which brought endless factions of Kibei from all the centers estranged him even from this category of persons. By now, he was by no means the most popular member of his small group of five. Their various sustaining interests in art, literature, or Japanese sports had left him far behind. At this point, without family and with only attenuated friendships left, we note a rapid crystallization of symptoms. He became lazy and slovenly in habits. His restlessness at night was noted, and he would fall asleep over a Japanese book in the daytime. His literary choices became more and more juvenile, with badly written collections of fairy tales and myths prominent. In comparison with his earlier tastes, there was greater tolerance of stories about vendetta and revenge.

The altercations with his father, on brief visits before their departure from the center, gradually died down. The family noted that he was becoming morose and distant. As the time for departure approached, they appealed for the right to take Jiro with them. His status was clouded as a Kibei as well as by the first qualified answer on citizenship rights. No Kibei in such status could go elsewhere. In Jiro's description, the fences closed in on him and fear took over.

Before departure, his father arranged to bring him to the hospital for observation, as his friends had obligingly and politely suggested. The father did so with a finally hopeless, passive, and mutely compliant Jiro in his wake. Lacking center facilities in this barracks town of almost twenty thousand people, even rudimentary therapeutic approaches to mental illness were reduced to the phrase, "for observation purposes." The choice of site for this purpose could only be in a private ward of a distinctly overcrowded community hospital on center grounds. There was enacted the scene with which this chapter opened.

THE OUTCOME

BREAK WITH REALITY.   Psychiatric examination disclosed that Jiro was confused, depressed, frightened, and inwardly hostile. When not mute, he referred to officialdom in uncomplimentary terms. He refused to answer personal questions. He was frightened enough to appear entirely tongue-tied, but a few phrases and syllables could be uttered here and there. Following family departure, he became completely mute. With the targets of primary hostility now hundreds of miles away, an awkward suicidal attempt quietly transpired.

There were no hallucinations reportable then or in later hospitalization. In the hospital, after two months of practically no speech—a few phrases in a week's period—Jiro could become voluble when he chose. His own account indicates that he was affectively confused, but at times afraid of being laughed at: "my words would not have made much sense anyway." A lack of confidence, a certainty of being confused and ineffective, and feelings of strangeness and isolation mark his accounts for this period.

Concerning periods when communication was better established, Jiro recalls suddenly occurring needs to talk with someone or to hear from someone. There was, at such times of breaking through, the feeling that if contact did not occur, everything would become worse and again be unbearable. Generally stiff and awkward, even by Kibei standards, there was evidence of greater rigidity and inability to relax in the period of illness. Besides shyness and lack of spontaneity, a major ingredient of the rigidity was an attempt to control a flood of hostile impulses, along with a fear that they were becoming, in fact, uncontrollable.

In one discussion, Jiro remembered the helpless rage that boiled up to the surface. It was at this point that he recalled the tearing at grass and leaves, the jealousy of siblings, and the anger at father and grandfather "for trying to get rid of me." The rages were everywhere aimed at events as well as attributed to feelings about people. "I was angry that my grandmother died, or that my mother was sick when I needed help." In the center one could add the massive angers attached to whole categories of persons. There were the Issei, even beyond the father image, lacking in wise and omnipotent guidance. There were the Nisei pre-empting the attractive roles of center life. There were the adolescents and post-adolescents with their studied rejection. Or, finally, there were the family members as a group, seen in vivid terms of separation, lack of real welcome, and final departure. Certainly, the years abroad had robbed him of more than citizenship. Together with the jarring experiences of relocation and the political embroilments of the center, he had become, like many Kibei, the doubly rejected.

CULTURE CONFLICT AND PERSONAL STRESS. It is interesting to speculate as to whether balances in this family, the actual roles influenced by culture conflict, would have reached some equilibrium had not relocation and the swift march of wartime events intervened. Ultimately, under center conditions, this situation was not merely the introducing of new strains into family structure, but the literal tearing apart of a cohesive pattern. As the center continued, and as segregation was heaped upon the inequities of relocation, more people became mentally ill, and a disproportionate number of these were Kibei. Moreover, Jiro's case does not stand alone. Others like him had periods of acute onset at times when center stresses were at their height and equally dramatic recoveries in hospitals outside center confines. Under hospitalization, Jiro himself indicated that the stresses which had magnified family conflicts into large-scale cultural conflicts disappeared in his attitudes and feelings in but a few months. A therapist could become like a different species of "father," serene, untroubled, and supportive. Staff were, in certain persons, likened to "the family I never had." For a time, other patients were frightening, but later, as in Buddhist tenets, one learns "to help one another."

RELIEF AND RESTITUTION. A final visit to Jiro following remission, and in connection with later field work, disclosed that other Kibei and relocation center acquaintances were friendly to him despite his hospitalization. The old communities were re-establishing in California. Several had revived in the valley, and now, for once, there was a sense of common experiences, ineradicable, of former center life. Center Kibei who were younger, like his former roommate, were again selected as friends, no doubt because one could compete somewhat more successfully with them or at least tolerate comparisons. With time, it was recognized that not all Kibei are fallen stars and not all of life an endless series of disappointments.

Remission had come rapidly in Jiro's case. The six months of hospitalization were calmer than the four years of relocation history. The great wave of Kibei immigration before the war had contained few with as much repetitive and traumatic experiences as Jiro. He was now ready to call it bad luck, rather than helpless and hopeless fears. Since the family, in turn, can now plan without being held in official duress, they are fully aware of pitfalls in his fears of rejection, his awkward shyness, and his rigid controls of impulse. They have responded to his quest for equal rights, not only in citizenship, but in achievement and recognition. A whole second generation is now coming into its own, and the first generation, while nostalgic, is today more gracefully accepting the shift in authority and responsibility.

Projective data by test instruments were unavailable at the time of Jiro's acute illness, and his remission was almost too rapid to come within hospital testing programs. As one would guess, he showed a rather weak ego integration with a good deal of compensatory fantasy and concern about impulse control. Those traits have vastly diminished, and Jiro lives today in his family setting in which all members have learned much about their cultural identities, their changing pattern, and their need for cohesiveness. While no symptomatology is markedly in evidence in Jiro or in others of the family, the father's authoritarian attitudes, buttressed by older Japanese standards, were hard to soften in his own deprived existence. In this cultural group, the second generation, youthful at the time of World War II, has now taken firm root. With the passage of years, the mother's hypochondriacal defenses and "crisis illnesses" are gone. In this family, as in any other, we see how the illness of one affects the health of each member. In the group, uprooted by relocation, we discern the marks of overwhelming stress. But the Japanese family is ideally built for unified solidity over generations. A second generation, unmolested and given time, can put down roots deep in American soil.

14

An Aging Issei Anticipates Rejection

Trent E. Bessent

COMMITMENT

THE PATIENT'S STORY. The patient, Aki, a fifty-seven-year-old married Japanese, arrived at a State Hospital in the spring of 1956. Previous to his commitment he was described as seclusive and withdrawn, but pleasant and cooperative when interviewed. He admitted hearing voices but was unable to tell what they said. His affect was considered to be flat.

When admitted to the State Hospital he readily reported that he had thought somebody had been following him for the past three years and that he was getting into trouble for not paying enough federal income tax. He said, "Sometimes I have had feeling, someone gonna kill me or I'm gonna die. I don't want to kill myself. I'm afraid to die because I have children, all small children." Before coming to the hospital he said he drank one or two cups of *sake* every night "which might have been too much for me" and under its influence "I might have threatened to kill my wife." He thought he might have a "little head or mental trouble." He appeared to be preoccupied and absorbed in his inner thoughts and would sit and stare during the interview and on the ward. He did not volunteer information, but would answer questions readily.

In the opinion of the interviewing psychiatrist the patient's thoughts were not disorganized, intellectual faculties

317

were preserved, some insight was present but his affect was dull. Physical examination was essentially negative except for a cyst on his forehead and severe malnutrition. The patient had been losing weight for the six months prior to hospitalization. The presence of symptoms of agitation and depression, along with delusional ideation, led to the final psychiatric diagnosis of involutional psychotic reaction, paranoid type.

BACKGROUND

IN JAPAN. Through interviews with Aki and his wife it was learned that the patient had been born in Japan in 1899 as the second child in his family. At his birth, there was one older brother in the family. His parents reportedly got along well with each other, were both Japanese, raised in "similar environments." His mother was approximately twenty-three at his birth and his father about twenty-five. Both parents were considered to have had an "average" education for that period.

Aki's father and mother jointly operated a small tobacco stand and lived in an urban area. He described them as "nice parents," but was unable to specify their characteristics further. In discussing his father he said, "My father drank too much 'sake,' I was told, but can not remember. I was small." Regarding his mother he said, "Mother is nice; she did not drink." He did recall that she never spanked him, but disciplined him by talking to him or just "looking" at him. While being disciplined he held his head downward to avoid seeing his mother's face. He vaguely remembered his paternal grandfather as a man not averse to drinking. He recalled that as a family they were very poor and lived under crowded conditions. He was raised in the Buddhist religion, but has never been actively religious.

After his birth, four additional siblings were born, two brothers and two sisters. When the boy was about three years of age his mother sent him to live in a foster home because of her difficulty in "handling six children together." The other children remained with the mother. The patient was unable to describe his experience in the foster home and could not remember the events leading up to his having been sent there. He did recall returning to live at his mother's home when he was about seven years of age, but he was unable to give any detailed description of his life at that time. The child attended grammar school in Japan and reportedly "got along fair." During this period his father traveled to the United States and worked in California. When the patient was about twelve years of age his father returned to his family in Japan.

IN THE UNITED STATES. After a short visit in Japan his father again returned to the United States taking Aki, now about thirteen years of age, with him. The boy lived with his father in California for a short period. While attending school, he obtained employment as a house boy, doing kitchen work and house cleaning. He continued school for about two years in California, after which he began full-time employment.

His father returned to his family in Japan, but the patient remained in California by himself. During his adolescent and young adult years Aki worked in homes, on farms, in lumber camps, and in the produce market. He lived, worked and traveled by himself or occasionally with three or four other single Japanese men.

FAMILY RELATIONSHIPS. The patient was regarded as a "devoted son" sending "valuable gifts" to his parents and siblings, all of whom continued to live in Japan. As his savings allowed, he made several trips to Japan to visit his family but always returned to the West Coast of the United States. During his last visit in 1939-40 his father died of a "stomach ailment." His mother, who is now over eighty, continues to live in Japan. One of his brothers is "an alcoholic"; another, a doctor. Except for excessive smoking the patient's habits have always been moderate and he has spent most of his life working hard.

MARRIED LIFE

MARRIAGE ARRANGEMENTS. As a young man, Aki did not marry since he regarded himself as "too poor to support a wife." His sexual activity had been limited, coitus occurring initially at about age twenty-eight and at infrequent intervals thereafter. Before his father's death, however, arrangements were made for his marriage, which was performed according to Buddhist rites when he was forty-one years old. His wife, fifteen years his junior, had been born in the United States, but had gone back to Japan with her family while still a child. The newly married couple came to the United States in 1941. Because of her American birth, his wife returned as an American citizen under her maiden name, and they were remarried in a civil ceremony.

RELOCATION AND REVERSES. Shortly after their marriage his wife became ill with a fever contracted during the trip and their plans for starting a small produce market were blocked. Later they purchased property in his wife's name, but before they could establish themselves Japan entered World War II and they were sent to a Japanese relocation camp. While at the camp, their first three daughters were born, now aged fourteen, thirteen, and eleven. His wife was described as a very "devout mother," understanding and faithful.

Aki and his family left the internment camp in September, 1945 and returned to a California city. They met considerable resistance and hostility from the community, but were able to live in one room of a house owned by a Japanese family. Eventually they purchased an old house in his wife's name, located in an area of the city predominantly occupied by Negro families, several Mexican families, and a sparse distribution of Japanese families. The patient said that he felt hurt by the rejection from the people in the city, but realized that they were still angry because of the war so he "did not hold it against them." Two years after leaving the camp, his first son, now aged nine, was born.

REACTIONS TO SOCIAL STRESS

MARITAL FEARS.   During the period shortly after the son's birth the patient first began to fear that his wife might separate from him. A friend of his wife's had divorced her husband and the patient felt that his wife might do likewise. He was told that his wife would not divorce him because of the children, so he believed that his wife remained "only because of the children." Although he loved his wife, he was unable to tell her so. He worked hard during the day as a self-employed gardener and was tired by evening, so there was little conversation or activity between the patient and his wife. He never talked with his wife about his early experiences.

SOCIAL WITHDRAWAL.   A family friend described Aki as "very devoted to his immediate family." He did not participate in social life, had no specific hobby, and his chief interest was the welfare of his wife and children. On his days off from work his primary concern was with the upkeep of his working equipment, such as power mowers, edgers, and other gardening tools. He complained of headaches about once a week, but took no medication. In describing himself, the patient said that he had developed the "habit" of never speaking up on his own behalf. If he did not understand something his wife or anyone else said, he would never ask a question. He tended to take "gossip" as the truth, found it difficult to make a decision, and frequently felt confused in relations with people. He did not like arguments. He expressed concern because his adolescent daughters were openly critical of him.

His wife described him as "quick tempered," but added that "he gets over it quickly." The patient had planned to apply for United States citizenship, but had continually put off making the initial application. His knowledge about United States government and history came from his children's homework exercises. He expressed a strong desire for his children to have a good education so they could get ahead. Spending money on others rather than on himself, he tried to help anyone who came to him for assistance.

PERSECUTORY IDEAS. Approximately three years prior to his hospitalization he became anxious lest his federal income tax return, which had been filed by his attorney, was an incorrect account of his earnings. He began to fear that all his possessions would be confiscated and that his immediate family would be left to starve. His delusions included ideas that the "Gestapo" were following him and members of his family. He became extremely sensitive to the attitudes of people who employed him to do yard work, and if they were critical or not friendly he would quit his job.

Aki's fears and suspicions became progressively worse, and prior to hospitalization he talked constantly of the FBI being after him. He was suspicious of everyone, believing that the telephone had been tapped, that the house was wired, and that he was watched and spied upon twenty-four hours a day. He would awaken in the middle of the night convinced that a car driving by was after him. He talked of suicide, threatening to buy poison and kill himself. He reported a vivid dream in which his mother was sick and crying for him and saying, "I want to see you, I want to see you." It was his opinion that his wife had boy friends, and under the influence of alcohol he threatened to kill her and their children as well as himself. When he developed the notion that he and his wife had not been married legally or that she had obtained a divorce, he was admitted to the County Hospital and subsequently committed to the State Hospital.

HOSPITALIZATION

THERAPEUTIC PROGRESS. After the patient's arrival at the State Hospital he was given the tranquilizing drug "Sparine" for a brief period. His agitation was reduced, but his depression persisted. He appeared to be sufficiently intact, however, to benefit from industrial therapy and was accordingly placed on the gardening detail. By late spring he was working regularly and going to recreation. His delusional ideas regarding the federal government had been reduced and he appeared less suspicious.

In the late spring he voluntarily asked to join the psychotherapy group on his ward in order to "straighten out a few things on my mind." He attended the group regularly, and although he appeared interested, he remained essentially quiet. He expressed the view that hearing the problems experienced by other members present helped him to change some of his opinions. Ego strengthening, rather than uncovering, was the goal in the group psychotherapy. The majority of the patients in the group had experienced or were experiencing paranoid symptoms.

The delusional ideas which persisted involved the thoughts that he and his wife were not legally married, that she had other men friends, and that she had divorced him or would leave him shortly. Meanwhile his wife had obtained employment and the family had been getting along well without him. His wife visited him regularly on week ends and attempted to reassure him that they were married and that she did not plan to leave him. On July 30th the patient had the idea that he and his wife would be married again. He reasoned that he had lived with his wife fifteen years and she with him for fifteen years, making a total of thirty, therefore they would be married on the 30th.

Each week Aki anticipated that his wife would not come to see him the following week end, yet she appeared regularly. Although he began to trust her not to divorce him, the feeling that she would leave him would return suddenly at times. During her visits at the hospital, he found himself becoming tense and experiencing "peculiar" thoughts when she "looked" at him in what appeared to be an "angry" manner.

Although some of the statements his wife made had confused him, he had not asked her for clarification. Through support of the group, he began the technique of asking questions until he could understand the situation clearly.

He recognized that he had accepted the gossip of patients on the ward as the truth, and was constantly attempting to obtain advice from them. Before coming to the State Hospital, he had been told that he would have to spend the rest of his life there. He found it difficult to make his own decisions and tended to be confused by the many conflicting stories and opinions of others.

By autumn he had been able to leave the hospital on brief visits home where he now felt more at ease with his family and experienced less fear of rejection. He reasoned that he would not be sent away to his mother and siblings in Japan since he was the second son and had no home in Japan. His real home was with his own wife and children. It began to seem unlikely that his wife would divorce him. At his request she checked with the Hall of Records to prove to him that their marriage had been correctly recorded.

While on the ward in the hospital he now participated in games with the other patients. At times he appeared somewhat more hostile and aggressive toward other patients, but this behavior did not lead to any significant disturbance in his interpersonal relationships. Throughout his hospitalization he remained blocked as far as being able to offer any description of his parents or his feelings toward them except that they were "nice."

PSYCHOLOGICAL EXAMINATION. At the time of Aki's entry into the psychotherapy group in the late spring he was given the booklet form of the Minnesota Multiphasic Personality Inventory. His measured attitudes, as reflected in the test scores shown in Fig. 14–1, were in line with the agitated depression noted upon his arrival at the hospital; the Depression scale standard score was elevated to 82 and the Psychasthenia scale score to 77. Thinly disguised resentment toward society characterized his answers which brought the Psychopathic Deviate scale score to 83. Strong feelings of resentment because of frustrated passive dependent needs were reflected in a Sexual Deviation scale [1] score

---

[1] Marsh, *et al.*, 1955, A sexual deviation scale for the MMPI, *J. consult. Psychol.*, 19, 55-57.

of 84. High scores on this latter scale have been reported for patients with alcoholic and narcotic addiction, as well as for sexual offenders. A general hypothesis regarding the patient's disorder which could be developed from these test scores was that he experienced considerable resentment toward society for failure to provide satisfaction for his oral dependency needs. The threatened breakthrough of his unacceptable aggressive impulses led to symptoms of anxiety, depression, and projection of his hostility.

Because of his obvious use of either suppression or repression in dealing with his earlier childhood memories it was felt that additional psychological testing would be of value in working with this patient in group psychotherapy. In the summer he was given the Bender Gestalt, the Rorschach, and the Draw-A-Person tests. Throughout the psychological examination he expressed feelings of impotence such as "I give up," "Can't figure," "I missed that one maybe," and the general thought that he could not come up to expectations. It became obvious that the expressions of impotency reflected feelings toward himself rather than significant organic involvement when, for example, he was able to reproduce the Bender Gestalt figures accurately and directly (see Fig. 14–2).

His depressive reactions were reflected on the Rorschach (Test Summary A) in the paucity of responses ($R = 11$) and constriction ($F = 64$ per cent, $A = 54$ per cent). Moreover, there was only one M, and the only color was "blood" on II. His reaction times were generally prolonged and self-criticisms were frequent. His meager and self-critical responses indicated a retardation of perceptual and associative processes, an emotional inhibition, and general feelings of inadequacy and worthlessness, all pointing to depressed affect.

On the other hand, the patient showed a tendency to emphasize popular responses which suggested an over-compliant conventionality as a character defense. His one response which differed from the popular or conventional responses was to Card II after fifty-five seconds, "This is

sex . . . mm . . . I don't know, some blood is coming out
or something like that. I can't figure this out." On inquiry
it developed that the lower center *D* was a woman menstruating. It could be hypothesized that the blood reflected
sadistic and destructive impulses which he found unacceptable and disturbing. This sexual response together with his
failure on Card VI suggested a disruptive problem in sexual
adjustment with an inadequate heterosexual pattern, and
the possibility that destructive impulses were associated
with women.

An additional indication that he may have had difficulty
in identifying comfortably with an adult masculine role was
suggested by his response to the Draw-A-Person technique
(see Figs. 14–3 and 14–4). The figures of the "man" and
"woman" were essentially identical, with no sexual differences noted. The figure called a "man" was described by
the patient as a "dummy" and "selfish," while the figure
called a "woman" was described as a "nice person, understandable."

ROLE OF CULTURE IN AKI'S DYNAMICS

EARLY LIFE. The influence of his early Japanese culture
was clearly evident in his attitudes and behavior. The ob-
servance of a strict code of family duty was reflected in his
repeated dutiful return to his family in Japan, the sending
of gifts, and possibly his later emphasis upon "duty" toward
his wife and children. His suppression of any description
of his parents other than "nice" may have been a reflection
of his effort to preserve family honor. It can be hypothesized that any attempt at an uncovering form of psychotherapy, in which his ambivalent feelings toward his parents
might appear, would tend to precipitate considerable conflict.

One significant variation from the cultural pattern in his
childhood experiences was the separation from his family
at an early age and placement in a foster home. In the typ-

ical Japanese family the mother continues to be a constant source of food and love, even to the point where the child may appear "spoiled," with later stern school discipline introducing the first rude denial. For this patient there appeared to be an atypical early separation and a loss of his role in his family. An assumption may be made that this experience represented a rejection by his early love objects.

LATER DEVELOPMENT. His life during his adolescent and young adult years appeared to have been isolated and characterized by a general denial of need satisfaction. He continued the ritual role of dutiful son, but avoided all strong object relationships until his marriage in later life. After his marriage, and during the years in the relocation camp, his new role of father was not threatened, and there was no evidence of symptom formation.

Upon the family's return to the city his masculine roles of the father, husband, and head of the family began to meet with difficulty. Property was in his wife's name and there were not strong cultural ties to the community. After the birth of his first son the feeling that he might lose his wife and family increased. He had been replaced by others in his original family, and with his role as the father in the family unsure, he was in danger of another rejection.

SYMPTOM FORMATION. His behavior suggested that he had only limited ways of satisfying his need for object relationships that would assure him complete acceptance. When complete acceptance was not forthcoming, he projected his retaliatory impulses in the form of persecutory ideas toward a government that he felt had failed to accept him and toward a wife who also failed him by bearing a son who threatened his masculine role. His paranoid symptoms may reflect a striving to regain a lost relationship with some object, possibly a father symbol. His delusions regarding the government may serve the further purpose of protecting him from passive-homosexual temptation, originating in his infantile attitude toward his father. In line with this, his jealousy of his wife's imaginary lovers may have irritated him not merely because of the supposed interest of other men in his wife, but also because the other men paid attention to her and not to him.

His delusions of persecution by the federal government presumably involve the Japanese cultural emphasis on subordination to authority. His anticipated rejection and loss of status as the father in the family may have stimulated his unacceptable destructive impulses and, through projection, led to anticipated punishment by the authority figure. At a dynamic level closer to the surface, the anticipation of persecution by the government may be associated with the experienced rejection of being placed in the relocation camp during the war. He had experienced earlier direct discrimination against himself and his family by the government, so in later dealings with the government he again anticipated punishment.

Test Summary

A. RORSCHACH PROTOCOL

Response   *Inquiry*

CARD I. 4″

1. ∧ This is a bat, looks like a bat   1. The whole card.
to me. This is the top? > ∨ < ∧
Or a butterfly, a bat or a butterfly. That's all I can think of. I
can't think of anything else.

W   F   A   P

CARD II. 55″ ∧ < ∨ ∧ I don't know,
mmm, < ∨ >.

1. ∧ This is sex? mmm. I don't   1. Menstruating, this red.
know. Some blood is coming out
or something like that, I can't
figure this out.

D   mF, cF   Blood, Sex

Response	*Inquiry*

CARD III. 30″ < ∨ > mmm, oh.

1. ∧ Two men pulling something out of the ground, it looks like to me. I see the red and black colors on this, that is all I see. I can't see nothing else.

    1. Here's the head, arms, legs, hands. mmm—got pointed noses, long neck, this is standing, and leg here.

W˟   M   H   P

CARD IV. 16″ < ∨ > .

1. ∧ Some kind of insect, this one is (sighs). Black color, that is all I see.

    1. Whole thing looks like insect. Doesn't look like much.

W   F   A

CARD V. 10″

1. ∧ That looks like, let me see— what kind of animal this must be, I don't know. A bat or a butter- fly > ∨ < I can't name it. Some kind of animal, and black color.

W   F   A   P

CARD VI.

    > ∨ < mmm, this is hard. I don't know this one. I don't know what this is.

    I don't know.

    (Rejects)

CARD VII. 25″

1. ∨ That looks like a woman's hair. mmm—turn around, can't figure, I don't know what this one is.

    1. Woman's hair, outline of hair, that is all.

W   F   Hd

CARD VIII. 5″

1. ∧ Well, this got two animals, I don't know the name of these animals, got the color there, I can't tell you the color.

    1. Climbing up some place there, all I can see.

D   FM   A   P

Response	*Inquiry*
2. ∧ May be in center, look like a flower to me—that all I can figure. Got two animals and look like a flower.	2. Like Hibiscus flower. Color similar to it.

     D   CF   Pl

CARD IX. 45″   > ∨ < ∧

1. ∧ Don't know that in center, a violin or mandolin. Shape of in center. That all I can see.	1. Looks like strings in center. Shape of it.

     D   F   Obj

CARD X. 80″

I give up, I can't find anything there
—I give up—I can't   ∧ < ∨ < ∧

1. ∧ Looks like two crabs, but I give up.	1. (Popular)

     D   F   A   P

2. ∧ May be deer here. That all I can find, I can't think of anything else.	2. Deer or moose, big horn on it. About all I can see.

     D   F   A

RORSCHACH PROFILE

						R	11
W	5	M	1	H	1	F	64%
D	6	FM	1	Hd	1	A	54%
	11	m	1	A	6	P	5
		F	7	Obj	1	Sum C	1
		CF	1 + 1	Pl	1	M:Sum C	1:1
			11	Blood	1	CR	45%
					11	W:M	5:1

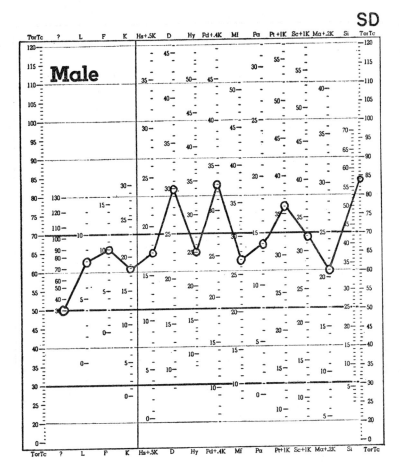

FIGURE 14–1. Minnesota Multiphasic Personality Inventory.

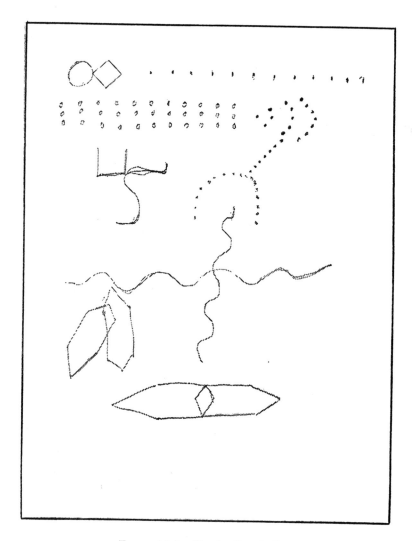

FIGURE 14–2. Bender Gestalt Test.

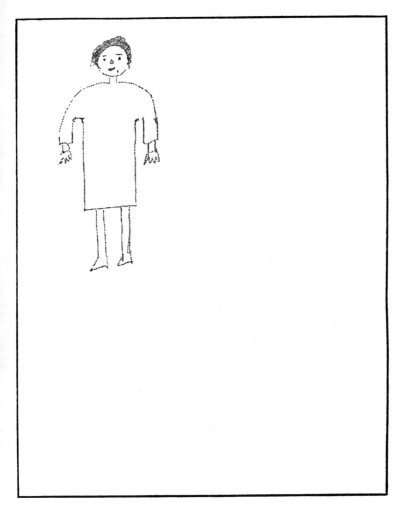

FIGURE 14–3. Draw-A-Person Test: Man.

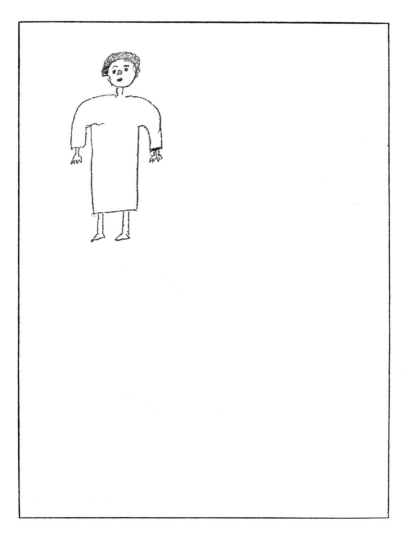

FIGURE 14–4. Draw-A-Person Test: Woman.

15

A Nisei Woman Attacks by Suicide

Norman L. Farberow and *Edwin S. Shneidman*

INTRODUCTION

While in a West Coast medical hospital, recovering from a suicidal overdose of Doriden, Mrs. Yosida Harada, a thirty-eight-year-old American-born Japanese (Nisei) woman, was asked the three "Make Believe" questions below to which she gave the following responses:

1. Make believe that you could tell now what you will be doing five years from today. Tell what you expect will take place during the course of the day, one day five years from now. You might describe where you will be, what you will be doing, what you will be thinking about at that time, how you will be feeling, or anything else you wish to say.

Five years from now, I'll probably be owning my own home, happy with my own family, regretting what I have done today but better for what I have done. I think the relationship between my husband and myself will be that much more deep.

2. Make believe that you are thinking of taking your own life. Indicate, in your own words, the note that you would write if you were going to take your own life. Make your note sound as real as you possibly can. Indicate what you think you would write if you were planning to commit suicide.

The note I did write to my husband was: "Dear Tom: I'm sorry but I have to do it this way. Please take care of the children. I leave everything to you." I didn't even sign it. I think I got groggy before I signed it.

3. Make believe that you have just inherited or won one million dollars. Indicate what you would do with all this money.

I would go out in the country and buy a big lot and build a beautiful home for the aged, just for the Japanese, and run it just for the Japanese. I would build something that no state government, not even the United States Government would come and condemn.

To most Occidentals, especially those who have never come into first-hand contact with Orientals, the culture of the Japanese presents many strange, fantastic, and unfathomable customs. For the Japanese who has been exposed directly to both oriental and occidental cultures, there are sometimes many difficult gaps to bridge, difficulties which may seem insurmountable and capable of being resolved only by such desperate measures as that attempted by our subject.

CONFLICT BETWEEN EAST AND WEST. Our subject, Mrs. Yosida Harada, was reared by a combination of strict old-world Japanese foster father and an impoverished orphanage until she was eighteen. Already exposed to the mores and traditions of the East by her foster father and the Japanese community, she spent a year in Japan, followed by six more years of schooling and hard work in the United States. She then went back to the Orient, this time to China, to run a mission and a children's orphanage. Five years later she married a Japanese businessman living in China, started her family, and spent the next six years in Japan before finally returning to the United States. She had spent approximately thirteen years in the Orient, teaching oriental culture to her charges in her school.

However, even greater conflict occurred maritally on introducing her husband to occidental culture, with its accent on masculine aggressiveness and apparent independence. The patient developed such severe guilt feelings and depression that she attempted suicide as a way of solving her own and her husband's problems.

APPEARANCE AND ATTITUDE. Mrs. Harada was seen on a ward the day after she had been admitted to the hospital for Doriden intoxication. She was a thin woman with a drawn face, who appeared moderately to severely depressed and who gave the general impression, as she talked, of a suffering person trying to do the right thing but aware that there were certain personal interests which conflicted with her ideas of what was right. She cooperated readily and seemed of above-average intelligence. There was apparently nothing organic interfering with her functioning at the time she was interviewed. The following account presents this woman's history in detail, most of it related in her own words as they were taken down in the interviews with a psychiatrist and a clinical psychologist.

THE SUICIDE ATTEMPT

RATIONALIZED MOTIVE.   As Mrs. Harada clearly indicates, the factors underlying her suicide attempt were of long-standing origin. She started by saying, "I'm only here because I thought that in this way my husband can go to Japan. He's not happy here and has not been in the past six years since we've lived here." She explained that she and her husband had been married for ten years. They met in China and spent the first years of their married life in Japan, where she was not particularly happy and was very glad to leave. Her husband, however, was

. . . of a different type, who doesn't understand what the thinking of the Nisei is like. He only knows the old ways, and he's very unhappy here, and always wants to go back to Japan. He never forces it on me but he always speaks wistfully of how he would like to return to the old country, and I feel very bad that he can't understand my not wanting to go there. So I thought that by killing myself I might be out of the way so that he could do what he wanted to.

Mrs. Harada then described what happened during the earlier part of the month.

I had a breakdown on the 10th of October. The doctor told me it was hepatitis and also that I had a slight heart attack. It was the first time that I ever had a heart attack. It really doesn't matter for me but I am very concerned about my children, what would happen to them if they didn't have their mother. I have worked real hard.

My husband has a job as a gardener. That's all he can do because he doesn't speak English, but he makes good money and pays all the bills. I have been running an orphanage of a kind but we had to turn it over to the old owners because the city inspectors claimed that it was deficient in many ways, fire, and safety, etc. Also, we had lost our cook. So I gave it up. There's another place that I manage in which people who have arrested TB take care of themselves. I work very hard, many hours each day, but I don't mind it; anything to keep busy.

SUPPRESSED HOSTILITY. The patient's husband had had hepatitis and had been instructed by his physicians to keep away from liquor. On the night of the suicide attempt,

. . . he came in very unhappy and again it was about the question of where we are going to live. Doctors had told him not to drink and I told him also that he wasn't to drink. But he went ahead and drank some beer that we always keep around the house for friends. I thought he would get into trouble but I didn't care any more. Isn't that terrible that I feel that way? He came home about eleven after having drunk a lot. I asked him what he was going to do. He told me to go to bed and not to wait for him. But it is a Japanese custom for the wife to wait for the husband, so I did. Then when he got home for the second time I took the 15 Doriden tablets. I called the neighbor right away and told him to take care of the kids, and that's the last thing I remember. The next thing, I was in the hospital. I just thought it couldn't go on. My husband is normally understanding and good. He is a fine man, but in this one area we have strong differences of opinion, although we have never argued about it.

Mrs. Harada went on with further discussion about her husband, pointing out how he had good qualities, but that they were the kind of qualities—the old-fashioned qualities —that were not appreciated in America, although she could appreciate them because of her own Japanese ancestry. She also pointed out how in many ways her husband was not capable of being extremely strong and aggressive since he could not speak English and she had to take care of his business for him. With no protests about her own problems, she repeated over and over again how much it hurt her to see him have such a great need for the old country.

PREVIOUS ATTEMPT.   There was a history of one previous suicidal attempt, which she had made when she was fifteen years old.

My father was a welfare worker. He was a sort of a wonderful person who worked with the Japanese in California. He had a children's home which took care of foundlings and orphans. I was raised there and treated just like the others. There was no difference. I felt very lonesome and hurt that my father did not have any more time or interest in me. It's not that he didn't care. He cared for me very much, but he didn't show it, and I didn't know it. I was sick at the time that I made this attempt. I had recently heard of a friend who had died because of taking too many aspirin and I was depressed, so I took some. It really wasn't serious. I just took a few and just got sick to my stomach. I felt very ashamed of myself afterwards that I had caused trouble for him.

SOCIAL HISTORY

EARLY MEMORIES.   The patient never knew her real parents. She was raised by Mr. S., the head of the orphans' home described above, and looked upon him as her father. She says of him:

My father was a very stern man. He expected me to do even more than other children were expected to do at the school. If anything went wrong, I was blamed. The children of course were very nice to me; they never blamed me for anything. I was their big sister. I sewed and cooked for them and took them out on trips. My father was almost a saint. He gave his life for that orphanage. He was the founder of the first humane society for the Japanese people and also he took care of the "picture brides." [1] He was a very sickly man and had tuberculosis at times and also had attacks of asthma. He returned to Japan on the second repatriation ship during the war. He was very disappointed over his treatment in this country because he felt that he had done so much for America and then he had been put in a concentration camp—so he returned to Japan in 1944, and

---

[1] The picture brides were girls who came from Japan to marry some of the men who had come over earlier. In letters to the girls in Japan the men would frequently create an impression that did not conform exactly to the facts and when the girls came over they were often disappointed at what they found. But they were really lost in the new country, and the patient's father founded this home where they could stay until they got settled.

then died a year later in 1945. He was very sick during the entire period that he was in Japan. I was in China at the time and didn't even know of his death until several months following it when I got a letter. I was very fond of my father. He was my only parent. I just couldn't believe that he was dead. Finally I got to the place where he was buried and then it dawned on me that he was gone.

I don't know who my real parents are. When I was just a baby my mother abandoned me to a Mexican family. After I had been with the family for about a month, Mr. S. heard that there was a child who looked Japanese who was living with a Mexican family. He visited me and decided from my appearance that I was Japanese and took me away from them before I was a year old. By that time I had already lost my fingers and some of my toes. Nobody knows for sure what caused it but the doctors said that it must have been a burn. Mr. S. tried to find my parents for me. He put an ad in the Japanese paper once a month for five years and in this way everyone in the Japanese community got to know about me and how Mr. S. had been my benefactor. Actually I was the first one that he took care of. After that when people heard and knew of some other child who had been deserted, they would call him and he would take care of them. I don't remember much about my childhood. It seems to me like I have been working all my life. I grew up feeling that I was taken care of by the Japanese community and that I must repay them.

The first memory I have is of the time when I was around five. Someone gave me a Momma doll and I left it outside and someone stole it. All my memories about childhood seem to be unpleasant. I lived with my father until I was five years old but I have no memories at all about that time. Then when I was five, Mr. S. became ill with tuberculosis and had to go to a sanatorium, and I lived at a Christian Home for Girls. It was pleasant, but it wasn't home. It seemed that the cook and the matron were always changing. I was the youngest of all the girls so everyone babied me. I remember how it was at that home. We would sit at the tables and eat our meals and they made us eat everything. There were a lot of prayers and singing of hymns. The singing was okay, but sometimes the prayers and other duties were just unpleasant chores, but we always did it. Sunday the only thing that we could do was go to church. First we would go to the Japanese church and then we would go to the American church. There was a backyard to play in, but I couldn't play much because of my age. The other girls were doing things like playing baseball and volley ball, but I was too young. The main thing I liked to do was play with dolls. I would make many, many doll clothes. They were always of the same kind. Just a little smock that would fit over the doll's head, but as long as there was a different kind of cloth around I would make a new one.

I made some good friends among the girls. The girl that I liked best was two years older and knew how to play the piano. Of course I couldn't play because of my hands but I would love to sit at her side and she would like to have me, and I would listen to her for as long as she played. The only real enjoyment I have had in terms of doing something myself was my singing. I sang religious songs, and sang in some of the choirs, and I sang in a glee club. I like to sing even now. But I didn't like the idea of being pointed out and I hated to be a soloist. I can remember the long trips to church on Sunday, even when I was a little older and some of the other kids were playing or going on dates, but I didn't mind because singing was something that I could really do.

I felt very unwanted. I was longing for someone of my own. I always hoped that some day I might find a parent. No one ever came to see me and I remember the other kids would talk about their experiences that they had with their parents. Many times they were bad ones consisting of scoldings and beatings, but I envied them even the bad ones because it meant that they had someone. Mr. S. was in the sanatorium at this time and I didn't even know of him or write to him. I expect that he was paying for me at the school and was probably writing to inquire about me, but I knew nothing of him.

There was never any sex education and I remember when I started to menstruate at the age of 11, I didn't know anything about what was happening. It seemed like no one had ever spoken to me about it before. I had seen some of the rags that the older girls hung out sometimes, but I thought that maybe they had just dirtied a lot of handkerchiefs. I remember I was playing a game and every time I would strike at the ball and miss they would notice that I was bleeding and they pointed it out to me and I thought something drastic had happened. I was very afraid to tell the matron about it, so I just went up and changed my clothes. Then after a while I had used all my clothes and so I had to tell the matron. Then she explained to me about menstruation and I was very relieved and never worried about it again. I used to get some cramps with menstruation but that changed after I was married.

I had never had any relationship with a boy until I went to China. Just before I left for China I had one date. He had some tickets for a play and I guess his date must have turned him down, so that was why he took me out. Boys never asked me out and I guess I never looked for it. I was very self-conscious and felt that I was ugly because of my hands and feet. Until I was five, I would stand in a corner or next to a wall whenever I was with a group of people that I didn't know, and if anyone would come near me I would say,

"No, no" and hide my hands behind my back. At the age of seven or eight, I was in the hospital for a whole year for operations on my hands. I had many operations but they really did no good. After that I used to go to summer school all the time to make up for the classes that I missed. It was the matron at the home who arranged for the operations and the summer school.

Then when I was 12, Mr. S. got out of the sanatorium and I moved to his house. Life was just one toil after another. I was very happy when I heard I was going to live with Mr. S. because I thought I was going to have a home, but instead he took me to this welfare school that he was running and I was a staff member. I had to iron and to cut hair. I was much younger than the other staff members so they used me as an errand girl also. I didn't mind because I felt useful when I was doing something, but I did feel very lonesome at night. Father and I had a cottage. I had my room next to his. Of course other members of the staff lived here also. I would finish with my day's work first and then go up to study. He was always out and when he did come back it seemed as if there were things that he had to do, so we never had enough time together. He was very good to me materially. He gave me a quarter each day for lunch and all the other things that I asked for, but he didn't show much affection. You know the Japanese people are like that, but I wanted affection very much. I wanted him to put his arms around me and I wanted to put mine around him.

Until I was 18 I helped at the school. My own recreation was very limited. Twice a month I went to the theater, and once a month, downtown shopping. I would go to the Five-and-Ten, my favorite store, and buy things for the children. Then I'd have lunch and take in a matinee. I used to go to the newsreel theaters and watch all the different news of the day, and then go back home. In school I was average. I was not outstanding but I really didn't have much trouble.

JOURNEY TO JAPAN.   Then came the patient's great adventure:

I had saved money enough to pay for a whole year in Japan. It was an obsession with me. I wanted so much to go back there. I was so self-conscious, I felt I needed something. I thought that maybe I would know my people better. It wasn't even that I could speak Japanese well because I couldn't, but I thought that there might be something about going there. It was about this time that I had to go to court to establish my American nationality because there was no documentary proof of it. Up to this time I never was sure of my relationship to Mr. S. People would tell me he wasn't my father. I would ask him about it but he would laugh it off. He would say, "How do they know? Were they there at the time?" So I would stop asking him, but when I had to go to court it was horrible. There were people swearing who I was and that they knew me and that they knew that Mr. S. was my father, but he told me at that time that I really wasn't his daughter. Then he told me about my early life. Mr. S. got a lawyer to prove that I was his legal daughter. You see he did do that for me; he thought that much of me. If I hadn't wanted to go to Japan, I probably wouldn't have records to this day and probably couldn't even have gotten married.

During my year in Japan, I traveled every place, saw sights, and I went to my father's birthplace and visited his relatives. I was accepted there, could talk to others; for the first time in my life I wasn't shy and I made friends, and it was wonderful. But I did want to come back to this country and go to school.

I came back to the institution and worked there and I went to junior college. I wanted to be a welfare worker, so that I could help my father and do work like he did. I took an academic course, child psychology, and things like that. Coming back to my former surroundings I was a different person. I could talk to everybody and hold my head up, but when I went to school with people that I didn't know, I was very seclusive. It was a little different, however, because I didn't have time to talk to others, but if I had to I could. I went around in the same circles as before. I never had an opportunity to mix with younger people. Again my life seemed to be mainly study and work. After I had finished the two years at the junior college I wanted to go on to complete my work, but I couldn't afford it. I asked my father for the money but he said he couldn't give it to me, that it wouldn't be fair to give it to one and not another, and that I would have to work my way through school. I borrowed the money from my father and finished nurses' school. Then I worked for another year at the institution and took the check for my wages to pay my Dad back. It had taken me a year to do it. I had to work very hard that year and I lost weight.

CHINESE INCIDENT.   The patient was twenty-four years old when a pastor from China came to lecture on the Chinese Incident.

Of course people like my father were very opposed to Japanese aggression and felt it was terrible and that the rest of us Christians would have to do something about it. This pastor was here for a long time and lived with us. He wanted to found a children's home in China to offset the Japanese brutality. He convinced my father that the need was there. One night my father came to my room and asked me to go in his place. He said that he was too old and that his work was really here in this country. I told him that I couldn't do it without finances, and he said I didn't have to worry about that; that the Japanese community would support it. There was a lot in the paper about it. A couple in the country wrote in to the paper and said that I was their daughter. One of my friends told me about it. At the time I was so interested in the work that I was going to do that I didn't take time to look them up. Afterwards I wanted to, but nobody knew where they were. *You know, I feel very funny about living to an old age.*[2] I get this feeling when I am working with old people which I often do. Sometimes I have the feeling that I might be helping my own parents without either of us knowing it and that scares the life out of me. I don't want to get old and have no one to care for me.

I went to China, and I had to build the place myself. I had the plans and I called in some people, contractors, carpenters, and so forth, had it built just the way I wanted it. We had 57 children. I had taken a lot of American clothing for the children, but they would trade off these clothes with the other kids in the neighborhood. So we had to build a school right in the institution. I was very happy but the year after we got there our funds were frozen. We couldn't get money from this country so I had to solicit funds among the Japanese there and we got enough to get by on. Then I got malaria and was sick for two months and during this time my assistant took over.

My experiences in China were very pleasant and I enjoyed the kind of work I was doing. Four years after I started, the government decided that all Chinese property was to be returned and we considered that the school was Chinese property, so I turned it over to the government. That was the end of my time in China. I became very friendly with the Japanese community in the city near my orphanage and knew them very well.

In 1944 we went to Shanghai and I started a school for children there. I couldn't return to America. I had lost my American citizenship because I was in the Orient. I had not known about it at the time, but the U.S. Government had passed a law saying that any Orientals who remained in the Orient past a certain period would lose their citizenship. I really did not mind when I found out about it, nor was I mad at the government. I was so devoted to my work. To me that was enough to make up for it. We had about 100 children in our school, and it was at about that time that I met my husband.

---

[2] Italics supplied.

COURTSHIP AND MARRIAGE. The patient was asked whether she loved her husband. After pausing for a long time, she said:

Well, I'm not too sure. Our courtship was typical Japanese style. We would go out together, to movies, to concerts, and for walks, but I didn't think too seriously of it. However, at that time my father came from America on repatriation, and because he encouraged the marriage I decided to get married. He felt that I was getting older (I was 29 at the time), and that if I got to be 30 it would be too late, so I said "all right." *Also I had a thought of not wanting to live too long.*[3] I thought at that time that I would just as soon live fast and die at 30. Actually, that was the first time I had ever had a home.

We had a normal kind of life, but it wasn't like in the fairy stories; things weren't perfect. However, I took what I had and made the best of it. I continued with my work because we had the plan at that time of returning to this country, and my husband's earnings were not enough. Two weeks after we were married a General of the nearby garrison called me in and told me that there was a young foundling whose mother had died and whose father was too busy to take care of it, and that this child had to have a home. He said he was asking me if I would take it and I could hardly refuse. He had the child there and practically handed it to me, so I took the baby home, and my husband was very angry at me for having done this. This was because the child cried most of the night and disturbed us quite a bit, and I had to give the child a great deal of attention. [The patient was smiling when she talked about this.] My husband was angry because my first thoughts were about the baby. However, we became very attached to the child and decided that we wanted one of our own.

Taking the baby was one of the few times that my husband and I disagreed. Although he was against my taking the baby, I did it anyway. Usually the way we deal with things is that he asks me what I want. If *he* doesn't want it, I usually won't go ahead and insist, but sometimes I do make decisions in spite of what he has to say. For example, I made the decision to take the baby home. Also I made a decision to take on an old folks home recently, even though my husband was against it. I did this because I am the only one in the city who does this kind of work and knows how to, and because of my interest in the Japanese people.

---

[3] Italics supplied.

I lived in Shanghai from 1944 to 1946. In 1945 when the war was over we gave up the school since it was no longer needed. At that time I found myself pregnant. We wanted a child of our own badly. I was having trouble with my appendix and went to a hospital, where I had an appendectomy. The scar wouldn't heal well because my belly was expanding all the time and it was a very difficult period. My husband was away a good deal of the time at his work, but my assistant who had studied with me after the school folded up was there to help me. She was my constant companion.

In 1946 we returned to Japan and one week later I had the child. We were living with my father's relatives at that time and were very unhappy. This was because they felt that they ought to give me certain parts of the family estate but didn't want to. We only stayed there until my daughter was two months old and I could travel. Then we went to visit my husband's parents, but they didn't want us there either. Finally we left them and went to Kioto where my husband worked as a real estate agent and I worked as an interpreter with the Occupation Forces. We both had to work because during the previous years we had accumulated tremendous debts, and also we were still working to get back to the U.S.A. I enjoyed my work even though I couldn't spend much time with my child. We stayed there until December, 1952. At that time a special bill was passed through Congress allowing us to return to the United States.

We got here in 1953. Previous to this time my second child, a son, had been born in 1948. He was a wanted child. My husband was particularly anxious because the first child had been a girl. He would like many more children but I feel that two are enough and I feel that since I have given him a son I have fulfilled my obligation. Again, after my son was born I only stayed with him for two months and then went to work. We had to do this in order to make ends meet. We came back to Los Angeles. I found a job and my husband started working as a gardener's assistant. He has never learned English, even though I have tried to teach him. Also he never did manual labor before [she laughs as she says this]. It was a blow to him to have to take on this kind of work.

HUSBAND'S JEALOUSY. When the patient was asked about the husband's having a job inferior to hers, she said:

He doesn't resent it. At the beginning it was a burden for him to keep up my father's name.[4] I always made an attempt not to be haughty, but he is very tense at times. My friends don't enjoy com-

---

[4] Since her father had had no son while the husband's family had another one, it was decided according to Japanese custom that her husband take her family name. See footnote, p. 300, on *yoshi* marriage.

ing over because if we start speaking English he gets hurt and walks out of the room, so all that we have seen during the past year or so are his friends. We have both been getting tired of our many activities.

On October 10, I had a slight heart attack and I had to give up one of our homes. My husband was supposed to take care of things but he didn't do very well, so I got someone else to help out. It was a young student and my husband resented this very much. He felt left out because I did so much work with the student and was very rude. He would be silent or go to bed early. We had just moved into a larger place. There was much activity. We were painting every night and my husband was under a strain. The student had offered to paint the bathroom ceiling but my husband didn't want him to. I told my husband I didn't think that it was very nice, and then I left the room and apologized to the student for my husband. My husband was very mad and went on a drunken spree. He felt, even though there was nothing in it, that I was going to have a love affair with the student.

SUICIDAL RETALIATION. So I thought that since his great ambition was to go back to Japan that if I killed myself he would have an opportunity to do this.

Asked what would happen to the children, she said, "They are closer to my husband than they are to me, so I think that he would be able to take care of them."

PSYCHOLOGICAL TEST DATA

The diagnostic test battery administered to Mrs. Harada on admission, included the Rorschach, Thematic Apperception, Sentence Completion Test,[5] and the three Make Believe Situations discussed in the opening paragraphs.

RORSCHACH. (See Test Summary A.) From a structural point of view, the patient's low productivity (nine responses only) was the main clue to her depression.

Her feelings of guilt over her attempted suicide were focused on her children who would have been left motherless had she succeeded. Her preoccupation with this idea is reflected in the content of five of her nine responses that

---

[5] The Sentence Completion Test used was developed by Dr. Carl Saxe (see List of Contributors).

concerned children or animals at play. Moreover, during the test she interrupted several times to remark on how terribly she felt about what she had done because of the implications for her children.

An interesting feature of this patient's record is its autobiographical flavor suggested by the Japanese stove seen on Card III.[6] The writers have often noted analogous autobiographical material in other cases of attempted suicide.

In terms of good form integration, lack of constriction, and evidence of creative imagination, Mrs. Harada's protocol is altogether normal.

TAT. One of the dominant themes emerging from the thematic material is the presence of a deep-seated hostility which is very carefully repressed by this patient (see Test Summary B). For example, on Card 1, the boy is seen in conflict regarding the use of a saw against parental prohibitions. This conflict between self-assertion and need to comply with authority appears to be a core conflict with the patient. The same theme is repeated on cards 2 and 3BM, which express feelings of guilt and shame on the part of the girl who, in attempting to assert and improve herself, is concerned over her responsibilities and duties toward the respected elders. Card 13MF suggests that her suicide attempt may have represented for her a breakthrough of the underlying hostility which she subverted onto herself. Cards 6BM and 7BM suggest that one of the factors contributing to her conflict was the difficulty caused by her need to play the maternal role for all, including her husband, while at the same time she wished her husband to be the warm, affectionate, fatherly figure who would understand her and let her act out this role. Her inability to solve this conflict may have contributed as a precipitating factor to the suicide attempt.

---

[6] Dr. Gertrude Baker (see List of Contributors) has suggested that the patient is trying to thaw out herself and her relations with others in front of a stove that is strictly Japanese—as a way out of her culture conflict.

SENTENCE COMPLETION. (See Test Summary C.) Despite the use of evasion and repression manifested by the patient's blocking on sixteen of the items, clues emerge which confirm impressions from the TAT and Rorschach.

Having no parents, she apparently attempts to overcompensate for this lack through preoccupation with her maternal role. Her attempt at suicide thus brings out more guilt because she would indeed have made her children motherless as she herself was. The deep repression of hostility which broke through in the suicide attempt is suggested in the following: *When I lost my temper* I tried to commit suicide. This item suggests that hostility for her must be repressed; any expression of anger might become dangerous, particularly against herself.

A suggestion that there were doubts as to whether the suicide attempt would really solve her conflict is noted in her response: *I suppose I want to* die. If it could be as simple as that, I would like to die. Other inferences suggest that her need to hold on to her love object is so great that when a threat of separation such as her husband's leaving her occurs, she becomes so depressed that she feels worthless, hopeless, and angry—all of which leads to aggression against herself.

MAKE-BELIEVE SITUATIONS. This test contains some strikingly optimistic notes. She expresses the feeling that in five years her family will be enjoying better relationships, and despite her regret over her suicide attempt, she feels that perhaps this may be responsible for a deeper understanding between her husband and herself. She again demonstrates her concern over her children and reflects a maternal tone in the suicidal note she actually had written. The "million dollar" wishes denote again her counterphobic need to work for elderly people.

Inferences from this material suggest that feeling deprived of parents she has dedicated much of her life to working for the benefit of parental figures. When this work was halted by outside authority her overdetermined needs in this direction were frustrated, thereby contributing to her growing feelings of depression and worthlessness.

SUMMARY. Mrs. Harada is very sensitive and of superior intelligence. While she manifests some insight into the source of her conflicts, she makes fairly effective use of repression to keep certain of her basic feelings from awareness. A very capable woman with extremely marked longings for the role of mother, she can function adequately when this concept is left untrammeled. Her voluntary comments in the Make-Believe test, regarding the precipitating factor in her present depression, suggest that when not permitted to play this all-caring, self-sacrificing role, she becomes guilty, feels worthless, and her self concept is crushed.

The test materials suggest that these strong maternal feelings stem from an overcompensation for her own feelings of being motherless. With strong guilt feelings and concomitant shame, the patient attempts to make her way in the world by being mother to others. The other dominant feeling which emerges from the test material is one of duty. This is in part a factor arising from her need to be a mother and in part a cultural factor stemming from mores in which filial duty is important.

A strong, effective woman, she must feel superior to her husband, whom she probably relates to in a mother-son relationship. Inferences from this suggest that his leaving America for Japan would be impossible for her because it would again represent a reversal of this position, which she could not readily assume.

Her attempt at suicide, then, could be interpreted as: (1) a method of giving in to the deep-seated hostility which has been repressed in the past, and (2) a resolution of her core conflict. With her husband threatening departure, and her overcompensatory maternal activities stopped by outside authority, her maternal self concept which is so crucial to her is crushed, leaving her with intolerable feelings of shame, guilt, and hostility.

PSYCHODYNAMIC FORMULATION FROM THE CASE
HISTORY

This is a case in which both cultural and individual factors have contributed in the production of a masochistic, self-denying, but extremely striving woman. The patient's early experiences which first amounted to total rejection, followed by relative rejection, in which she never had constant or strong parental figures, form a scar which is the basis of her subsequent activity. The intense anger and resentment which must have been experienced as a result of the early rejections had to be repressed because repression was necessary for survival. In reaction formation against the fundamental, angry passion which must have raged through her, she became the moralistic, giving kind of person that she superficially seems to be. Working together with this were the cultural factors of the Japanese civilization and the religious welfare community of the Japanese Christians who raised her. It is her identification with this group and, more specifically, with her father, which accounts for the strength which has enabled her to overcome personal and physical handicaps to a certain degree.

Although this patient would like to be loving and kind, it is difficult for her actually to be so. Because of her deprived childhood she cannot really dare to love others. To her they always present a threatening aspect; they can hurt and deprive. The main way in which it has been possible for her to relate to other people has been to assume the role either of a hurt, helpless child who must be helped, or of the helper to someone else who has been deprived and is relatively helpless. Only in this way has she been able to prevent the fear of being deserted from becoming overwhelming. Yet even in her relations with her own children and her husband, a return of the repressed hostility manifests itself. In regard to her children this is borne out by her constant rejection of them through being too busy to take care of them; in regard to her husband, by relegating him and the culture he represents to a secondary position. She compensates for the guilt to which such hostility gives rise by continuing her practice of being a welfare worker.

PSYCHODYNAMICS OF THE SUICIDE

Mrs. Harada's suicide attempt can be looked upon in one sense as an attempt to escape the tension occasioned by her becoming aware of hostility toward her husband. As she continued her practice of demeaning her husband in subtle, indirect ways, numerous rationalizations were open to her. These were that her husband did not understand English, that the other people with whom she associated needed a certain part of her time, etc. But to a certain extent these rationalizations were dependent upon the husband's accepting his inferior position. When he did not do this, when he complained and when he acted hurt, it became harder for her to convince herself that she actually was not hostile toward him. Finally, his statement that she should not wait up for him, which was contrary to Japanese mores and had some of the implications of a threat to leave, made it impossible for her to deny that there was hostility toward him.

There are other symbolic implications of the suicide. This patient expressed herself much of the time in passive ways. It has always been necessary for her to deny that she has had desires which must be fulfilled or that she has had passions which must be satisfied. So, too, in the expression of anger she has always been passive, and in the supreme expression of anger and hate toward her husband she could not at this time allow the feeling openly, but rather expressed it passively in an attack upon herself. Thus, she makes her husband suffer through her self-punishment. But in a way she also punishes her husband more directly, not only because he feels sorry for her, but because she threatens him with what has always been regarded by her as her greatest fear, the fear of being deserted. By dying she will desert her husband and leave him a helpless child.

It is possible that were this woman seen at some other time, she would not be considered psychiatrically ill. However, the dynamics of passive aggression seem to be quite clear and one could call her a passive aggressive character.

CONCLUSION

It is regrettable that no follow-up was possible for this unfortunate woman. Subjected as she was to the demands and pressures of her conflicting cultural mores and her own intrapsychic needs, it is difficult to foresee a happy life in the years to come. With her defenses already so well established and her character structure so firmly molded, her "success" in life seems to depend on whether or not she can re-establish her repressive mechanisms to the level of their former effectiveness so that she can again achieve some measure of joy through toil and pleasure through suffering. It is interesting to speculate that her exposure to the self-effacing doctrines of her oriental culture has to some extent been useful in helping her to achieve the required degree of effective repression of her own intrapsychic demands and feelings. Thus, her bicultural heritage has been for her both a facilitating factor and reservoir of strength and adaptive techniques, as well as a source of ambivalence and conflict.

The oriental doctrines of feminine submissiveness and de-emphasis of the individual have aided her in submerging herself in her work, enabling her to be the all-giving mother figure either to the very young or the very old. But her oriental mores did not equip her for interaction with her peers, and her difficulty evolved as her husband finally rebelled against the childish position into which she had gradually been forcing him. In the Orient he probably had not been very much aware of this, but in the United States his growing resentment gives clear evidence that he was rebelling against the role that she had subtly been imposing on him.

Mrs. Harada left the hospital to go back to this same situation, with the pressures still there, the conflicts still basically unresolved, and the resentments still smoldering. Over this total situation is again drawn the cloak of repression based on many long years of training by foster father, orphanage, and the oriental outlook on life. For Mrs. Harada, it seems like an uneasy truce.

Test Summary

A. RORSCHACH PROTOCOL

Response	Inquiry

CARD I. 2″

1. A cat.

    1. (Center D) (Q) Eyes—mouth, ears, cheeks.

CARD II. 3″

1. Halloween.

    1. Black and orange hats, black costume, orange shoes. (People?) Children at play. (Q) Children want Halloween costume.

CARD III. 2″

1. Eating in front of Hibashi.

    1. (Patient explained Hibashi is a stove in Japan.) We used to sit in front of the Hibashi—only not in that fashion. We used to sit on our knees. (Patient then described in some detail how they used to sit in the winter around the stove while they ate.) (Anything else?) No—used only this part of the blot (Black).

CARD IV. 3″

1. A bat.

    1. I guess I have Halloween on my mind. Not really like a bat—just resembles it a bit.

CARD V. 2″

1. That's a real bat.

    1. This is like a bat. (Q) Wings, tail. (How see?) Flying. (Anything else?) No (*sadly*). Am I mentally ill? (Examiner reassured patient at this time.)

Response	*Inquiry*

CARD VI. 6″

1. Skin of some sort.

1. Skin pinned out to dry. Never seen it but that's the way it looks like in pictures. I haven't my glasses. (How much?) (Bottom D) (Q) Seems like it's pinned in various places to keep it stretched out.

CARD VII. 18″

This doesn't remind me of anything. (Rejects)

I don't see anything in this. (Now?)

Add. 1. Maybe little children playing. (Q) Just these two—playing in the water. This head (upper D)—this (center D) portion out of water. (Sex?) Either one.

CARD VIII. (very long pause) **32″**

1. Don't think I can see anything here—guess it could be a flower.

1. I don't know name of flower—very beautiful, comes out in A.M., goes back at night. (How much?) (outer D) (Q) We had one like that in garden. (Anything else?) I don't know; I guess they call it passion flower.

CARD IX. 8″

1. Seahorse.

1. (Top part) (Q) This top—playing in the water. I don't know whether this is fountain or not but seems as if they're playing around water.

CARD X.

1. Crabs at play.

1. (P)—These and they're also playing on the seashore. (Red D) (Seashore?) The rocks. (Crabs?) My husband is so fond of crabs.

Test Summary

B.   THEMATIC APPERCEPTION TEST

CARD 1.

(Strains to look at card.) A little child looking at instrument. Doesn't know what it's all about but would like to use it if he could.

Is it a saw? (Whatever you think it is.) I can't see very well. (Feeling?) He wants to use it but doesn't know—and has been prohibited to use it.

O: I think he'll try it. T: "The Forbidden Tool."

CARD 2.

(Very long pause.) A girl on way to school and she watches as her mother and father toil on the field. She feels bad because she wants to help them instead of going to school. (Father and mother feel?) They want her to continue going to school.

O: She'll go to school. T: (holds chest in pain) I don't know.

CARD 3BM.

That's a little girl which probably has been punished. (Q) She's crying—she's probably forgotten to do her task or something.

O: She'll be forgiven. T: Don't know.

CARD 6BM.

That's a mother and son and the son is very unhappy with mother and the mother is probably very unhappy with him over something he has done or said. He's leaving (starts to cry).

O: She'll forgive him. T: "The Parting" (sobs).

CARD 7BM.

Father and a son who understand so well (rubs eyes with hand). (What does father understand?) The father and son have had a disagreement but they understand now and all is forgiven. No title.

CARD 13MF.

Man and wife. Husband is stricken because wife is ill. (Husband feeling or thinking?) He does not know what to do.

O: She'll probably go to the hospital and she'll get well. T: "A Moment of Despair."

CARD 18GF.

(Very long pause.) A woman and a man at the foot of the stairs, I guess. They're very fond of each other. They must be teen age—romance.

O: They'll probably get married. T: "Love in Bloom."

CARD 16.

Doesn't remind me of anything. (Story?) (Shakes head.) I want to see my children—I shouldn't have done this to them. (Cries.)

Test Summary

C. SENTENCE COMPLETION TEST

1. *I pleased my friends when* I did little things for them.
2. *My secret desire is* to run.
3. *Even though I loved him, he* wants to return.
4. *I thought of myself as* selfish.
5. *A wife has a right to* love.
6. *I would make enemies if* . . . (shakes head).
7. *I don't like men who* drink.
8. *I gave in because* . . .
9. *I could not love him because* . . .
10. *I wish my friends would* understand.
11. *My body is* . . .
12. *When he refused me, it meant* . . .
13. *I like women who* . . .
14. *My friends don't understand* that I need work.
15. *Sometimes sex* never appeals to me.
16. *When nobody cares, I* don't care.
17. *I like myself when* my children are around.
18. *I was really loved by* my husband.
19. *Sometimes marriage* too big of a burden.
20. *I was annoyed by people who* drank.
21. *I feel worse if* . . .
22. *When he began flirting with me, I* . . . (shakes head).
23. *Making friends is hard if* it isn't hard.
24. *It isn't right for a child to* be deprived of a parent.
25. *I wanted my mother to* I've never known of a mother.
26. *When I was punished, I usually* cried.
27. *I don't like to* cry, I guess.
28. *I almost lost hope when* my husband left.
29. *Nobody could force me to* . . . (in great pain).
30. *When my parents argued* I've never had any parents.
31. *What I have to do is* make it up to my children.
32. *When I lost my temper* I tried to commit suicide.
33. *My father annoyed me when* . . .
34. *I always worried about* my children.
35. *If only my mother* . . .
36. *I would get better if* I knew my children were well.
37. *I am scared by* fire.
38. *My father should have* . . .
39. *When something worries me, I* get panicky.
40. *Being told what to do* is a relief.

41. *My mother annoyed me when* . . .
42. *I was undecided so* . . .
43. *I watch people for* . . .
44. *I wanted my father to* . . .
45. *I was criticized when I* . . .
46. *My mother should have* . . .
47. *I would feel lost if* my husband left me.
48. *When upset, I* don't know what to do.
49. *The worst thing about getting older is* I've seen so many old people, I don't want to get old.
50. *I suppose I want to* die. If it could be as simple as that, I would like to die.

16

The Divided Path: "Psychocultural" Neurosis in a Nisei Man

Leonard B. Olinger and *Vita S. Sommers* [1]

THE PROBLEM OF IDENTIFICATION

In attempts to understand the etiology, significance, and treatment possibilities of the various behavior disorders, attention has been sufficiently directed to the roles played by anxiety, other specific symptoms, and the overly harsh superego. It is only within recent years that the problem of ego identification has been more systematically examined and its prominence recognized in psychopathology. The case under study in this paper is one in which the centrality of the identity factor is plain; the roots of this patient's symptoms could be found in the tangled skein of his own "unrootedness."

It has been said that an individual may have numerous identities. He is the person he thinks he is, the person he hopes he is, and the person he wants to be. He is the person others see, the person he wants others to see, the person he is afraid others see. He takes one role with respect to some people, another with respect to others, and so on. And he may change these roles and self-perceptions at different times and in different settings. The identity of each of us varies in its definiteness partly as a function of our limited self-knowledge and partly as a result of its constantly shifting character, however imperceptible these

---

[1] The junior author served as psychotherapist.

shifts may be. Inasmuch as we have all evolved from infancy into various stages of maturity and have been exposed to a wide variety of situations defining our role or identity in some way, we have been afforded greater or lesser opportunities to accept (or introject or incorporate) or to reject (or repress, inhibit, or deny) aspects of the environment and characteristics, values, or attitudes of those with whom we come into contact. The multi-facetedness of the identification process is a logical result.

When particular cultural factors are introduced into this highly complex developmental picture, an intricately interwoven pattern is designed in the fabric of the personality. And when these cultural factors are not restricted to a single dimension but are plural in character, as well as conflicting and perplexing, the ground is laid for confusion and doubt. It was such split identifications that had harassed and tormented our patient, Ichiro, for many years before he was able to deal with them through the increased understanding and maturity which psychotherapy made possible.

THE PATIENT

Ichiro is a Nisei, handsome, and intellectually very alert. Aged thirty-four, married, and the father of a five-year-old boy, he is a member of two widely different cultures. Reared in the spirit of oriental ideology, he later adopted and assimilated occidental thought, customs, values, and behavior. Linguistically, too, his was a double exposure; he spoke Japanese at home and English on the outside. Religiously he similarly had a basis for confusion since his mother had been educated in a Methodist missionary school, whereas his father remained Buddhist. And his dual national allegiance, while not an uncommon one for children of immigrant parents, became in his case a potent factor in his breakdown when, as a result of World War II, his conflictual feelings threatened to engulf and overwhelm him.

His presenting symptoms were ulcers, aggravated by spells of depression with suicidal thoughts, sleeplessness, and fear of losing his mind. Ever since he had been medically discharged from military service, he had been in and out of jobs, working variously as vegetable clerk, waiter, migratory farm helper, and elementary school teacher. At the time he entered therapy, Ichiro was earning his living as an insurance salesman and was deeply in debt financially.

It was after eighteen months of treatment that he secured a job as an English teacher at a high school. About a year later he received an appointment to teach English at an Eastern university. His treatment lasted approximately three and one-half years, covering more than three hundred sessions. Some pertinent case history material may be helpful in pointing up this patient's salient conflicts.

CASE HISTORY

Ichiro is the oldest son in a family of eight children born to parents who migrated to the United States. The father had made numerous unsuccessful attempts to obtain engineering work for which he had been well trained in Japan, so he settled as a farmer. However, he was nicknamed the "philosopher and poet" by the other farmers because he thought more about poetry than potatoes, more about Confucius than crops. The patient described his father as harsh and volatile, a narrow, opinionated man with a brilliant intellect and a stoic philosophy; the patient feared him "more than anyone or anything in the world" and as a boy had felt deeply ashamed of him. He resented not only his foreign manner, sloppy appearance, and poor English, but also his lack of appreciation for boyish pleasure and play. He felt that his father made a virtue of being different, and the more he stressed the difference, the more eager Ichiro seemed to overconform to American thoughts and customs, "hating everything Japanese." He all but disowned his father because he considered him a hindrance to the development of an American personality. His mother, he felt, was puritanical and disciplining; the children were never allowed to smoke, drink, or play cards and the patient felt as though he had "one foot in hell" whenever tempted to touch his genitals. Emotionally his mother was "warm in a distant way only; she was more prone to criticize than to praise." He thought of his mother as unsupportive in his conflicts with his father.

As a very young child, Ichiro remembers, his father used to employ "shock treatment" to force the boy to overcome his fears. In later years, the conflicts were intensified between boy and father as their lack of understanding reached new peaks. There were, however, hardly ever any arguments between the father and the other sons, who were "tactful, diplomatic, and subservient." Ichiro resisted "giving in." He played ball when he should have been feeding the horses; he read when he should have been cleaning the stables. When these derelictions were discovered, Ichiro tried to lie or make excuses and often would be "beaten to the ground" for lying. Yet, "the more brutally I was treated, the more obstinate and defiant I became; and the more I feared my father, the more I hated him."

In view of the unquestioning obedience to the father expected in Japanese culture, Ichiro's defiance was not comfortable and resulted in tormenting fear and consuming guilt which caused him frequently to be afraid he would break under the strain.

FIRST RORSCHACH APPRAISAL OF PATIENT

Perhaps it ought to be stressed at the outset that in order to use the Rorschach effectively as a "validating" instrument for the study of personal and social adjustment in individuals from different cultural backgrounds, not only would a thorough inquiry seem essential, but it would appear equally important to obtain, wherever possible, associative material to the Rorschach content, so that it might be seen how specific responses may be related *symbolically* to the culture. In the present case, this was done in the testing procedure as well as in therapy sessions, when the patient would discuss from time to time his test responses. The results were analyzed in terms of personal, interpersonal, and cultural reactions.

In the second month of therapy, the first projective evaluation was made. In assessing the Rorschach (see Test Summary A), one is struck by the patient's initial reaction to the ink blots. The opening response in a record is customarily regarded as setting the theme for the entire Rorschach, as well as reflecting the subject's mood, concerns, and preoccupations. Ichiro's first response, ". . . X-ray of the stomach, the intestines," suggests anxiety and somatization tendencies, which were, in fact, prominent among his presenting symptoms. In keeping with this trend, the second response, "gray moth," is most likely a reflection of Ichiro's dysphoria.

The content of the two M responses in this record (figure of Mephistopheles on Card I, and "grotesquely masqueraded figures with mutilated legs" on Card II) points to the emotional forces at work in the patient—his massive fears associated with rage and guilt. In his associations to the first M, the patient declares that he feels "sinful and guilty" about defying his father. The second M seems to display his castration anxiety and fear of destruction. The response reads: ". . . grotesquely masqueraded characters playing some kind of a game . . . (pause) . . . I think a person shouldn't look too long . . . (longer pause) . . . That stump of a leg bothers me . . . as if it were shattered."

The absence of the popular M on Card III reflects the deficiencies in both his early object relationships and his consequently poor interpersonal relationships at the time of testing. On IV (the "Father Card"), the patient sees "a deep sea creature, stingaree with a double stinger." This percept indicates what is probably the specific object of his castration fear. He finds Card VII, which is frequently regarded as the "Mother Card," as "the least suggestive, interesting, and meaningful picture." It merely reminds him of a "microscopic slide of yeast or something like that . . . not a very interesting thing." This response suggests that he does not really know his mother, does not see her as she is. The presence of *Fc* and *cF* in this percept may mirror the patient's desire for affectional expression and his acceptance of the idea that a woman is capable of providing it, but he does not seem able to tolerate the fact that he needs it; this would lower him too much according to adult masculine standards, especially in the Japanese version.

Card II, which, as has been pointed out, highlights some of the patient's fears, seems also to be telling us something about Ichiro's self-perception. One response reads, in part, ". . . a strange configuration. One is a mirror reflection of the other. He is pressing against a wall, trying to get at something and all he sees is his own reflection." The experienced Rorschach analyst recognizes this as a highly idiosyncratic response. It is as if Ichiro were saying: "No matter how much I look at myself in the mirror, I cannot change; it is the same old Ichiro—my face is that of an Oriental. I want to be Caucasian, accepted and comfortable, but when I look at myself honestly, I must face the painful reality that I am a Japanese, a member of a minority group which I reject, and I hate it."

His response on the same card, "Looks like a man's or woman's pelvic section upside down—looks both male and female. Sort of an empty, empty void in there . . . Whole thing—ambivalent—sexually male and female," has obviously important implications. It exhibits not only Ichiro's sexual confusion, but suggests, as sexual confusion often does, a more general confusion, as his word "ambivalence" confirms.

Card III, previously mentioned because of the absence of the popular *M*, underscores the extent of subtle inroads into Ichiro's ideational processes. His reference to the colon, with its anal implications, ends with the question: "Did they pick these (Rorschach cards) because I had a stomach condition?" This kind of pre-paranoid thinking gives a clue as to the character and depth of his fears and uncertainties which necessitate the development and employment of paranoid mechanisms.

It is on Card V that Ichiro makes his first allusion to the symmetrical aspect of the ink blots, an allusion which he thereafter makes to several cards in this record and to almost every card in the succeeding Rorschach protocols. The implications of "symmetry" comments are discussed below. It need be recorded here only that they were present from the beginning, which, in view of this man's intense struggle with opposing parts of himself, is perhaps not surprising. As his percept (No. 3) on Card X implies, symmetry is important in order to keep balance and avoid the precarious situation of falling. Ichiro's constant need to walk the tightrope between the areas on both sides of him, one of which he rejected, the other of which rejected him, kept him in constant turmoil, tearing him apart as the tightrope forked off in two directions. And, unable to choose either of the two paths which his limited perceptions offered, he was, like his percept on VI, being vertically split open.

TAT INTERPRETATION

The first TAT (Test Summary E) shows clearly this patient's distinctly opposite concepts of what male and female, father and mother, are. His identification, although predominantly masculine, seems conflictual in that he fears (1) that he cannot measure up to his father's very high standards and (2) that any exhibition of passive dependency might be indicative of feminine tendencies within him. Apparently, this conflict, which is not atypical for boys in their developmental sequence, has been reinforced by his cultural problem as a Japanese-American. This cultural problem heightens the struggle between ego identity and superego. He wonders consciously whether he should dutifully acquiesce passively and submissively to the parental Japanese culture or whether he should rebel, assert himself, and accept American ideology. Several of his TAT stories illustrate this dilemma. For example, on Card 1, he predicts that the outcome of the story will be "either complete acquiescence or open rebellion." Card 2 suggests to him "a conflict in the mind of two young people . . ." with the question, ". . . shall I follow the age-old tradition or shall I break away and assert myself?" This theme runs through nearly all his plots. On the unconscious level, however, the conflict is sharper because it is complicated by self-splitting ambivalence. It is apparent that Ichiro is torn between a desire for freedom and a fear of independence, between angry and hateful feelings alienating him from others and the pressing need for love and emotional support.

In therapy, the pattern of his life unfolded. It became apparent to the therapist, although not at first to the patient, that whenever Ichiro felt unable to cope with mounting frustrations and challenges and the maelstrom of emotional reactions they evoked, he would take refuge in illness where he could surrender to his various infantile and passive needs without being further weighted down by guilt or risking an open break. The TAT highlights his conflicts, and the Rorschach, abounding in anatomical responses associatively linked up with major illnesses, reveals his primary defense mechanisms. It was the inadequacy of these defenses, since they left him depleted, anxious, and continually oppressed, which brought him into treatment.

TREATMENT OBJECTIVES

Superior intelligence and introspective capacity, combined with flexibility, sensitivity, a genuine motivation for help, and a sense of responsibility for guiding and altering his life, were all promising features in the prognostic picture. Knowing who one is has been shown to be an essential part of learning how to be effective in dealing not only with other persons but with the various internal pressures. Ichiro had no clearly defined notion of who he was or how he ought to behave. He did not know whether he was oriental or occidental, adult or child; he was torn between rebellion and conformity, love and hate; he could not be sure whether to act independently or follow passively, to reason everything out logically or allow himself to feel emotions honestly. In short, his social, personal, spiritual, and physical selves took divided paths.

In view of the noted ambivalence, it is perhaps not surprising that three years of indecision passed between the patient's initial referral for psychological treatment and his actually contacting the clinic. In accordance with Japanese attitudes, Ichiro regarded accepting help as "a sign of weakness," especially when this help was to come from a woman therapist.

A major goal in therapy as it is conducted in the Western world is to free the individual; the usual method is to attempt to lessen the harshness of an overly strict superego, to strengthen the patient's ego, and to increase his power of self-determination. This is a goal which is at variance with Japanese traditions of filial piety and self-effacing respect for Father, Emperor, and God. Violations of these *mores* merit self-punishment, which in Japanese ideology finds its extreme expression in *harikiri*. Ichiro's self-punishment, which was manifested in his florid symptomatology, may have derived partly from this kind of cultural mandate. If so, the objective of superego alleviation would seem to be one of the main therapy goals.

A second objective, perhaps more important than the first and yet closely related to it, was the clearer definition of the self, or what has been called clarification of ego identity. In the present state of our knowledge, this goal is best accomplished by enabling the patient to look at himself and thus to learn not only who he is and to modify or alter what he wishes to, but at the same time to accept whatever in himself he cannot change. In the present case, the patient needed help in examining all aspects of himself, particularly the painful ones which he had so long postponed facing. For Ichiro, this meant countenancing frankly all the feelings raging or stagnating within him, which were driving him relentlessly.

In the initial months of therapy, the patient fought battles
of rage and rebellion with the therapist, as he had with his
father. He repeatedly tried to maneuver the therapist into
being a restricting, withholding, and prohibitive authority
figure like his father. He called her "illogical" when she
pointed to his feelings; "evasive" and "inscrutable" when
questions were reflected back to him; a "liar" when she
denied she was angry at him, and an "unbashful female"
when she referred to sex. He had to work for a number of
months before the anger and fear, and the consequent guilt
and depression, were alleviated sufficiently to allow the
positive and tender feelings to emerge in the transference
situation. His frequently expressed goal then became to
"reconcile with my parents as easily as I can with you" (the
therapist).

He paid tribute to women, heretofore described as inferior, as "the more stable people in my life." He came to
recognize two kinds of feelings toward them—admiration
and resentment, which, he began to understand, stemmed
from relationships with his two older sisters who were academically more successful, more athletic, less fearful than
he. He came to feel that his mother had been sturdier than
his father, and he expressed the feeling that his wife's stability was like a "Rock of Gibraltar." As he mellowed in the
newly discovered appreciation of his mother, his ventilated
anger permitted him to recognize his admiration and sympathy for his father and his own responsibility for many of
the conflict-incidents between himself "and the old man."

It took him six months in therapy to realize that he had
all these years been equating compliance and humility with
"giving in" and "admitting being wrong." He learned that
he had been equating tender feelings with weakness and
thus had been having to deny in himself feelings that were
as real and warm as the emotional climate he had been
seeking in his parents.

In what might be called the second phase of therapy,
Ichiro reported reading his first book on Japan, which gave
him a widened vista and new respect for things Japanese.

Prior to this, he had read only American books about Americans, and had identified wholly with American ideals and values. It was for this reason that, after Pearl Harbor, his psychocultural conflicts were so intensified; although in the American Army, he felt he was still a Japanese and did not "belong." Thus, he now felt rejected by America just as he himself had previously rejected everything related to Nippon. He was, in this sense, on the threshold of nowhere, with no trustworthy guideposts or supports; he was, in the words of a poet whom he quoted, "wandering between two worlds, one dead, the other powerless to be born."

With the gradual change in his self concept, deriving from greater appreciation of his resources and understanding of his reaction patterns, came the realization that he had been harsher in judging himself than his father had ever been. This insight relieved his guilt and anxiety, made possible a more comfortable identification with his father, and reduced his symptoms.

To gauge his level of tolerance for frustration and anxiety, and to re-evaluate his ego strength in general, Ichiro, in his eleventh month of therapy, was referred for retesting.

SECOND PSYCHODIAGNOSTIC TESTING

Only the Rorschach was administered on this second evaluation of Ichiro (see Test Summary B). Analysis of these data shows interesting, although no startling, changes. All in all, the therapeutic gains appear to have affected the total personality picture very little. The responses suggest that the emotional immaturity and affective imbalance into which the patient can be easily thrown when faced with anxiety and frustration are still in evidence, though much reduced. The center of reference is still himself, but he can now bring out feelings which help him to identify with, and also understand, other people. Of this he had previously been incapable.

This second Rorschach is interesting in several ways. Firstly, it points to the general consistency of personality, as evidenced by the essential similarity of this to the first record. Secondly, it reflects the subtle changes occurring as a result of the forces which psychotherapeutic explorations seem to have set into motion. Thirdly, the character of these changes appears to be paralleling the progress in treatment. For example, the symmetrical and anatomical features previously alluded to are repeated and elaborated. The Mephistophelian percept is again given, and the castration symbol on Card II of the first protocol remains, although here mentioned in the Inquiry rather than in the performance proper. It is augmented, however, by response 2 of Card VI, where he sees ". . . some tubular organ-like structure that has been shattered and exposed. . . ."

The first Rorschach yielded only one "flowers" percept—a response generally associated with passivity. On this second administration, colored flowers appear on VIII, IX, and X, perhaps attesting to the increased awareness of Ichiro's underlying passivity, which contrasts so markedly with his rebellious assertiveness on the conscious level. Repeated, but only as an additional on the second Rorschach, is his ice cream percept, a response clinicians tend to interpret as indicative of oral-dependent cravings.

Most striking, perhaps, is his response to Card VII. Here, he sees a Pacific Island, and also, "two baboons looking at each other." This suggests the bare beginnings of a more realistic acceptance by him of his Eastern origins, reconciliation with which is still far from comfortable.

As Ichiro is learning to understand his relationship to others, he seems to be making tentative overtures to interact with the world outside himself, of which he is becoming more conscious. There appears little in this record reflecting any changes directly connected with the patient's psychocultural difficulties. Rather, what one observes seems to be related to the intra-individual differentiation and development that must precede the rapprochement between himself and the forces of conflicting allegiances and claims on him that he needs to continue holding at bay.

ICHIRO'S DREAMS

It took more than two years of therapy before the patient was able to get a clearer understanding and clarification of his feelings and attitudes toward women. At first he had used membership in his culture as the "excuse" for his perception of women as "an inferior breed." He admitted that his admiration of the therapist was mixed with feelings of contempt. Part of his disdain for women he attributed to the fact that one could not fight with them as with men because "women start to cry, while with men you can fight it out." In reviewing his relationship with his wife and the part that their son played in it, particularly as he noted the young boy's jealousy of the parental affection, he uncovered the part his pronounced jealousy had played in his very disturbed relationship with his own parents.

His dreams reflected many of his fears, wishes, and feelings. In the initial phases of treatment, he reported recurrent dreams. Their content consisted of ghosts and beastly animals, or his mother weeping and his father glaring with a reprimanding grimace. As therapy proceeded, he found his nocturnal fantasies peopled with women of doubtful reputation and himself in their company, in settings such as burlesque shows, taverns, brothels, etc. Many of his dreams related to the Oedipal situation. Others involved pursuit by dangerous animals where, on one occasion, he finally fell down exhausted but was surprisingly unharmed by the pursuers; instead, these hounds became like puppies whom his wife was stroking. In his interpretations he likened the bloodhounds to his fears which struck terror into him, whereas they were playful puppies to those who knew how to handle them. In relating these fears to his father, Ichiro recognized as his guilt was dissipated in this area that his father's "rejection" of him in childhood had been influenced by his own personal and cultural conflict.

Another dream which Ichiro reported depicted him wor-
shipping at a shrine with Caucasians. In his associations
to this dream, he spoke of his "worship" of things American,
of his over-Westernization, and he bitterly had to acknowl-
edge that his oriental facial features would forever set him
apart from the dominant culture with which he so desperately sought to identify. The more he became conscious of
his conflict, the more accepting he could become of his race
and culture. His subsequent dreams reflected the gradual
rapprochement.

RORSCHACH III

The Rorschach on third administration reveals an improvement in form-level (see Test Summary C). Nevertheless, the obsessive features persist and, together with Ichiro's
preoccupation with the bilateral symmetry of the blots, are
of considerable importance in understanding him. The latter are often interpreted by clinicians as defensive intellectualizing maneuvers calculated to belittle or otherwise control the affect associated with the perceptions in the ink
blots. Ichiro's anxious, fearful feelings are mirrored in his
references, once again, to the Mephistophelian cape and
wings (Card I) and in both responses to Card II. In the
first response to Card III, however, the patient seeks a retreat from the emotionally disturbing stimuli in preoccupation with the formal characteristics of the blots. Here this
otherwise intellectually gifted subject has difficulty decid-
ing whether the blot could be a butterfly or a bow tie.

The references to bilateral symmetry in the first part of
the record are repeated in cards VII and IX, where they
occur in connection with the so-called feminine symbols.
In this respect the Rorschach would seem to be corroborat-
ing the clinical material regarding conflict over women—
a conflict that, as has been noted, had been intensified by
cultural attitudes. Since a further interpretation of these
references to symmetry suggests that the subject is external-
izing strong feelings of ambivalence, the persistence of

these conflicting cultural attitudes is highlighted. Such ambivalence, clinicians recognize, almost invariably carries with it equally pronounced feelings of guilt. This, then, focusses on one aspect of Ichiro's dilemma: To renounce his heritage engendered guilt; he felt guilty about deserting the Japanese culture. Yet he did not know who he was, and he was afraid of who he would become, if he could, indeed, become anyone.

What other changes does the Rorschach reflect? The excellent recovery which Ichiro shows in responses 2 and 3 after the initial one in Card IV echoes the desire to come to grips with the authority (i.e., father) problem. It is as if he were still fearful of the dangers surrounding the problem, while simultaneously seeking to master them. Such mastery would, of course, mean more comfortable, effective self-assertion, but, as the "fireman's boots" percept may indicate, this continues to remain a hot issue. Ichiro has not yet recognized that his father had been unwittingly inflicting the fruits of his own conflicts and disappointments on the patient, and he needs to handle the entire area gently.

And how fare the women in his life? Cards VII and VIII, when viewed serially, present an interesting composite picture. What is immediately striking is the introduction of a new concept, the ginger root, which probably mirrors his acceptance of, and identification with, things Japanese. In elaborating this percept, Ichiro explains that "the Japanese use this root a lot, that it has a nice taste." But, more than that, this concept suggests the emergence of very tender feelings toward his mother (and the therapist). The immediately following response (map of Pacific Islands) conveys the impression of apprehensive, yet nostalgic, feelings for her (and the "motherland?") The "symmetry" and "reflection" remarks in response 3 could represent the retreat into logical thinking in order to escape the Oedipal implications of the previous percepts, while the references to the Negroid face (Card III) and "ape-like faces" (VII, 3) may reflect the continued difficulties in accepting himself as a Japanese. His guilt and ambivalence seem now to be asserted with further vigor in the "fungus" concept (response 4). The word "reminiscence" which Ichiro uses here supports the notion of nostalgia for the mother. Further, the word "multiplying" lends a feminine-reproductive aspect to the flavor of his productions, and appears to express his sentiments concerning women as a "low form of life." The guilt associated with both the Oedipal wishes and the ambivalent feelings toward his mother as a parent and as a Japanese is probably exacerbated because in therapy he must, yet is afraid to, examine his feelings toward her "under a microscope"; this he dreads, lest not only his illusions but his misconceptions and prejudices be shattered.

The nostalgic feelings are given further significance in the light of responses 2 and 2A on Card VIII. The "desert" concept carries the implication of a sense of isolation and, in conjunction with being "posed on a rock," hints that Ichiro may be thinking of leaving therapy. On the other hand, the "ice cream" percept may be expressing the continuing dependency on both mother and therapist, which he simultaneously craves and fights. Since the patient is married, it may be assumed that the strong cross-currents of emotion which whip and cut across the relationship of the patient to the significant female figures in his life would also carry over to the marital situation; the cross-cultural attitudes regarding women would require some re-examination. This would seem all the more true in view of the differing attitudes of Japanese and Americans regarding the expression and experiencing of tender feelings, such as love.

This third Rorschach, then, establishes that some forward moves have been made. In therapy, the patient reported a progressive diminution in the physical symptomatology, and these changes are paralleled in the testing. Although there is no significant change in the total number of responses from the first to the third Rorschach, there is a successive decrease in the number of anatomical concepts, from ten to six to three, a trend continued in the fourth Rorschach. These are replaced with less stereotyped, more individually relevant and personalized responses and, in this sense, represent an increased productivity. Thus, the personality may be said to have changed from a primarily psychosomatic to a largely psychoneurotic orientation; Ichiro no longer needs to be sick to escape unpleasant or fearful situations.

TAT II

And what does an analysis of Ichiro's TAT productions reveal? An interval of more than two years separates the two TAT protocols which the patient gave. In Card 1 of the first TAT (Test Summary E), Ichiro deals with the stimulus material by projecting a "disgusted" boy who must take violin lessons; the issue is acquiescence versus rebellion. In the second TAT (Test Summary F), on the same card, Ichiro views the boy as "discontented" and resenting having to practice, but the urgent matter of a decision to be made between revolt and submission is absent. Both protocols show similar differences on Card 2. Here, reflecting once again the cultural influence, the tradition-versus-progress theme is retained and elaborated, but it has ceased to be a compelling issue.

The differences in 6BM are interesting in that the assent-versus-opposition theme is repeated, although here the overtones pipe out the independence-dependency conflict as well. In the first record the vacillation of the hero leads to no stated decision on the part of the patient as to what course the hero will follow. In the second record he is resolute and assertive, making the forthright decision to break away, and this without tension, hesitation, or remorse.

On the first testing, Card 12M elicits a story of two brothers (different parts or identities of the patient?), one of whom is succumbing to an incurable illness while the other looks on helplessly. On the second testing, this same cards brings forth the story of a father who prays successfully for the restoration to health of his sick son. Cards 7BM and 13MF change in their feeling tone from the first to the second administration; there is a marked decrease in dysphoria, to which the Rorschach has also attested. Over-all comparison of the two protocols reflects diminished conflict, despondency, and hypercriticism on the patient's part, and more comfortable acceptance of himself and others. In short, as conflict is reduced in all spheres his ego identity is clarified and integrated, and his anxiety is lessened to manageable proportions.

The plot for the blank, Card 16, portrays his thoughts and feelings in the fourth phase of treatment, which he entered in the third year of therapy. Entitled "Snowbound," it tells of a tired, hungry man returning home after a long journey "into the unknown reaches of emotional isolation from all that he loved and cared for." During this fourth phase of therapy, Ichiro apparently continued to explore his feelings and attitudes regarding his relationship to others, and he broadened his inquiry to a more intensive examination of sex. Once again, he learned to understand what he had previously tried to ignore, and once again he experienced relief from tension and new emotional growth.

Twenty-one months after his third Rorschach, in the concluding phases of his treatment, Rorschach IV was administered.

FOURTH RORSCHACH

Lest the impression be gained that Rorschach III and TAT II confirm that Ichiro, thanks to therapy, lives happily ever after, the fourth Rorschach should be inspected. This record is striking in several ways. Productivity is significantly up: previous protocols consisting of nineteen to twenty-two responses are now more than doubled, as Ichiro gives forty-nine main responses and one additional. The shift in the psychogram from right to left in successive Rorschachs remains largely stable, and, despite the 150-per cent increase in R, the number of Anatomy responses drops from three to two. The $W:M$ ratio shows some improvement (18:1, 11:1, 15:1, 45:1), and the Manner of

Approach shifts from a preponderance of W per cent (82 to 58 to 75 to 37) to an increase in D per cent (from 14 to 27 to 20 to 43). In terms of quantitative Rorschach rationale, Ichiro thus seems to be becoming more earthbound, less needful to escape into compulsive overorganization, and more comfortable in perceiving the world in many respects as others do—at least as other Americans do.

In content (see Test Summary D) he continues to show some concern with the symmetrical aspects of the blots, suggesting a continuing ambivalence and the likelihood that many doubts remain unresolved despite a lessening of his discomfort in facing them. Perhaps the complete resolution of all doubts and conflicts would be too optimistic an expectation under even the best treatment and tutelage.

The patient seems also to be interacting more with the examiner than heretofore. Although these interactions are partly defensive, there are indications that he feels freer to speak what is on his mind, to channel off some of his anxiety. Somewhat self-conscious about his responses and their possible significance, he is, nevertheless, able to verbalize these candidly now. In the past, when he has seen sexual percepts, he admits that he labeled these "pelvises" in order to hide from the examiner his sexual thoughts; this would account, in part, for the fewer anatomical responses found in Rorschach IV. He is also able to speak more of the violence which he projects into the blots without, apparently, the fear that formerly inhibited him. He also is aware that his productivity is markedly higher than on previous testings and he observes that it probably will "get better as time goes on."

By way of confirmation of the above, an excerpt from a letter which Ichiro wrote to the therapist in his third year of therapy might be pertinent. He states: "Without realizing it, I have harbored an unusual dread of mental tests. And through therapy I find that it goes back to my mother's calling me *baka* (crazy) when, as a little boy, I would cry after experiencing a frustrating incident at the hands of my

father. I was afraid that somehow the tests would sub-
stantiate my being *baka*."

On many of the responses Ichiro's inquiry is longer, too,
as he seems more relaxed and ready to give associations.
Although many of these responses have been given previously, he elaborates them. For example, on Card VII, he
repeats the "ginger root" concept, stating: "If you've seen
ginger root, it has this irregular, swollen shape . . . and you
almost feel there is a certain sponginess texture—almost solid,
but could give if you squeezed it hard . . . Has a pungent
odor and taste. Japanese in particular love it; they grate
it and eat it with fish, sometimes pickle it, use it with a
leaf which gives it a brilliant red color, use it in various
ways in their cookery." Ichiro seems to be "returning
home."

The importance of associations is underscored because
of the differing attitudes and practices regarding human
feelings and their expression. For example, the Japanese,
like the Indians and other Asiatic peoples, do not kiss in
public; the connotations of words like love, caressing, holding, etc., would then have different cultural significance.
The kinds of responses which we would get from persons
with cultural backgrounds foreign to our own need to be
evaluated differently from the way in which we assess the
content of records given by individuals reared in the ways
of the West.

Part of the psychological report written on the basis of
Rorschach IV, but integrating it with all the previous test
data, reads as follows:

> In the past, when the patient could not tolerate the fact that he
> felt rejected, because of his fear that the accompanying anger was
> too dangerous, he pretty much had to avoid seeing women as sexual
> objects. Shy in their presence, he tried to keep his sexual impulses
> out of awareness as he had his aggressive ones. Now that he can
> permit himself more impulse expression, his interest in women as
> sexual objects is growing. He still tends to demean them, but is
> much more involved on an emotional level and less so from an in-
> tellectual point of view. And yet, because hostility related to feel-
> ings of rejection is so interwoven with his sexual feelings, an expres-

sion of his sexual desires produces anxiety. For him, the only comfortable sexual role is a passive one. He has identified masculinity as authoritarian, tyrannical, vain, reprehensible, and ultimately dangerous, because it would turn people against him, just as he had turned against his father. In order to preserve the affection of important figures, he has developed a passive, feminine orientation. In connection with this passive self concept, he wants to be a "kind and generous" father in contrast to the one he has felt his own father was. A very important step he needs to take if therapy is to produce stable results is to learn to understand that it is possible to be an assertive male without being a destructive one. This may enable him to develop the kind of impulse expression which should make further somatization less necessary, as well as to help him to express his anger appropriately without feeling that every outburst is, as his father's had been to him, cruel and unacceptable.

EPILOGUE

It was Ichiro's acute identity-diffusion crisis as a result of the war that eventually led him to seek psychological treatment. In therapy, he learned to understand his feelings better and to gain a greater appreciation of his heritage and his resources. There continue, of course, to be unresolved problems, but the emergency character of his previously more pressing ones have lost their catastrophically threatening implications. We have seen that the sexual area is one of these unresolved foci and that there are continuing conflicts of identification, but their destructive edges have been blunted. The scar of the dual cultural exposure is still a little raw, but the distress it formerly engendered has largely vanished.

The tests carry home the point that this problem of ego identity smolders, but the patient's defenses have apparently become more workable and no longer paralyzing. The test productions in the latter part of treatment, in contrast to the conflict-laden ones during the early period of therapy, reflect the much more satisfactory adjustment which Ichiro has made to the demands that the culture makes on him and that he makes on himself. In the beginning it was apparent that he rejected everything Japanese and overdeveloped his American attitudes and values;

now, he is leaning in the opposite direction. During his Sabbatical year, he plans to go to Japan to study how English is being taught there. Perhaps this is a way in which he will eventually arrive at a middle road which he can travel comfortably, a road he can find and follow more easily with the better acceptance of the reality that there is no all-or-none solution to his problems.

By way of confirmation, significant psychological test impressions—excerpts from several paragraphs written to the therapist toward the end of treatment—might be of value. He says:

> . . . I have been more like my father (whom 1 feared and resented) than I realized. I understood things intellectually but not emotionally. Through therapy I have re-lived, re-experienced, and re-evaluated the past. The process was excruciatingly painful, but out of that pain has come a new understanding (that) is gradually changing my life. Once again I am able to use my mind, my body, and, most important, my emotions constructively and creatively . . . I never realized how totally blind I was to myself . . . I can see that my parents were not solely to blame and that I too had a very vital role in the problem. And perhaps the greatest blind spot I had was that I didn't realize I had a special problem concerning my mother; I thought it was solely my relationship with my father that caused my difficulties. That I had a woman therapist was most fortunate; I almost cancelled my appointment when I learned that instead of a man I was to be treated by a female psychologist . . . I still have periods when I am not fully able to cope with my own powerful emotions, but these are of shorter duration . . . and . . . I can act as my own therapist more now . . . I am making progress in the right direction . . ."

Out of the many hours, months, and years of painful soul-searching, Ichiro has emerged stronger, surer of who he is, and more confident of where he is heading. More self-directed and productive, less rebellious and confused, this man appears to have achieved, as a result of several years of intensive therapy, greater freedom from a harsh, be-devilling, and punitive superego and a larger measure of self-knowledge, self-realization, and emotional tranquillity than he has ever known. He is no longer driven along a divided path.

Test Summary

A. RORSCHACH PROTOCOL I

Response	*Inquiry*

CARD I. 7″

1. That looks like the intestines to me. Sort of like an X-ray of the stomach, the intestines.

1. Entire blot—spinal column—white areas—organs and black and white—grey—suggests another X-ray effect.

W,S   Fk   At

2. Also looks like a gray moth.

2. Markings on wings—feelers here.

W   FC',Fc   A   P

3. Looks like an old-fashioned wood-cut of Mephistopheles. But I think the X-ray is best—spinal column, intestines.

3. The devil in the black and with tremendous wings and in that posture — hands outstretched — demonstrates. (Woodcut?) Simplicity of line. (Black?) Sure black, associated with deviltry.

W   F→M,FC' (H)

CARD II. 23″

1. Looks like identical grotesquely masqueraded characters playing some kind of a game.

1. Seems like—pressing against a mirror—body in black—red head. The mutilated leg is somewhat disturbing. (See the mirror?) No. (Mutilated?) Because fragmentary ends and the startling red in contrast to black.

W   M,FC   (H)

I think a person shouldn't look too long. There are many things. (long pause)
That stump of a leg bothers me. As if it were shattered.
That's a strange configuration. One is a mirror reflection of the other.
He is pressing against a wall, trying to get at something and all he sees is his own reflection.

Part of 1.

Part of 1.

2. V Looks like a man's or woman's pelvic section upside down—looks both male and female. Sort of an empty, empty void in there.

2. Whole thing — ambivalent — sexually male and female.

W,S   F   Sex

Response	*Inquiry*

CARD III. 17″

1. They all have that configuration of the pelvic region with a big colon and something suspended beneath—kidneys—makes me think of an anatomical chart. Did they pick these because I had a stomach condition?

     W   F   At

1. Spinal column, pelvic region—big intestine. Kidneys (center D). What this is suggestion of I don't know. (Kidneys?) Kidney shaped. (Else?) Well, general location but should be higher.

CARD IV. 18″ ⊙

1. ∨ This looks like one of those deep sea creatures—fantastic looking creature, a stingaree I think. Not a pleasant thing.

     W   F   A

1. Doesn't have much meaning unless taken as a whole. (Q) It was similar—had one stinger but this one has a double stinger. One on each side—flappers to propel it through the water; head, eyes. (Being propelled?) No.

It looks like some little known sea animal, eyes, head, two flappers.

Same as 1.

2. It does look like a fragment of animal tissue.

     W   Fc,mF   At

2. (Q) It looks like some organ. The convolution of a tissue. (About?) The shading. It seems like a cylindrical thing split this way (demonstrates).

CARD V. 7″ ∨

1. ∨ Looks like a flying bat. Kind of a moth or butterfly, not a very interesting or pleasant thing to look at. It does have symmetry.

     W   FM   A   P

1. Distantly apparent either way ∧ more bat ∨ more moth.

CARD VI. 8″

1. ∨ Looks like the pelt of some animal.

     W   Fc   A obj   P

1. ∨ Neck region, legs—tail portion here and spotted coloring reminds me of fur.

2. Yet dark straight line looks like some valvular organ that's been split open this way (indicates).

     W   cF,mF   At

2. Same description as IV-2.

Response   *Inquiry*

CARD VII. 13″ V

That doesn't remind me of much. I suppose if a person were to look at it a long time he could get various associations.

1. Looks like a microscopic slide of yeast or something like that (laughs) not a very interesting thing.

   1. Seemed to me—courses in botany —all divisions are something like potato bulbs—one on the other, shading somewhat.

W   cF   Pl

CARD VIII. 30″

1. I think these were all made to suggest some anatomical structure. The right and left symmetry and the color enhances that.

   1. Chart—but also color of organs.

W   C/F→CF   At

2. It looks like two lizards clinging to a rock.

   2. (Usual)

D   FM   A   P

3. Almost like the circulatory system in there.

   3. Artery—blue portion the vein. The artery—exchange of blood (moves hands).

W✕   CF,m   At

4. V This top half up here reminds me of some mixture of ice cream. Strange thought. But I think an anatomical thought is suggestive in all of them.

   4. Bottom D—Scoops of ice cream, orange and strawberries.

D   CF   Food

CARD IX. 40″ V ∧

1. This has that anatomical structure. Spinal column in back and organs suspended on either side.

   1. (Color?) More presentation of the organ, organ with column like vertebrae in the back.

W   CF,mF   At

2. V∧V This part looks like some kind of exposed flesh of some kind.

   2. Just coloring here (bottom D).

D   CF   At

Response	*Inquiry*
3. Just a blot of colored ink—yet there's a column on which these things are suspended (m) some look male and some look female.	3. (Can't) (Male and female?) No, don't remember.

    W   CF   Art,Des

CARD X. 3″ ∨

1. ∨ Like some exotic flower on a stem.	1. Whole thing—like an iris—shape and color—of course no flower has 4 or 5 shades of color—a sectional view.

    W   CF   Pl

2. ∨ Just still suggestive of anatomy. In this case. I think female.	2. (Female?) Pelvic bone and this portion here (top gray).

    W   F   At

3. ∨ This portion, some strangely colored sheep's head—mouth, nose, eyes, horns, ram's head. Symmetry makes them suggestive of so many things. The symmetry gives it whatever significance it has. Otherwise it would be chaotic. Just dabs of color.	3. ∨ Just here—horn (green), eyes (yellow lion); harness over nose (blue); nose (wishbone), and whiskers down here—white color.

    dr,S   F,FC′   Ad

The whole series, something to do with anatomy. The symmetry and the organ. The stomach and intestine region, the lower pelvic region. Some suggest male and female. Some male or female. That's just a generalization. Without the symmetry it wouldn't have much significance. All of these have balance which is pleasing. It doesn't look precarious. This idea of a sheep's head persists. A sort of fiery, angered look.

TESTING THE LIMITS

Best?: X. Very interesting color—symmetry—color composition, more possibilities.

Response	*Inquiry*

Least?: VII. Least suggestive, interesting, meaningful.
Two stacks—by color.
Only part of blot:

III. Some individual bending over a pot.
II. Not much significance (Butterfly?) Not particularly. (People see). Red portion.
V. Not very well (Woman's leg?) Saw okay.
IV. Boot.
VI. Sort of like a pistil < or a turtle (top D).

Test Summary

B. Rorschach Protocol II

Response	*Inquiry*

Card I. 18″

1. In the last test I said it looked something like a spinal column going through.

    W   Fk, FC′   At

2. Also some figure with batlike wings—I don't think it is a very interesting design from a design standpoint. Same symmetry through the card.

    W   F→M,FC′   (H)

1. Suggestion of ribs in through there—the color is like an X-ray negative. (Color?) Films always are gray and black.

2. Small hands—wings—extended—here the body, feet down here—you see some odd pictures of Mephistopheles. I've seen some old woodcuts—sort of dark angel—suggestive of person with wings and outstretched arms. An artist's color of Mephistopheles.

Card II. 15″ I don't know what to think—

1. As I remember quite vividly—looks as if—faint suggestion of pelvic structure in human body. Red portion looks like female anatomy. I would say interesting design.

    W   F   At,sex

2. Mere reflection of some grotesque figure leaning against reflection of itself in the mirror.

    W   M,FC   (H)

1. The whole thing sort of anatomical structure—could be some organ—kidney, or organ with similiar structure on both sides—female genitals here. (What helps give that impression?) The design in this part here.

2. Like some red hooded figures pointing up against its reflection—the foot is shattered here. (Shattered?) Yes, it looks shattered.

Response	*Inquiry*

Card III. 5″

1. All of them faintly suggestive of   1. This part here.
pelvic region. Same symmetry
of design as all of them do.

   W   kF   At

Add. 1.

   W   M,Fm   H   P

Add. 1. Does look like two figures leaning across this fashion sort of mirrored effect—X-ray—red portion could be internal organs but wouldn't come out red on X-ray. 3 figures almost tugging at something in center—girls for some reason. (Q) High heel shoes and fringes of dress —wind is blowing fringe of dress.

Card IV. 5″

1. Like a squid—some deep sea animal.

   W   FC′   A

1. Like some deep sea figure. (What gives the impression?) I recall 10 years ago being on the pier and seeing my brother-in-law bring up something like this—barbed tail—coloration and suggestive outline—just a squid or stingaree—sea turtle maybe.

2. Also looks like some hide from some animal.

   W   FC,FC′   A obj

2. Head, tail, two legs, peeled in that position and looking directly down upon it. (What else helps?) Color too—I've seen fur that color.

Again the horizontal symmetry
or design as all do.

Card V. 3″

1. That looks like some flying object. Could be a bat or some dark moth maybe—doesn't matter which way—upside down. Like some nocturnal insect of some kind.

   W   FM,FC′   A   P

1. Some black moth or flying bat. (Flying?) Yeah.

Card VI. 8″

1. ∧∨ Like the hide from some animal.

   W   Fc   A obj

1. From top—tail down—here—the leg part. (What else helps?)

Response	*Inquiry*
2. ∧ Looks like some tubular organ-like structure that has been shattered and exposed—like mucous membrane in there.	2. This part in here looks like mucous membrane.

D Fc At

Add. 1:

D Fc obj

Add. 1: This is like some feathers, Indian design hung up for display. (Feathers?) Dark tipped.

Add. 2:

Ⱳ FC′,Fc obj

Add. 2: Looks like a fur coat with zipper down center. (Fur?) Dark, gray black coloring—feeling of furriness.

CARD VII. 15″

1. Looks like a map of some island.

 W F Geo.

1. Map of some Pacific island—Borneo or Philippines. (What helps?) (With finger patient marks around the edge of the blot) As I recall my geography it's Borneo or French Indochina.

2. The two figures on the side—faces like two baboons looking at each other from opposite sides—like reflections.

 D FM, FC′ Ad

2. Dark faces. (Dark?) Could be pigmentation.

CARD VIII. 13″

1. These look like two horny toads looking at each other—like some lizard or desert animal.

 D FM A P

1. Except for color look like lizards. (Color?) Just the shape is suggestive.

2. All these ink blots have same column effect as if anatomical in structure. You can get some interesting designs out of ink blot can't you? Almost like a flower design if looked at from a distance, color a little bit off.

2. This part like orchids I've seen in Hawaii.

Add. 1. The consistency here is like scoops of ice cream.

FC Pl   D   D cF, CF food

Response	*Inquiry*

CARD IX. 10"

1. That has a floral design in there —a sectional viewpoint.

   Dr   FC   Pl

1. Cut in section—see the inside of the flower. (Q) Cross section—the pistil, stamens. (In previous one it was color that helped). Yeah, color helps—sure.

2. Again anatomical effect here as of dark ridges.

   Dr   F   At

2. This part in here. (Q) Looks like others do.

3. These two are like kidneys.

   D   F   At

3. These two—the shape.

CARD X. 3"

1. ∧∨ This is a kind of beautiful design—like the composite of various beautiful flowers.

   W   CF   Pl

I think from an artistic standpoint this is the most pleasing in design and color.

1. Exotic flowers you see in tropics— huge flower—various colors. (Parts?) Stem, whole effect—flower effect— pistil — stamens — petals, different colors.

2. ∨ Like some camel's head—nostril and harness.

   S,Dr   FC   Ad

2. Harness coming over the eyes, two yellow eyes and nostrils. (Yellow?) Yeah.

TESTING THE LIMITS

Color on II?: (Shattered feet, blood?) Yes. (Woman's organs?) Don't know.

Texture on IV, VI: No more than given.

Like most: X. (Q) Most colorful.

Like least: IV and VII. (Pick one of these) IV. (Q) Ugly.

Division: II and III, anatomical, others, non-anatomical—flowers, animals, insects, like that.

Sex? No. Male sex organs? No.

Test Summary

C. RORSCHACH PROTOCOL III

Response	*Inquiry*

CARD I. The trouble is (laughing) I remember these very well. 20"

Response	*Inquiry*
1. Looks like a moth. The thing that's amazing is that it's meaningless . . . just one side . . . but the bilateral symmetry gives it meaning.	1. The design as a whole. Definite wings and beginnings of antenna. Spots on back that moths usually have . . . these dark and light here.

W   Fc   A   P

2. (Laughing) I've seen pictures of this as Mephistopheles with this cape—sort of flying figure.

W   M   (H)

2. Hands going like that—not much of a head, but body pretty well defined, and these could be flapping wings there. (Flying?) No, legs together—standing—ready for flight. Add. 1. Does (laughs) look like an X-ray. This light and dark.

W   Fk   At

CARD II. Doesn't matter which way I look at it, does it? 45" ⊖ ⊙ ∧ < ∨ ∧ ∨

1.   This does look like the pelvic region (smiles)—kidneys or something. Anatomic structure anyway.
∧ > ∨ Don't think it's a very pleasing design—just red on black —kind of grotesque.

W   F→FC   At

(Holds back of neck as in pain.)

1. This does look like a human pelvis through there. This red suggests something like organs with much blood supply, although (laughs) that would be a funny place for kidneys.

Add. 1. Taking it this way, it looks (∧) like some grotesque figure pressing against his own image. Something (laughs) must have happened to its foot. I suppose (chuckles) that you can see a lot if you look at it long enough.

W   M   H

CARD III. 25"

1. The red looks like a butterfly— bow tie or butterfly.

D   FC   A   P

2. I think if you look at the entire composition, it looks like an anatomical chart. Intestines coming down thru here. Some organs here on the sides. Seems to me I like to look at it as a whole rather (smiles) than a

1. I think I see some kind of moth or butterfly. (Which?) Possibly a butterfly because it's more brilliant in color.

2. Then again whole composition looks like X-ray of human body, although in X-ray, color doesn't show. (Hums)

Response

Inquiry

particular part of it. Do you want me to spend more time on it—or what?

W   F   At

Add. 1. This could be Negroid face∨ prominent occipital region and head bulging in back. (Q) May be wrong, but looks like dark kinky hair. (Kinky?) More shape of head than anything else, and flattened nose there.

D   F   Hd

CARD IV. 20″

1. ∨ This looks like one of those stingarees (stinger rays?) that my brother and I once caught by mistake in Long Beach.

W   F   A

1. I called these stingarees—I'm not sure—this has two tails, but should have only one. I was gonna grab it and I was warned not to.

2. ∧ Some kind of sea animal.

D   F   A

2. See the nose, eyes. Head is very clear.

3. Then, again, looks like a pelt—some sort of animal skin.

W   Fc   A obj

3. The whole thing. Hind and fore legs. (Skin?) Texture—fur-like texture. (Fur?) Lines across—dark and gray and white texture of the whole.

4. Looks like a pair of fireman's boots (chuckles).

D   F   obj

4. Here. General shape is the only thing.

CARD V. 10″

1. ∨ This looks like a moth—some kind of flying creature—antennae. I've seen organisms like this under the microscope—half of it. Not a pleasing design (laughs).

W   FM   A   P

1. I think it's a flying creature. Could be a bat or moth. Might be a bat. I see wings across here, legs and antenna. Or do moths have antenna? Bats don't. Or—do they? Never seen bats up close. Maybe thinking more of pictures of bats I've seen (hums). (Flying?) Suggestion of flight—there's movement there.

CARD VI. 26″

1. This looks like some kind of animal skin—like kind of work Indians do in the Southwest, this on bottom being some kind of headdress. Looks like tacked on

1. Hunters usually cut down the belly and expose it. Almost feels like furry texture. This could be a tail very well; I guess it could be. And the headfeathers are behind it.

Response

a wall for an exhibition or something like that. (Hums).

W   Fc   A obj   P

Inquiry

I have tendency to see things in wholes (laughs). (Feathers?) Have seen these tacked up in Grand Canyon lodges on walls. (Imp?) Dark tips and lighter consistencies as you go down.

CARD VII. 37"

1. ∨ I've seen ginger root that looks like that. Japanese use that—has a very nice taste (smiles). That's how ginger root looks.

W   F   Pl

1. Sort of formless root that has this kind of texture. (Texture?) Sort of smooth—outline irregular, but surface smooth. (Smooth?) Not too much contrast of light and dark as you would see in that (VI). (Used?) The whole thing.

2. ∧ This part looks like Pacific Islands. I've got a little headache this afternoon—stayed up too early—I'm a confirmed night-owl.

W   F   Geo

2. Map of the South Seas. Japan or the Philippines—string of islands. Could be part of Hawaiian Islands, where I was for some time.

3. ∧ Looks like sort of apelike faces (smiles) facing each other.

D   FM   Ad

3. Just this part here . . . small bee-like eyes, nose and mouth. Looks like reflection as all these blots (laughs) do, because of their symmetry. (Facing?) Yes, maybe looking at each other.

4. ∧ This looks like some kind of organism you see under a microscope—fungus growth or something. (Hits back of neck as if head aches.)

W   Fm   Pl

4. Remembering some lab courses I've taken—some look like that under the microscope, under a slide. Yeast plant looks like that, though not so irregular. Sort of reminiscent (chuckles). Looks like some low form of life under a microscope. (Used?) Whole thing, because these look like several cells in process of multiplying.

CARD VIII. I think this is the nicest from the standpoint of design. 25"

1. ∨ Looks like some kind of tropical flower—that shape, but not quite the same color I've seen in Hawaii. Usually tropical flower more brilliant.

W   FC   Pl

1. Again looking at the whole thing. The stem would come through like that.

Response	*Inquiry*

2. ∧ Looks like lizards or horny toads that you see out on Nevada desert.

W   FM   A   P

2. Just this half here. See that creature up there—four legs and suggestion of face. (How seen?) Seems posed on rock of some kind. Of course see same thing here. (Rock?) Lizard suggested rocks.

Add. 1. Consistency of color reminds me (laughs) of ice cream—combination of orange and strawberry.

D   CF   Food

Add. 2. Looks like ostrich feathers up here—this orange part—feathery look. (Feathery?) Plumes, like folded toward you. (Q) Color, like on women's hats in Gay Nineties.

D   CF→FC   Obj

CARD IX. 9″

1. This looks like a flower also—a cross-section, cut down the center, so you can see the pistil and stamen.

W   FC   Pl

It is interesting what symmetry can do; you can see so many things (laughs). Symmetry's such a wonderful thing: seems to work meaning into something that isn't there. I think the color combination is something not too appealing.

1. Exotic tropical flower—dissected so you can see the pistil and stamen. (Q) Color as well as shape of the part—color primarily I think; this in center suggests stem. This would be petals, stem, colors of stamen.

CARD X. 10″

1. V Looks like some kind of ornate flower—I'm talking about the whole composition, not any particular part. Then, too, it also looks like it's dissected and you can see the pistil and stamen.

W   FC   Pl

1. This one again looks like some very gaudy tropical flower—again sliced through the middle. There (bottom), these at the base, could be embryonic seeds. Fancy multi-colored petals with stamens and pistils showing here.

2. V And in here, camel's head, with eyes, nose, and harness over its nose (laughs).

dr   F   A   O

2. Nostrils, bridle fitting over nose, head gear. This (green) might be fitting over the forehead, too.

TESTING THE LIMITS

Best? This (X) one. (Why?) Because it reminds me of exotic tropical flower and I have many pleasant associations with Honolulu and the Hawaiian Islands.

Least? Well, that's tough. Seems to me this one (II) I liked least. It's suggestive of violence. You do have that blood color and you do have that shattered look there (laughs), as if bleeding (vaginal area of II), and it does look unpleasant.

Humans? Well this (I) Mephistophelean figure here. (Other?) Two figures leaning across, here, maybe tugging (III) at something. And these apelike figures (VII) could by a stretch of the imagination be human.

Sex organs? Oh—this (II) could very well be. The red. And this part (middle D on II) could be almost like the male organ there. I guess that's the only ones that are. (VI?) This long part might conceivably be. (VII?) Not too much. (Vaginal area VII?) I suppose it could be with stretch of the imagination. (What would it be?) More suggestive of female than male I guess, though it gives both suggestions.

Test Summary

D. RORSCHACH PROTOCOL IV

Response	*Inquiry*
CARD I. 25″ Trouble is I see about the same thing.	
1. V Seems like a beetle of some kind—or a moth.	1. Whole. (How do you see it?) As I say, there is symmetry—these could be wings—these conceivably could be the antenna—very short but nevertheless suggestive of one.
W F A P	
∧ The thing that gets me about the Rorschach is that while they are just blots, the fact that because they are symmetrical, there seems to be more—because of the bilateral symmetry—seems to be more than just the blot.	
2. ∧ Looks like a bat in some ways. (Pause.)	2. (Something special about the blot made it look like a bat?) I suppose the color—suppose there's a lot of feeling goes with colors and black is associated with bats. (Don't you like bats?) I don't recall any experience with bats but I guess something you pick up from reading—associated with darkness, dimness, mystery.
W FC′ A P	
＞∨☺ I suppose if you looked at this for any length of time, you could see anything.	

Response

3. Looks like these are little musical notes around here (laughs, points) somehow—

dd   F→FC'   Art

This Rorschach is an interesting test (laughs). You're projecting yourself into something here.

Inquiry

3. (FC' only additional.) If I see something else, I can mention it? (Do you see anything else?) Add.: I see a female figure—legs here—hips—body. Seems she has her hands up in this fashion (gestures). (Which way is she facing?) With her back towards us—and her hands like this. These are her thumbs— only this doesn't look like her head (laugh). Could be wearing a cape (gestures a high collar) like the nuns wear.

D   M   H, Clothes

CARD II. 15"

1. You know the simple contrast between the black and the red—it seems to—it seems to convey a feeling of violence somehow (laughs) of blood.

W   Csym→   Blood, H
          CF, M

(Puts card flat on table.)

1. (Was this a concept or just a comment—you mentioned blood?) Yes—suggestion of blood—and this part (pointing to red lower area) looks almost like a bleeding wound of some kind—these (covers half of the blot) could be human figures— red head—crushed here. (Do you mean the head is crushed?) No, down here. (The red head then is just to locate the head and not blood on the head?) Yes. (How do you see the figure?) Actually two figures —actually grotesque, but with a stretch of the imagination—could look like human figures. (Any kind of . . . ?) One foot raised (raises his foot), hand up.

2. This part here (pointing) looks like a moth or butterfly.

D   FC   A

2. (Butterfly or moth?) This is the suggestion of wings. (Shape then?) And color—butterflies are more brilliant than moths.

3. ∧ Like the skin of animals— somehow (pointing to the two black areas).

WX   Fc,FC'   A obj

3. (Animal skins?) General shape— texture. (Texture?) This murky black—and white—black and gray (uses FC' black and silver as well as Fc, but can't tell which is more prominent).

4. > This does look like the human pelvis in through here. (Studies

4. (Pelvis?) This looks like the pelvic bone and this looks like the

Response	*Inquiry*
card for a long time.) I think a person could read too much into these things (laughs). W⁺,S F At→Sex	area where . . . (pointing to white space in center). This looks like the hip bone. (Just the shape?) Yes— (Does this have anything to do with it—lower D?) Well, this is funny— it's a female pelvis this way (upright), and male this way (upside down). And this could be some internal organs (color denied).

CARD III.   8″ V

1. ∧ Looks sort of like a bow tie here (laughs).

    D   F→FC   Clothes   P

1. Shape only, though could be a red bow tie.

2. This portion here looks sort of like a negroid head (laughs). Two of them.

    D   FC′   Hd

2. Shape as well as color—I may be mistaken but it seems to be large in the back—is that characteristic? (I don't know.) Seems to be rather large—melon-shape—that may not be true at all.

∧ 30″ > V ∧

3. ∧ Looks like two women somehow—facing each other—I suppose we could look at the whole as well as part, can't we? (Hm Hm) Whatever—(holds card at distance, turns it around, puts on desk).

    W⁺   M,Fm   H, Clothes P

3. (Tell me about it.) Well, they're . . . hard to say what they're doing —suggestion of a head—suggestion of a body—leg—skirt—shoes. (How do you see it?) Seems like a terrific wind blowing from the back. (What do you mean?) Like they're bracing themselves from the wind, skirt blowing.

4. V This part here looks something like a gopher—some kind of animal.

    dr   F   Ad

4. Where did I see that? (Studies card.) That part there—hmmmm— can you conceive of an animal head there? (Shows card to me.)

5. This portion here looks something like an X-ray, you know.

    D,S   kF   X-ray

5. (X-ray?) Oh—X-rays are usually black and white and gray (outlines with white spaces).

6. ☉ ∧ Looks like a mask somehow— when you look at it from a . . .

    W, S   F   Mask

6. (Mask?) Now this is going to take some imagination. I'm taking all this in its entirety (the white ground). These could be suggestion of eyes—this nose—this mouth,

Response

Inquiry

Maybe I'm taking too much time on these. (Don't push yourself to see things, but take as much time as you need.) I think I feel a little more comfortable than the other times—was more in a rush the other times.

huh? (Yes.) This could be outline of head—way you look at it.

CARD IV. 13″ > ∨ > ∧

1. ∧ This is like an animal fur of some kind.

1. Whole—shape, texture.

   W   Fc   A obj

2. ∨ This (runs fingers several times around the center lower D) is some kind of a head—could be reptile, could be animals.

2. Can see the eyes—the suggestions of the nose here.

   D   F   Ad

(Studies card, turns it several times.)

3. ∧ Looks like a boot (studies card). I can't (laughs) tell much more about that . . .

3. Well, the boot portion is—doesn't look much like a boot but could be —I suppose.

   D   F   Clothes

CARD V. 5″ ∨ ′

1. ∨ Now this looks like an insect flying of some kind—moth—bat— looks like the antenna of some kind of an insect (shows me card briefly).

   W   FM,FC′   A   P

2. ∧ Looks like the drumstick (laughs) of a chicken here (covers all of the blot except the lateral extension.)

2. (Shape.)

   d   F   Food

3. Like a pair of tweezers in here.

3. (Shape.)

   d   F   obj

Response

4. **>** Looks like kind of a laughing man with a goatee (laughs), if you look at it from this angle.

D   M   Hd

I suppose you can cut off sections and look at it, can't you? (Yes.) I have a tendency to see things in their entirety. Profile of a man with a Roman nose, a high-bridged nose. Seems to have a long, flowing beard.

CARD VI. 8″ ☺

1. This looks like the skin of some animal. (Covers lower part.) Like the feathers of some bird up here. Somehow reminds me of a hunting lodge—skin stretched on the wall, some kind of a trophy, huh?

W   Fc   A obj   P

2. (Covers part.) This looks like a jacket with a zipper up the front (rubs card with finger). This has sort of a fleecy texture—like wool.

Fc   Clothes

3. Like a puppy's head up here.

d   F   Ad

4. **V** (Laughs) Could look like a scarecrow in a field.

W   F   (H)

(You have a good imagination.) Not good enough, I think. (It's much better than it was at the time of the other tests. I should think it would get better as time goes on.)

CARD VII. 25″ **V∧** (Patient talks with me about the indefinite form and how it promotes associations.)

Inquiry

4. (Goatee—shape only.)

1. Whole, and the texture. (Feathers?) They do look like feathers—and in hunting lodges when people want to boast—display their trophies—they have stuffed birds on them.

2. Just the line is important for the zipper.

3. Let's see (a little difficulty finding it but ultimately does.)

4. (Holds card at distance.) Using imagination—have a pole with old clothes stuck on it—like some farmers do in the Mid-West.

Response	*Inquiry*

1. Λ This looks like a map of some islands here.

    D   Fk   Map

1. (One-half the blot is covered.) Could be map of the Philippines—or Hawaiian Islands—Japan—just looks like an aerial view there.

2. Looks like some monkeys (laughs) facing each other.

    dr   Fc   Ad

2. (Covers all but the faces.) (Monkeys rather than people?) Bulging eyes—dark muzzle—like fur instead of skin—hair instead of skin.

3. Two people with coonskin hats on (laughs).

    D   M,Fc   Hd,Clothes

3. (Furry caps—how did you see it?) Substituting people for baboons or monkeys—tail of the cap flipped up. (Flipped up by movement of the people or wind like on the other one?) No suggestion of wind here—nodding of the head.

4. V Looks like two can-can dancers doing an act here (laughs).

    W   M   H

5. When I look at this, I get the feeling it's bitter cold somehow—can see these little icicles hanging down (laughs).

    d   F→Fm   Ice

5. (Icicles?) For instance, I lived in Chicago for a couple of years—as the day warms up, they start to drip. (Hang?) Solidly fixed—no danger of small ones like that falling off. (What about this one, the large one?) Large one—broken off with little ones forming on it. If these were the eaves of the house, I think these would be pretty solidly attached.

6. > Look at it this way—looks like an elephant—with trunk.

    D   F   Ad

6. Suggestion of an eye here and trunk here.

Maybe I see too much animals, huh? (No.) (Some card turning and then after 50″:)

7. < You go in these oriental stores —you see dried ginger root—this looks like portions of dried ginger root.

    W   Fc   Food

7. Whole. If you've seen ginger root, it has this irregular, swollen shape. (Shape then?) Shape, and you almost feel there is a certain sponginess—texture—almost solid but could give if you squeezed it hard.

Response	*Inquiry*
	(What do you think of in connection with ginger root?) Ginger root has a pungent odor and taste; Japanese in particular love it—they grate it and eat it with fish, sometimes pickle it—use it with a leaf which gives it a brilliant red color —use it in various ways in their cookery.
8. This portion looks like a Scottish terrier of some kind.	8. (Form only.) Could be one here, too (pointing to lower center section). (Are they related in some way?) Two distinct forms.
D F A	

CARD VIII. 30″ Some card turning. It's amazing what the introduction of color does on an ink blot like this.

1. Looks like an exotic flower that I see in the Hawaiian Islands.

   W   CF   Pl

2. On top looks like ostrich feathers.	2. This has that feathery quality— up here (flicks card). (What do you mean?) Combination of color —and density of color.
D FC,Fc A obj	

3. > Looks like some kind of an animal, doesn't it? (Yes.) Ready to spring—like some red-furred animal—if there is such a thing.

   D   FM   A   P

4. Parts look like coral that you see in the islands.	4. Particularly in here—you see this colored coral in various parts of the country. (FC and Fc.)
D FC,Fc N	

5. In through there looks like the skeleton of a fish.

   D,S   F   AAt

6. (Laughs.) Seems funny but this has texture of raspberry sherbet —mixed with orange sherbet—up here—has that kind of texture.	6. If you've ever scooped it out of a bowl—it has that consistency— gives a sort of dippled (*sic*) effect.
D CF,cf Food	

Response   *Inquiry*

You know, it's amazing—you look at it from the side—get something different when you turn it around. This Rorschach test is an ingenious device. Maybe a person tells more about himself than he realizes, huh? (Laughs.) (Patient looks at watch.) (Do you have an apointment?) No, am I taking too much time? (No —not at all.) Thought maybe you had something else to do.

CARD IX. 14″

1. This portion—this looks like a flower that's been cut through— see the pistils and the stamens here (shows me card). Looks like a big tropical flower of some kind.

    W,S   CF   Pl

2. Bits of coral.

    dr   CF   N

3. (Points to upper D) This looks like parts of a lobster—boiled lobster color but not that vivid.

    d   FC   Food

4. In here looks like a crocodile—in sort of a marshy place.

    D   FK,CF   Ad

5. V>V Seems like I see something like—what kind of bird you call it—a crane maybe—tilted—with its neck tilted back.

    D   FM   A

CARD X. 15″ V This is—this is kind of an interesting design.

1. V Looks almost like an iris—like an exotic iris in through here.

    W   FC   Pl

1. (Stamens and pistils?) Here and here—suggestion of seeds in here.

2. Places like this (green upper edge)—they're jagged. This could be that pinkish coral (orange D).

3. Primarily this part (extensions). Color and shape, huh?

4. (Marshy?) I associate sort of a gray-green with marshland—decayed gray-green vegetation. (Laughs.) Brown, stagnant water.

5. Where did I see that? This is the claw—this the breast—and the head somewhere in here—tilted back (tilts head).

1. Whole thing. (The whole thing looks like an iris?) I shouldn't say iris—some large—bloom—hardly see a flower with so many colors in it.

Response	*Inquiry*
2. Looks like blue crabs of some kind (laughs).	2. (Have you seen blue crabs?) No (laughs). (That's kind of whimsical—they just happen to be blue, huh?) Yes—don't know if anybody else has seen blue crabs either (laughs). They're in the same class as pink elephants. I think.
D F A P	

3. $>\wedge$ See some kind of a camel here—(shows me). Eyes here—something here (blue D in center) —nose here—nostrils.

S,dr   F   Ad

4. These yellow look like some kind of flower I've seen in Hawaii.

D   FC   Pl

4. Yellow flower here and here (all four yellow areas) coming out— horny leaf-like structure which encloses the bud and the flower just beginning to bloom.

5. This green part looks like parts of a flower—foliage of some kind.

D   CF   Pl

6. Looking at it from here (holds card at arm's length), looks like a lot of marine animals climbing up a coral reef. These look like blue crabs—sea horses—jelly fish. (Puts card down.)

W   FM,FC,Fc N

6. Sea horses. These are indefinite shapes—could be some kind of sea creature without definite form (referring to jelly fish).

This is the most interesting of the group. (Why?) It's more complex in design. Instead of one or two colors, you have five colors here—instead of all together it's spread out and yet you have the bilateral symmetry so it gives a complex design. (Picks card up again.) You know I never noticed what an effect simple symmetry has on a person—you have design. There is purpose— and then the working in of the colors. Interesting thing, this Rorschach test—a progression from simplicity to complexity.

Response   *Inquiry*

Do you always give them in this
order? I wonder if the intention
is to go from the least complex
to the most complex—from the
least colorful to the most colorful.

Testing the Limits

Least? (Long pause.) Well, this (V) is least interesting from the standpoint of design—lacks qualities which stir the imagination—simple black.
(Also pushed together into the solid form?) Yes—these are diffuse, capable
of being looked at from various points—this doesn't offer much to the
imagination.

Test Summary

E. Thematic Apperception Test I

Card 1.

He's very disgusted that he has to play the violin. I think . . . he's
looking . . . he doesn't know whether to be happy or sad in this
situation . . . that he has to study the violin. Possible the mother
and father had musical ambitions when they were young and tried
to project their ambitions onto the boy. The outcome will be either
complete acquiescence or open rebellion. (Most likely?) Equally
likely. It would depend on the kid's personality. If he's a serene
acquiescing nature he will probably continue lessons; if defiant, he
will stop. (Which is he?) He looks like the acquiescent type to me.

Card 2.

It seems to me that this tells the story of two childhood friends . . .
girls who grew up to young womanhood and they . . . I think
. . . the setting is undoubtedly one in which most of the population followed the soil. When they grew up one followed the age-old
tradition of being a farmer's wife . . . raising her children in the
old tradition. The other girl was influenced by the modern times
and went to school. In the scene they meet rather unexpectedly.
The girl who follows the old folkways has a look of indifference . . .
mixed with a look of defiant haughtiness, I would say . . . and the
girl in the foreground looks more sorrowful and sad that old friendships have been broken up through no fault of her own. Sort of an
intelligent looking girl . . . emotionally stable I would say. Determined to follow her own bent. I think that if she leaves the country
and finds others who share her interests she will make a resounding

success. Otherwise I think she will end up mighty unhappy. The very rigidity of the furrows seems to suggest the age-old tradition out of which she springs. So I think basically the picture suggests a conflict in the minds of the two young people . . . "Shall I follow the age-old tradition or shall I break away and assert myself." I think one girl shows quiet acquiescence to her way of life with some pride in her husband tilling the soil. The other girl doesn't show any sign of disdain at her past life but only a sort of sadness that childhood friends have to have a parting of the ways sooner or later. A very powerful picture, I think. Who painted it? Grant Wood? Definitely European.

CARD 3BM.

A very poignant picture. This girl shows that she has had an immense capacity of suffering in silence. But years of suffering have been too much for her; she has reached the breaking point. She is about to commit suicide, but the pistol has dropped from her grasp as she suffers silent agony. But I feel that she will have the fortitude to emerge from this despair and resolve her dilemma.

CARD 4.

There is a definite melodramatic artificiality about this picture. Both are studying for effect. It is the typical screen hero, tempted by a seductress, but triumphs in the end. Not very impressive.

CARD 6BM.

This picture suggests that age-old idea of the Oedipus-complex—a grown man, torn between love and veneration for his mother and his own private desires and needs. He is a confused and unhappy young man. On the one hand he sees his aged and graying mother who disapproved of what he contemplates; on the other he feels that he must live his own life. The outcome is uncertain. He will openly rebel; he will acquiesce completely; or, he will attempt a half-hearted compromise which will prove to be unsatisfactory in the end.

CARD 7BM.

This story is basically the same as the one above, only the father is substituted for the mother.

CARD 8BM.

This picture can be interpreted in two different ways: (1) It is the story of wide-eyed youth. He has just graduated high school, and he contemplated a career of being a great doctor, a great humanitarian, who performs his deeds of mercy under the most adverse circumstances—and triumphs! (2) The other side of the picture is this: He dreams of a successful medical career. However, he is somewhat confused, although he is not quite conscious of his confusion. He sees himself brilliantly successful, but the gun in the foreground seems to suggest the painter's attempt to show the young man's dilemma. Instead of the youth being the successful surgeon; he might be the victim of modern warfare.

CARD 9BM.

This is a picture of lethargy. Grown and toughened men are seen resting after hard manual labor. They are like stolid animals. They have accepted their lot in life and do not attempt to better their condition. The youth in the left-hand corner sees the men in sleep. What does life hold for him—that is the question in his mind.

CARD 9GF.

This appears to be a picture from a modern short story, serialized in some woman's magazine. It is somewhat over-dramatized. The picture suggests a sort of moonlight rendezvous on the beach; all did not go well; the young lady departs in haste; another woman—possibly the wife of the man in question secretly witnesses the scene.

CARD 10.

A sort of artificial and posed love-making. Could be a still scene from a classic drama. On the other hand, it suggests a serene and mature love which comes from two people's sharing many experiences over a long life time.

CARD 11.

This picture is a little uncertain. It reminds me of a scene from an old myth. It seems that a monster of huge dimensions is emerging from a cave, causing men and horses to scatter in fright. It holds no particular appeal to me.

CARD 12M.

Here is a picture of two brothers, who apparently were very close to each other. The painter depicts the sorrow and despair of one brother, looking on helplessly as the other sinks down under an incurable illness.

CARD 13MF.

"And her bought red lips were sweet . . . but I have been faithful to thee, Cyanara, in my own fashion." Here is a youth—a student, who, it seems, was brought up in a rather puritanical manner. He has the natural curiosity concerning sex and women. His curiosity and desire are finally satiated, but instead of the glowing experience he thought it would be, he finds himself torn by remorse. This story would be plausible, but the woman concerned seems too static, too oblivious to his predicament. Could he have killed her?

CARD 13B.

Here is the typical Horatio Alger Jr. setting of from a log cabin to the White House. But I see only squalor and despair in the picture. The child's chances for a brilliant future seem to be foredoomed by his environment.

CARD 14.

A somewhat startling picture of contrast at first glance. I suppose it was the author's intention to show the hopes and desires of youth at the open window, while his surroundings are complete darkness.

CARD 15.

A very startling and interesting picture. This scene reminds me of the old story of Faustus. The tragedy of Faustus was that he desired power, wealth, beauty—everything that most men long for; he desired, above all, power over other people. This power gave him a greater sense of self-realization. But in his lust for power and wealth, he did not temper his desires with love. Thus, he not only caused his own downfall, but destroyed all those with whom he dealt. This picture could very well be Faustus in old age, viewing the many many lives he ruined, and in the ruining, he shackled his own growth and development. Thus, the painter dramatically shows an old man shackled by his own lovelessness, surrounded by those he destroyed.

CARD 17BM.

This picture has little appeal to me. It simply depicts a gymnast, climbing a rope in competition.

CARD 18GF.

A rather poignant picture. Here, it seems to me, we have a scene between mother and daughter. It is somewhat akin to the return of the Prodigal Son, only this is between erring daughter and forgiving mother. There is both sorrow and love etched in the pained face of the mother, and in the abject posture of the daughter, we see remorse, hopelessness, and yet a spark of hope in the forgiveness of the mother.

CARD 18BM.

This is a highly interesting picture, highly dramatized for effect. Here we see a youth apprehended. The youth has a sensitive, intelligent look. And his dress suggests that he is the poor-student, turned criminal sort of thing. Here is a youth who has much promise, but through perhaps his intellectual pretensions, he found it difficult to make proper adjustments. Thus, frustrated, he turns to crime. The picture shows his apprehension. His face shows both resignation and defiance.

Test Summary

F. THEMATIC APPERCEPTION TEST II

CARD 1. "Boyhood Discontent."

It seems that the boy in the picture is being forced to take violin lessons. He is a picture of discontent. Perhaps he is thinking of the fun the gang is having while he must stay in and absorb "culture." Perhaps he has parents who feel that inasmuch as they (the parents) lacked the opportunity and the leisure to take music lessons, they would like to see to it that their son would be given that which they were denied.

CARD 2. "Midwestern Primitive."

This picture seems to depict *tradition* vs. *progress* or to contrast two attitudes toward life: (1) An attempt to get away from the small rural areas, and (2) Pride in living like one's forebears—close to the soil. Two girls—possibly close friends pose each other. One, attending a college or university, looks on with mixed emotions; the other, haughty that she has the strength and stability of home, husband and land, looks askance at her sophisticated friend.

CARD 3BM. "The Well of Loneliness."

The girl seems to be suffering some great sorrow—so great that she must cry alone in her room. It reminds me of Radcliffe Hall's *Well of Loneliness* or Ilka Chase's *In Bed We Cry*. The pistol at her side shows that her despair is such that she even contemplates suicide.

CARD 4. "Jealousy."

It seems that the young man is filled with jealousy, or simply blind rage. At any rate, it seems that she is attempting to calm him down and persuade him to stay. Her carefully plucked eyebrows and artfully shaped lips suggest many things. Could she be a nurse? Actress? Prostitute? It is difficult to say, and the picture in the background is baffling.

CARD 3GF. "Despair."

This picture reminds me of a Biblical tract I still have in my possession. Many years ago I worked in a market at night, and I always transferred street cars on Fifth and Main Streets. I saw a gathering of people, and I elbowed myself to the front. A young Salvation Army worker handed me a tract. Automatically I put it in my pocket. The next day I found it and was about to throw it away, but a most lovely poem called "Beautiful Snow" arrested my attention. It told a poignant tale of a girl who had *fallen*—you know the rest. The picture depicts one of the fallen, it seems, and she staggers under the weight of shame and sorrow.

CARD 6BM. "Conflict."
This picture seems to indicate that the two—mother and son—have had some rather bitter words, and this is goodbye. The mother is a widow who sacrificed to send the young man through college. He has been a devoted son, but now he has decided that he will get married and live without her. She feels neglected and alone; he feels torn between love for his mother and love for his sweetheart. But he is resolute. He will leave, but provide for her necessities.

CARD 7BM. "Youth and Age."
It seems that the two might represent father and son. By the way the older man keeps his hair and trims his moustache, I'd say he is a European, born in Germany or perhaps France. The young man, of course, is American born. There is a chasm between them because of their different backgrounds and education. There have not been violent outbursts, but rather a series of disagreements extending over many years. However, as the son grows up he learns that underlying their many disagreements, is *love*. His reactions to his father have been magnified and distorted. Now he understands. *Schluss*.

CARD 12M. "The Believer."
It seems that a humble farmer's boy lies ill. The father, knowing nothing but a blind faith in God and God's ability to make all things work together for good, kneels in compassionate prayer for his son's recovery. And the humble, untutored father's prayers of faith are abundantly fulfilled. The son is healed.

CARD 13B.
It seems that this little boy's parents live in the South as sharecroppers. They live in very sordid surroundings. I would like to paint that golden picture of a typical Horatio Alger, Jr. here—"from rags to riches"—but this little boy is shaped by his environment. He will not leave his way of life. He will continue to live the life of toil and hardship which his parents knew.

CARD 13MF. "Lust for Life."
This is a sensitive young man who has ambition. He attends college away from home. Day after day he burns the midnight oil. Day after day he resists "the temptations of the flesh." But one night, right after a tough exam, he is walking in the crowded section of South Chicago, and he meets a girl. To his amazement he is saying and doing things which are entirely alien to his nature. He has invited her up to his apartment! After he has satisfied his longing, he is remorseful. He is tormented by pictures of sacrificing parents and brothers and sisters at home. He steadies himself. In the end, this

scene will fade; he will achieve success, but the memory of this evening will cause him qualms of guilt.

CARD 15. "The Lost Leaf."

This picture depicts a man who has long outlived his usefulness. He has also outlived all his friends and associates. Often he comes to the graveyard to mourn and reminisce over the graves of those whom he loved. His shackled hands suggest his slavery to the past and to past traditions and ideas. He is a symbol of a rigid, unchanging personality who clings desperately to old ideas and customs—not because he believes them to be true, but more because he is afraid of new things and new situations.

CARD 18GF. "Mother, Dear Mother."

The young lady in the picture seems to be quite alone in the world except for a little baby perhaps. She has lost her husband, and comes to her old mother for consolation and advice. The mother, who seems to be of old immigrant stock, and who has seen and experienced many tragic things, consoles her daughter. They decide to move away, forget the past, and begin again.

CARD 16. "Snowbound."

It seems that both earth and sky are filled with white, falling snow. Animate and inanimate objects are thickly covered with a thick blanket of new fallen snow. There is a muffled silence in the air, and on the totally white landscape, there is a figure walking briskly with back bent toward the storm. He is on his way home after a long, long journey. He is tired. He is hungry He is aching to see his loved ones on this Thanksgiving Day.

Night descends, and he is still trudging through the silent, dark night. And suddenly he sees a light! It comes from a comfortable cottage, surrounded by stately trees. He is home! The young man sees his little family through the windows. He knocks. They smother him with hugs and kisses. He is home, comfortable and safe, after a long and perilous journey into the unknown reaches of emotional isolation from all that he loved and cared for.

17

Personal and Cultural Factors in Treating a Nisei Man

Charlotte G. Babcock and *William Caudill* [1]

All men are in a sense the same, but the settings—both personal and cultural—in which they work out their problems are various, and hence their solutions to these problems differ. A somewhat more technical way of saying this is that the nature of psychological defenses and the integration of these within the personality exhibit a wide range of variation in all cultures, but the distribution of personality types within this range is differently patterned from one culture to another.

The case presented here is of a young man of Japanese-American background. The patient was referred for problems of apathy, loneliness, and depression. He was in psychoanalysis for two years. The rich and lengthy clinical material produced during treatment cannot be presented in all its many aspects here, and since this is a book on the effects of culture on psychopathology, less will be said about what this patient shared with all men, and more will be said about his personal version of the cultural background from which he came and how this entered into his treatment.

---

[1] The case material presented here was gathered as part of an inter-disciplinary study (mainly during 1947–51) of the personal and cultural adjustment of Japanese-Americans to life in Chicago, and reported elsewhere. The senior author served as psychotherapist for the patient in this study.

What follows is divided into three parts. First, we shall give something of the background of the Japanese-American group to which the patient belongs. Secondly, we shall present a summary of the case. Thirdly, some of the points referred to in the case summary will be taken up for more extended discussion in terms of the family, the relations between older and younger brothers, the patient as a person and his interpersonal life as an adult, and some aspects of the relations between the analyst and the patient. Within these limits, and without attempting to follow the conflicts presented to their ultimate resolution in the therapy, our discussion is meant to stimulate, rather than to exhaust, thinking in these areas.

CULTURAL BACKGROUND

The patient in whom we are interested here is a second generation Japanese-American, or Nisei. From his childhood, his family was somewhat better off than the average, and the patient himself more consciously determined in his struggle to find a satisfying and mature identity than was true for most Nisei. However, in many ways the structure and dynamics of this man's family can represent much of what would be found in any family composed of Issei parents and Nisei children. The life of the Japanese-American has its roots not only in the United States but also back in Japan itself. What is the history of this group?

EARLY ARRIVALS. The early Japanese immigrants arriving about the turn of the century began to call themselves *Issei* to distinguish themselves from their American-born children whom they called *Nisei*.

They did not come to the United States with permanent residence in mind. They intended to make money and return to Japan. By federal law they were ineligible for United States citizenship. Their own language was very different from English, which they had great difficulty with and felt no urgency to learn unless their occupation compelled them to do so. Even after many men acquired wives from Japan, often as "picture brides," and established a family, their eyes were turned toward Japan and they frequently sent their children back to Japan for education. These American-born, Japanese-educated children are known as the *Kibei* or "returned."

WAR RELOCATION. The United States entered World War II after the Japanese attack on Pearl Harbor at the close of 1941. Early in 1942 all persons of Japanese ancestry, alien Issei and American citizen Nisei, were hastily evacuated from the Pacific Coast and placed behind barbed wire in what certainly must have appeared to Japanese-Americans to be concentration camps. These people were the only ones singled out for such marked treatment as a group without any reference to their loyalty as individuals to the United States. A few families were able to avoid this experience by independently moving to inland cities and towns. The family of the patient discussed here was fortunate in being among these few.

CONGRUENT VALUES. After the war, many Nisei settled in the Chicago area where no precedent of prejudice had previously been established, and where they became extraordinarily successful in adapting themselves to the middle-class standards of the Caucasian population. Contrasting with the situation in many other minorities, there seems to be a significant compatibility, but by no means identity, in the value systems found in the culture of Japan and the value systems of the American middle class. This compatibility of values gives rise to a similarity in the psychological adaptive mechanisms which are most commonly used by individuals in the two societies as they go about the business of living. The Japanese and American middle-class cultures share the values of politeness, respect for authority and parental wishes, duty to community, diligence, cleanliness and neatness, emphasis on personal achievement of long-range goals, importance of keeping up appearances, etc.

There is no implication, however, that the social structure, customs, or religion of the two societies are similar.

They are not, and Japan and middle-class America differ greatly in these respects. Nor may we infer that the basic personality or character structure of Japanese and middle-class American individuals is similar. The main thing is that both Japanese and middle-class Americans characteristically utilize the adaptive mechanism of being highly sensitive to cues coming from the external world as to how they should act, and that they also adapt themselves to many situations by suppression of their real feelings, particularly desires for physical aggressiveness.

Given this sort of relationship between the two cultures, when they meet under conditions favorable for acculturation, Japanese-Americans acting in terms of their Japanese values and personality will behave in ways that are favorably evaluated by middle-class Americans. Nevertheless, because the values and adaptive mechanisms are only compatible (and not identical), and because the social structures and personalities of the two groups are different, there are many points of conflict as well as agreement for the Nisei individual attempting to achieve in American middle-class life.

CONTROLLING MECHANISMS. A common defense against anxiety was the mechanism of separation—the failure to make a contact rather than to betray anxiety or to cause oneself to lose face in any way. The Nisei client, pushed to the social agency under the stress of relocation, always thanked the worker for what she offered, but if he felt any embarrassment, which was often unrecognized by the worker, he simply did not return again. Thus, when the worker offered more than the individual could accept, namely put him under too great an obligation, the anxiety became so great that it was handled by breaking the contact. In many cases, because of the façade resulting from the value that feelings should not be shown openly since this would be a sign of weakness or lack of self-control, rather deep pathology was often overlooked. For example, in the case reported in this paper, it was only in the second year of analysis that the deep guilt compatible with the presenting problems came out in the open. This guilt was by no means entirely repressed. The patient knew about it consciously but the defenses were so strong, and the penalty of shame so great if he were to reveal what he really thought, that he could not talk about what was known to him sooner.

All Japanese-Americans must meet the problems of shame and rigid control of feelings, and the many sources of these patterns of behavior lie in the culture of Japan. The stress placed on close conformity to the rules for behavior in Japanese culture does not mean that the Japanese are an emotionless people. The Japanese have adequate emotional resources, but at the same time these feelings are ruthlessly suppressed in many areas of life. Emotions are freely, even ebulliently, expressed in recreational pursuits, but in the serious areas of life concerned with vocational and family matters, conformity to obligations and suppression of emotions are mandatory.

AGE AND SEX ROLES. In Japanese culture the individual is less the unit of society than the family, which is all important. In theory, the individual scarcely exists as such; he achieves his identity only as a member of certain larger groupings such as the family, school, community, or nation. In Japan there are many types of hierarchy but the most fundamental are those of age and sex. The authority of the parents tends to continue throughout life, and age carries with it great prestige and power. Women are subordinate to men and tend to follow the Chinese dictum that a woman obeys her father in her childhood, her husband in middle life, and her son in old age. This particular dictum will be seen to be crucial in understanding the role of the mother in both the psychological and cultural dynamics of the family of the patient discussed in this paper.

CHILD DISCIPLINE. Traditionally, in Japan, the discipline of the child is in the mother's hands, the father remaining a somewhat distant figure toward whom the child must learn to show respect. The main teaching and disciplinary techniques are teasing and ridicule—physical punishment is not often used. The oldest male child is the most favored because he must later carry the heaviest responsibility for the family. Male children in general are more favored, but, on the other hand, they are the ones who will later have the most direct contact with the outer world and who will be the most vulnerable. If there is no male child, the oldest daughter is often taught that she must, to a considerable extent, take on responsibility for the family as if she were a male.

As a child grows older he must learn an ever-increasing number of restraints which require subordinating his will to duties, to neighbors, to family, and to country. These obligations are communicated to the child by an extension of the pattern of babyhood teasing. If he has been disobedient at school, if he is criticized for mischief, his family becomes a solid front of accusation and rejection. Thus, in Japanese or in Japanese-American society, the approval of the outside world becomes exceedingly important, and an individual comes to feel that the eyes of the world are continually upon him. In such a situation, the best defense lies in a precise knowledge of exactly what is expected of one.

As stated here, this version of Japanese culture was the one the Issei brought with them when they immigrated to the United States during the first decades of this century. This older version of Japanese culture has, of course, been modified over the years in Japan itself, particularly since the end of World War II. However, it was this older version of Japanese culture that the Issei passed on to their Nisei children in America. With this cultural background in mind, let us turn to the problems of the Nisei as expressed by the patient in our case.

THE PATIENT AND HIS PROBLEM

As indicated earlier, the patient was a twenty-four-year-old, American-born, single male of Japanese ancestry. At the time of referral, he was a graduate student at a university in a large Midwestern city. He had been in the city for about six months when he was referred by a Caucasian friend, the brother of his girl-friend whose psychoanalyst informed him about the Japanese-American research project.

FEELINGS OF APATHY AND LONELINESS. The patient described his problem as an all pervasive one. It had been with him in varying degree since he was in high school. He was not interested in anything. He felt apathetic but not fatigued. He was able to get himself to work only by bribing himself by such devices as promising himself that once he worked he could then buy something he wanted or permit himself to spend a couple of hours on the week end "in some way that might be pleasant," such as going to a movie, going for a walk in a section of the city other than that where he lived, or possibly going into a bar for one drink. He had little wish to study although he did so. He did not know what his goals were and was uninterested in his academic field of political science. He considered the latter to be paradoxical because he was interested in politics, business, history, literature, and other cultural pursuits.

The patient described his feelings of uselessness, apathy, discontent, and loneliness as coming on gradually when he entered high school and found himself separated from his friends—the Caucasian children with whom he had played throughout his school days. He was raised in a large city on the West Coast of the United States and described himself as the only Japanese child in a middle-class Caucasian community. There were other Japanese families in the city, but they were widely scattered, and he saw the children of these families only on week ends. While his parents enjoyed these contacts with other Japanese, he did not. He got along well in grade school and was liked by the teachers because of his politeness and industry, but in the eighth grade a male teacher showed disinterest and was critical of him. When he entered high school he felt extremely isolated. It was within these two years that his symptoms became manifest and developed to an intensity which pervaded his whole being. Within a year after his entrance into high school, World War II began and his family shortly moved to an inland city, where they lived out the war.

Shortly after being graduated from high school the patient was drafted, and after his basic training he was sent as an interpreter to the Philippines and Japan. He was in service from 1943 to 1946. On returning from military duty he entered a university in the city on the West Coast where he had grown up and to which his parents had now returned and resumed business. Here he completed his work for his B.S. degree and after the summer came directly to the Midwestern university with fairly unformulated plans beyond the wish to obtain a Ph.D. degree in political science.

AMBIVALENT IDENTIFICATIONS. To each new experience following entrance into high school, the patient reacted with the symptoms earlier described. There were periods of considerable mood swing, but the prevailing affect throughout this entire period had been one of painful depression. He had feelings that he never "belonged" to either the Caucasian group or the Japanese group. He disliked the Nisei in the Midwest although he too was a Nisei, and he tended to feel "in revolt from them or to be revolted by them." He felt that they were not sufficiently intellectual, that they did not have the interests he did, that their attitudes toward life were not his, and that, like his parents, they were "very bourgeois." On the other hand, he found himself unable to make friends easily among the Caucasians and felt isolated from social groups. He had dated very little, either as a GI or as a civilian.

HIS FAMILY

BACKGROUND. Despite the fact that in the initial consultation the patient described himself as the only Japanese child in a world of Caucasian children, he was the second of three sons, having a brother four years older and one two years younger than himself. His family history differed from that of many Japanese in America in that the family had been of rather high social status in Japan and financially well off. His maternal grandfather lost his fortune in the land reforms following the Meiji regime and, coming to this country, set up a successful import-export business in the early part of this century. In the course of his business he communicated with an uncle of the patient's father in Japan. Through this business connection, the parents of the patient met.

Although both parents were reared in Japan, the mother initially had come to the United States with her own family. On their return to Japan, she was left in the United States in the care of a brother who died in his young manhood and about whom the patient felt there was considerable mystery in the family. Before his death, however, the patient's parents had met and were married. Thus, the mother was not a "picture bride." The marriage was arranged through the families according to traditional Japanese custom. The age difference between the parents was about five years; at the time of the patient's treatment the father was fifty-five and the mother "about fifty," the vagueness of her age being accounted for by her general tendency for secrecy about herself and her past.

REMOTENESS OF MOTHER. The mother was described in the early interviews in hostile, despairing terms by the patient: she was a good woman in her own eyes, very meticulous and concerned with order in the housekeeping; she was interested in only one living person, her eldest son, and was unaware of the rest of the family. Her other interests were in her dead brother and the "ancestors" in general. The picture of the mother changed very little as the treatment progressed. A hard-working, very proud woman, she was quiet, inhibited, and restricted, quite distant from her husband though caring for his physical needs, devoted to her eldest son, and interested in her younger sons only for their potential helpfulness to their father's business. In many ways she was more isolated in the culture of the

United States than the father and was the carrier of the earlier traditions. She carried these grimly, and more from her own need than from any overt sense of pleasure to herself in maintaining the "god-shelf" and other meaningful symbols, or from the joy in sharing these aspects of the culture with her family.

FATHER'S INFLUENCE. The father was described as a successful person. He was an importer of art objects until World War II interrupted his business. When he re-established himself after the war, he increased the range of material goods which he bought and sold. He was aggressive and skillful in his business and had a reputation for honesty as an Oriental and as a person. As the treatment progressed, the patient was better able to see both the strengths and weaknesses of the father and to experience some genuine admiration for his courage and persistence, as well as for his ability to modify his behavior toward his sons and this country. At home the father was quiet and passive, dominated there by the mother. He seemed submissive and, in the eyes of the patient, like a son to her. He did not interfere in her relationship to the eldest son, of whom he too was very fond. Although responsive to some of the patient's projects, he showed little personal interest in the younger sons. The father regarded his three sons as a business asset: "three brothers together are better than three separated." During the war, the father "sulked." The patient did not think he was depressed but rather very angry with good outward controls.

Both parents valued education and insisted on high academic standards for their sons, but the father was more active in reading literature, newspapers, and technical articles than was the mother. Occasionally the father showed interests in fishing and other sports. In these activities his attitude was more that the children should accompany him than that he was taking them with him for their pleasure. He recognized all three sons although he clearly preferred, trusted, and confided in the eldest son. His recognition of all three sons was in contrast to the behavior of the mother who loved only the eldest son and openly rejected the two younger boys.

THE FAVORITE ELDEST SON. The eldest brother, Joe, was always a successful student and was given many privileges as a child, including music lessons and receptive attention to his social interests. No one mentioned these things for the younger boys. Joe finished college on the West Coast and went on to take a Ph.D. at a famous Eastern university. The patient felt especially bitter because the parents attended all the graduation ceremonies of the eldest son including that for his Ph.D., but they attended none of his. They did not even come to his eighth-grade ceremonies, at which time the patient felt utterly deserted. Joe went into the business with his father as a partner soon after his education was finished. Prior to this, however, for many years he had been the father's confidant and had worked in the retail store and with the books, while the two younger sons were never permitted to wait on trade and were relegated regularly to menial tasks in the basement of the store or to hard labor in the warehouse. Joe married a Nisei girl when he finished his Ph.D. and brought his wife home to live in line with accepted Japanese custom. Shortly there ensued trouble between the wife and mother-in-law, and the mother was displeased with her eldest son because he was unable to quell the rebellion of his wife. This was the only time the patient could recall that the mother had shown any displeasure with her eldest son. Because of this trouble, Joe and his wife moved away for a few months, but after the arrival of the first child, a grandson, the mother and daughter-in-law were reconciled, and the mother became active again.

THE YOUNGEST BROTHER AS A BURDEN. Tom, the youngest brother, finished college in a desultory fashion and at the beginning of the patient's treatment was totally without goals. He appeared to the patient to be immature for his age both physically and psychologically. He was apathetic, irresponsible in his work and about his person, unresponsive to requests made to him, boastful about deeds not accomplished, and had been an increasingly poor student over the past three years. He and the patient had always been fairly close, had fought violently in competitive arguments for which they were both punished by the parents with instructions to the patient to prevent recurrences, and had sometimes felt a common bond in perpetrating some mischief. The patient felt nevertheless that Tom was very demanding of him, not considerate of his interests unless they were in the common cause of hatred against the parents and Joe, and at the same time altogether too dependent upon him. Within the first year of the patient's therapy, Tom had a brief but violent schizophrenic episode. For at least eight weeks before the episode, the patient was harassed by daily long distance telephone calls from his father, from Joe, and occasionally from Tom, for him to come home and take care of Tom or manage him. No thought was given to the interruption of the patient's life that this would entail. The patient finally gave in and went in time to witness Tom's violent destructive outburst at home. The patient arranged for hospitalization and psychiatric care for Tom while the family stood back helplessly and blamed him for Tom's illness.

DIAGNOSTIC IMPRESSION

On initial contacts with the patient he presented a picture of an asthenic young man of slight build and quiet manner. He showed much cringing submissive behavior but this was without withdrawal and included an ability for acute perceptivity about his surroundings. He did not talk freely although he answered questions and with effort volunteered a limited and guarded amount of information in carefully chosen words. He had a smile, both shy and cynical, which he used defensively and often too quickly, and he was self-depreciatory in gesture and speech. Areas of stress in the conversation, such as questions about his isolation from other Japanese, his father's "sulking," and his mother's denial of his presence, provoked moderately severe stuttering. He had a good grasp of general information and of his current situation and was aware of the realities he was facing although he confessed that he often sat either helplessly or stubbornly passive when he knew that other behavior, as in a classroom, was expected of him. He displayed superior intellectual capacities, including ability with conceptual and abstract thinking, and was able in some instances to introspect with insight despite his highly defended façade. There was adequate though very inhibited affect. A diagnosis of a passive-aggressive personality disorder with severe overt and covert anxiety was made and psychoanalytic treatment recommended.

PSYCHOTHERAPY

Fears and nightmares. The patient began his therapy promptly, and was seen regularly four times a week for two years. Early in treatment his bodily defenses against his intense anxious and depressive affect and his hostile and curious impulses became apparent. Fear and anger haunted him at every turn. He was shy, awkward, ill at ease, and immobilized in his physical behavior. He lay tensely on the couch more as though he were holding it together than it were supporting him, his arms and legs held as though bound to his torso. Long silences were broken by hesitating use of words and disjointed phrases, or by frank stuttering, and were accompanied by blushing, dripping hands and brow, and all of the physiological signs of anxiety. He complained of "freezing up" and of trying to make himself a part of his physical environment, wishing that he could come in an invisible form, or that he could become a part of the analytic couch.

His first hours were filled with bitter reminiscences, and the dreams first reported were recalled from his childhood. Presently he confessed that dreams of the same character had been a part of his nightly activity at frequent intervals for many months. They were often of nightmarish quality and almost all ended inconclusively. In most of them he

was alone or accompanied by a "guy" about his own age.
They were about such subjects as approaching a house or
some other building alone at night. He saw sinister men
approaching the house, or coming out from it, or finding
him coming toward it. They loomed in a menacing fashion
before him, or chased him through passageways; sometimes
the men were engaged in a great battle over a city or a
house in which he was caught in some way between the opposing forces, both of which wanted to destroy him in order
to get him out of the way. Occasionally in the dreams he
was armed, but usually ineffectively, and in a large majority
of instances he was totally undefended except for his ability to run and to hide. The first dream in which he was
openly the aggressor appeared in the third hour and was as
follows:

> It was in our home in X and there was a duck or a chicken or a
> dog sitting on the sofa. My mother was somewhere in the back-
> ground. She had placed the dog there. I knew what was going to
> happen. The animal was going to relieve itself. My mother was
> always in the background. She was approving of the dog on the
> sofa. I would put it outside. Then it was on the rug. Then it took
> a shit, right there on the rug, to use a vulgarism. It did a little, then
> a lot. It covered half the rug, yellowish-brown.

He associated immediately to the rug. His mother was
very fussy about the rug. They always had to take off their
shoes and put on their slippers when they came in. She
did not like to have him bring friends over because they
would dirty the rug. When he occasionally ventured to
bring a friend, he was always embarrassed because of the
shoe restrictions and felt very angry with his mother. He
thought that in the dream he was "just shitting on the rug
in defiance of my mother, to show my hostility. Yet she
was showing her approval of the animal. I didn't see why,
since they were my guests, she couldn't stand a little dirt
on her rugs." The mother never worked in the rooms that
had rugs, but swept them daily, sometimes oftener. She
did her sewing and other work on a table in the kitchen
which was covered with a long overhanging cloth. The

patient and Tom often played under the table for hours at a time but the mother never spoke to them while they were under there. Often the patient played or read there alone. When the mother was there he tried talking, in Japanese and later in English, about things he thought would either interest or anger her, but she did not respond. When infrequent callers, usually the Japanese minister whom the patient especially disliked, came to the house, or when the patient had been punished, he retired under the table where he read, fantasied, or played with simple toys noiselessly for hours. Sometimes he was not missed and slept there through the night.

REJECTION BY MOTHER. Historical antecedents which shed light on his symptomatology and behavior were gradually revealed. The mother emigrated from Tokyo when she was sixteen. Hers was a high-status family that had been in business for several generations. The father, however, came from a small village and his family did not belong to any *kenjinkai* (prefectural association). The mother was disappointed in the marriage because she wanted "a dashing suave city-bred man instead of a country fellow like my father is." However, true to her role as a Japanese woman she accepted the decisions of her family. She was pleased when her first-born was a son and from his birth was devoted to him. She belittled the father and expected him and the two younger sons to do the menial tasks. In contrast, her first son, Joe, whom she called "the boy," had to be well-dressed, well-educated, and the way for him to become a great person made easy, even at the sacrifice of the others. The mother wanted only one child. Joe was strong and active. From the time he started to school she washed for him daily, put money in his shirt pocket each morning, often slipped him extra money when the father refused it to him, brought him coffee and food when he studied in the evening, and never retired herself, even when in college he studied very late for exams, until he was asleep. The patient discovered early that she did not have a similar interest in him or in his younger brother. When the patient was very small, the mother dressed him as a girl and he did not have a boy's haircut until he was nearly five. The mother frankly expressed her wish that he had been a girl and he was assigned more household tasks such as washing dishes, sweeping, and cleaning than was the younger brother, Tom.

The patient resented the fact that his given Japanese name in its feminine form was a common name for a girl. Joe teased him unmercifully about this and about his small size, calling him the "female fugitive from kindergarten." In addition to making known her displeasure that the patient was not a girl, the mother punished him when he quarreled with Tom by calling him *moraigo* (adopted son). The patient felt that he was an adopted illegitimate child, and early he had strong feelings of inferiority and inadequacy. He was frequently told how much trouble he made his parents because he had rickets in his infancy and required expensive medical care. When he was in the eighth grade it was discovered on a routine school physical examination that he had a visual defect requiring glasses. He was terrified, lost his appetite for several days, did not dare to tell his parents because it would cost money, and finally prevailed upon the school nurse to explain to his father what he needed. "They always treated me as an interloper, an adopted son, so I could never demand anything. I must always be inconspicuous to my mother but even more to my older brother. I built up a lot of hostility toward him. I couldn't talk to him anymore."

EFFORT TO PLEASE FATHER. The father's past history also lent weight to the patient's unhappiness as a second son. Although the father protested the mother's efforts to push the patient into a girl's role, the father himself, as the eldest son in his own family, felt that the eldest son was the most important, belonged closest to the father, and should repay the parent with filial piety. The patient respected the father despite his mother's disparagement because he felt that the father was honest and hard working and had made a success of his business in this country. However, the father too was a victim of the mother's demands in that, after a working day of no less than twelve hours, he did many of the household tasks—dressed the children, tried to see that they ate adequately, and kept the property repaired. When he cleaned the yard or did similar tasks, he insisted on the help of the two younger children, while he required nothing of the elder brother, Joe, except that he work in the retail store.

The patient can remember no efforts that he ever made to please his mother. He obeyed her meticulously, was afraid of her, and felt very lonely and unloved. However, he early tried to please his father. He worked very hard about the yard and the house despite the disadvantage of his slight size. He set himself tasks that he thought would please the father such as chopping wood every day and piling it neatly so that the father could easily carry it into the house. He worried about the weeds in the lawn and not only picked the dandelion blossoms, row after row across the lawn, but forced Tom to do the same. In all this he hoped his father would notice his efforts.

His entrance into school was almost catastrophic for him. He was very frightened but did not dare show it, and for days was unable to eat or speak. Although Joe had been sent to nursery school and encouraged to play with Caucasian children, the patient had seen very few such children and could not speak a word of English upon entering school. A month after he started he developed a bad cold and blew his nose in his neatly folded handkerchief. The teacher said he should not do this, and told him to shake out his handkerchief. He had no idea what she was saying, thought she was scolding him, and worried about this for a long time. Despite this bad beginning, school shortly came to be a place of relief and some pleasure for him as long as he did not have to stand up before the class or in other ways display his awkwardness and smallness. His teachers thought him cute, encouraged his development, offered him praise for his efforts, and did not make fun of his shyness.

RITUALS AGAINST ANXIETY. Although he was a worried, anxious, and an "unhappy miserable runt," he managed to find some solace at school and with Tom in his early years. Despite this, he had many signs of, and defenses against, tremendous anxiety. He had frequent nightmares, often had trouble falling asleep, and developed many rituals. The neat piling of the chopped wood, the pulling of the heads of the dandelions in even rows, all had their magical meaning of tasks completed and something "accomplished." Such accomplishment was a requirement of the mother and of his own internalized controls. When he asked his mother to help him with his school work, or to stay with him while he studied as she did with Joe, the mother refused to comply.

She said I was talking rubbish when I said I would like to have her pay some attention to me. I should go to bed and let her sleep. In order to fight all of the things that I had to fight and that menaced me, I used to pray from 8:00 to 8:15. I couldn't get myself to sleep doing this but I would try. . . . I would say the Lord's prayer, ask for the protection of the family, name each one of the members of the family and all the relatives that I could think of and then begin to name the people up and down the street. I had rituals too. One ritual was connected with washing my face before going to bed; I would have the palm of my hand touch my ear three times. In going to sleep I would lie on my side, clap my hands together and open and close my mouth three times like my grandmother and mother used to do in front of the Shinto shrine. Actually I clapped my hands like they did in front of the shrine in order to ward off the evil spirits, but I opened my mouth too. I would pray for us not to be taken away, for the war not to develop, and for the family's business to improve. I had compulsions to do this. These compulsions were the worst around about 10 but some of them persisted until I was 12 or 13.

SCHOOL FRUSTRATIONS. In contrast to earlier school satisfactions, when he entered the eighth grade the situation was painfully altered in that the teacher, now a man, had a strong dislike for Orientals. When the patient would raise his hand, the teacher would stop and tell him to put his hand down. If the patient made an error in reciting the preamble to the Constitution, the teacher was angry, called him "dumb," and threatened to summon his parents to school. He was again terrified and, as on other similar occasions, could not eat for four days. The parents were not summoned, and the patient retreated into a passive, apathetic state. This became worse when his class was divided into sections and he was separated entirely from those two or three boys with whom he had felt comfortable.

WAR, WORK, AND DEPRESSION.   The following year brought the entrance of the United States into World War II and the patient and family moved to an inland city where the patient suffered discrimination because he was Japanese. As mentioned earlier, his depression became intense at this time. It was aggravated by his father's reaction to the war with his resulting withdrawal from any participation with the patient. The patient worked very hard during this period. He was a greens boy for the golf course, raised chickens on his own initiative, thought of various devices to establish credit for the family since money was not available even to pay the grocer, and in many ways was the mainstay of the family. Joe again escaped by being in college. Despite these efforts of the patient, his father took no notice of him, although he occasionally helped the patient with his chores.

The patient finally gave up completely and welcomed being drafted into the army, feeling that he would probably be killed and then the whole matter of his life would be settled. Somewhat to his surprise he was put into a group of Nisei. He did not like them and struggled considerably with the arduous training since he dared not do anything other than keep up with his companions. Yet, the patient managed. After basic training he was transferred to the intelligence service as an interpreter and sent to the Pacific Islands and later to Japan. Here for the first time in his life he felt valued for his own merit, and during these years was less "numb" but continued to be depressed. On his return from Japan where on his own initiative he had visited the families of both parents, he found that neither his father nor mother was interested in his observations. On the contrary, his parents were rather angry at his observations, feeling that these were depreciatory of their families. His depression returned and he decided his only escape would be through education. He returned to college and then moved toward his graduate degree.

"WRETCHED OFFENDER." The course of the analysis was punctuated with rich dreams and fantasies with which the patient struggled in an attempt to understand and bring to some realistic solution his intense and painful feelings of hostility and shame which made him impotent in matters of maturation and prevented his use of his identification with the shrewd, hard-working, and able businessman, his father. He struggled further to discover and establish his own identity, not only as an adult male but also as a Nisei in both a Nisei and a Caucasian culture. The childhood dreams of violence were played out again and again. An example that appeared in the first phase of treatment was as follows, and consisted of three fragments from a dream:

Fragment (a) Two short words buzzed in my head after a nap. They were "wretched offender."

Fragment (b) Two enemies tried to attack the family to kill us. I had a revolver loaded and shot at both of them. Then I put it under my belt and waited for the next attack to come. I should have released the revolver. I tried to take the bullet out of the chamber so that I could release it without firing. I did this with difficulty but couldn't find the bullet to return to my pistol. I was doing this from the dining room table. I asked mother where the enemy went. Mother was not helpful. She had some dress material on the table.

Fragment (c) I was in the back of the house with father and Joe and Tom. We were hiding from the enemy who were coming up in a gun boat. The machine gun was mounted on the desk. We were hiding behind the door. The door's upper half was a window. Everyone saw it and we could not get ourselves out of range. But he also could not come out to make a truce. So they called us to do so. I noticed that I was armed. I said I would come aboard if I could bring a member of the enemy with me.

To this dream he associated that he was the wretched offender. He brought back many memories of having been called a wretched or weak child by his mother. He went on to say that he was puzzled as to why he felt fairly comfortable with Caucasian women except where he was under direct attack for being an Oriental, as when white men were hostile to him when he took out a Caucasian girl. In contrast, he felt very ill at ease with Japanese women. His first girl-friend was a Caucasian woman about ten years his senior—a warm loving person who was very much interested in him and who mothered him without being sexually demanding of him. Later in his analysis it was apparent to him that he felt he should marry her, and that she wanted him to ask her, but that she would not be devastated if he did not. Eventually he was able to bring this relationship to a comfortable close. When reminded that he had been talking about his younger brother as a "wretched offender" also, he brought out both his anger at, and envy of, this brother since the brother in his disturbed state could act out against the family all the hostility that the patient had felt toward them. A great deal of his hostility against his father (here and elsewhere in the material) came out against Joe, the elder brother, but his feelings of being hurt, deprived, and unrecognized by his father were not displaced.

Enemies without and within. The dream fragments (b) and (c) appeared in many forms for months. The enemies varied from Caucasians who attacked the father's business or who humiliated the patient for his slight body and being Japanese, to Issei or Nisei who ignored or ridiculed him or handled him roughly, as he felt the Japanese doctor of his childhood had done. The analyst also appeared in his dreams as attacking him "from behind." He had many fanstasies about the analyst's "power" both as a woman and as a person whom he saw occupying a high status. He imagined that her word, like that of the Emperor of Japan, was absolute law. If one displeased this powerful person, suicide would be demanded. This justified his carrying the revolver as in the dream. But the carrying of the revolver was equally justified by the fierceness of the enemies who many times were clearly his father or his brothers, almost never his mother. His mother appeared repeatedly as "wretched" also and as "not helpful." He varied in his affect from absolute terror to the feeling that it was demanded of him (i.e., by both his parents and himself, and certainly by his professors) that he take the initiative despite his fear, master the enemies, and save the day. Rescue and peace-making fantasies appeared in profusion, but never without great anxiety both in his dreams and in his conscious thoughts and behavior. He felt he was really inadequate and improperly equipped—that his "pistol" was defective or that his "bullets" would be ineffectual. For months he suffered in the colloquia which were a part of the postgraduate program. He felt utterly paralyzed when called upon so that he either said nothing, but "smiled a crooked grin," or said much less than he thought appropriate. Despite the pain of this behavior he often out-thought his classmates and frequently felt that he could give the professor a "good argument which if I weren't so silly he would enjoy too." Some break in his flow of angry hostile dreams came when he began to recognize that a part of himself constituted the enemy and that he was terrified but yet fascinated with his own aggressive and hostile feelings and fantasies.

FEELING OUTCAST. Some resolution of these conflicts led to his feelings of sexual confusion and his notion as a child that he could never be sexually successful as a Nisei, but only as an "outcast." His mother wanted him to be a girl. This he knew he was not. His efforts at inspection of her genitals in the bath had led him to suspect that she did not have a penis. Further he had noticed when he was very young and bathed with his grandmother in the communal bath that she covered her genitals with a towel, while his mother "grew hair."

The patient felt that the only loved and accepted man in the family was the eldest brother. The father was useful for the business, but he and Tom were only important as errand boys or storeroom handlers and hence must be "outcasts." He had the constant feeling of being watched disapprovingly. For example, he said:

It was bad at home but especially at those Japanese picnics. The Association would put them on. I hated them. There were maybe 2,000 people there, people my mother knew. She seemed to like them and people talked to her but they never talked to Tom and me. My father took a Japanese newspaper to read and talked business with the men. He told me to go away and not bother them but he kept Joe right with him. I just wanted to hide and I wished my family would hide, just go to some spot in the park which was inconspicuous. The feeling of shame—not wanting to be seen, feeling ashamed. I couldn't do anything with the others or anything the others did. My father in some ways seemed to feel the same. There would be races in the afternoon. I couldn't run as fast as the other boys or do as well physically. Tom and I were both afraid. They would have concessions selling soft drinks. That made me feel ashamed and afraid. It was uncomfortable and awful. I have that kind of a feeling when Caucasians look at us. Really peculiar. I doubt if most of the Nisei really feel that way at picnics but I felt this way. I never played with any of these kids. I never knew anyone or where to stand. I knew I wouldn't be accepted and knew I would be teased and ridiculed.

IDENTIFICATION WITH BANTAM HEN. The patient's loneliness, his feelings of shame and disgrace, and his curiosities were somewhat relieved by his identification with and devotion to his bantam hen, which was his pet for several summers. His ability to care for this living thing encouraged him and provided the impetus during the war years for the flock of chickens by means of which he helped to take care of and feed the family in its great need, even enlisting the father's grudging help. Of this period the patient said:

I got along pretty well in school, up to the eighth grade that is. But at home I could only play or fight with Tom or sit under the table. I really didn't have any friends. The Caucasian boys thought we were queer and the girls just ignored me until I met Jane. But she was older and she wasn't afraid of me. But I did have my bantam hen. I was very curious about what women were like throughout my childhood and had lots of fantasies about the girls in my class, particularly the seventh and eighth grade. I would fantasy that they would undress and show me their genitals. I would look and look and think maybe my eyes were deformed, but I couldn't find out. . . . Then I had my bantam hen, and she was warm and liked me. She would follow me around the yard and be cheerful.

Sometimes I took her in my arms and walked down the creek with her and talked to her. But somehow she got pregnant. . . . I mean she laid an egg. I certainly felt guilty and I acted guilty when my bantam hen was having a baby. I had to hide the whole thing from Tom. It was forbidden and dirty. I knew the egg was under her too. It was something awful. I couldn't tell anyone. I could even fool my parents too. That bantam chicken was illegitimate. The rooster was not ours. And roosters often had two hens. I used to give all the hens human names and as a consequence I thought they should have the same morals.

THERAPEUTIC GAINS. In general, over the two-year period, the patient's therapy moved well as the unconscious concomitants of his conscious thought and behavior were explored in his daily events and through the repetition of meaningful life experiences in the transference. At the end of the first six months of therapy he was able to qualify for his Ph.D. Before the therapy terminated he had completed his thesis. He became increasingly more articulate with his professors and much more able in his contacts with them to see his role as a graduate student rather than as a depreciated little boy. As he gained strength in the area of education, an area similar to his first area of acceptance (the first seven grades of school), he was better able to deal with his problems concerning his brothers and father. Ultimately, he pointed out to his father that he could be of help in the business but that he would function in a different role from Joe. He became much more comfortable with Nisei men but remained somewhat indifferent to Nisei women, seeing them as sharper and on the whole less loving than Caucasian women. Ultimately he married a Caucasian girl. The patient's clarification of his own role as man rather than boy, his identification with his father's strengths, and his repudiation of his mother's rejection through his easier relationship with Caucasian women reinforced by the warmth shown him by his grade-school teachers, came to fruition in this marriage. Four years after analysis, the marriage is stable with two children. He is in partnership with his father and older brother, the younger brother having settled for a minor position in another firm.

He is doing very well financially and socially in both Caucasian and Japanese-American cultures. His mother has remained chronically depressed but seems relieved both by his ability to take care of himself and to be of help to his father. He feels that she still has little awareness of her role in his life and that her life is quite barren except for her attachment to the grandchildren, his own two children and the son and daughter of Joe.

PSYCHODYNAMICS: PERSONAL AND CULTURAL

CENTRAL PROBLEMS. In the very first hour the patient presented the major problems which were to occupy him for the subsequent hundred hours. In his presentation the central figures in his family situation were the mother and the elder brother. The father and the younger brother were really secondary and related.

A little later in therapy, the desires of the patient to please his father by producing something, and at the same time his anxiety about creation and growth, the relations among the siblings, the obligations the patient is expected to fulfill, and his characteristic ways of meeting problems were all developed further.

A NOSY MOTHER. Various aspects of the character of the mother continued to unfold as therapy went on. For example, the mother's efforts to influence the choice of a wife for the patient in such a way as to make her old age more secure came out during the fifty-second hour. The patient spoke of returning to this country after his military service. At this time his mother wrote him asking why he had not married in Japan. She made it clear that she would have preferred an Issei girl to a Nisei girl, and that a Caucasian girl was not suitable at all. Here we see, in the light of the patient's subsequent marriage to Ruth who was Caucasian, some of his rebellion against his family. Equally we see both the personal and cultural aspects of the desires of the mother in that she would have preferred as Japanese a wife for her son as was possible. This would have enabled her to exercise more control over the wife—the most control over a girl from Japan, less over a Nisei girl, and least of all over a Caucasian wife.

During the 113th hour the patient returned again to the question of his mother's cleanliness in terms of his associations to a dream. He said the dream was like his mother, who would worry if the bathroom wasn't clean, and that she scrubbed the bathroom continuously. He said, "Come to think of it, she was scrubbing something all the time." This statement is interesting in the light of the earlier remarks made about the cultural context and meaning of cleaning in Japan, one aspect of which is its use by the mother or wife as an indirect expression of anger. During this same hour the patient indicated how he expressed his hostility towards his mother by dirtying things, particularly in the struggles around bowel movements. There is no space here for an extended discussion of the point but the patient's desires to make a relation, even a hostile one, to his mother, and the connections early in life between the balance of the evaluations placed by parents and children on simple childhood tasks as, in the case of our patient, chopping wood, producing feces (and their relation to money), and the ability later in life to work and produce are all present as part of the content and meaning of what the patient went on to say in the same hour:

The bathroom is the worst possible embarrassment—going to the bathroom. It is like going to school with my slippers on or doing something else of that kind. [Analyst asks why excretion is so embarrassing.] I see my mother with chopsticks hunting in the feces for the pennies we swallowed. It was horrible. She just couldn't stand it. She just abhorred it. And I think we must have swallowed pennies sometimes just to make her handle the feces. The cleanest room in the whole house was the bathroom, and as soon as we had made stool or anything, she rushed right in and cleaned it up. This always made me angry. [Analyst says perhaps he felt his mother wasn't interested in what he produced.] I can't sit down to work. I just can't sit down and do something. They are going to make fun of me. It just wastes my time. I am lost before I start. If I do something on my thesis, they won't appreciate it. That is the way I felt about her. She just didn't appreciate it. She just made me angry.

They aren't going to appreciate any work I do for them. My excretions made work for my mother. Washing diapers was the worst type of work possible. She hated it. And she had to work and work to get them immaculately clean. If anyone forgot to flush the toilet, they got the very devil. I never will forget her embarrassment and how she would make everyone keep the place clean for her. She wasn't concerned about anything I did for her or for my father. They would very seldom command me but I always knew what they expected me to do. They never praised me even when I cleaned up the basement or chopped wood. I tried to do lots of cleaning to get her interested. . . . I would get excited and chop and chop and sometimes my father would like it. I just can't do anything for myself. I just can't. I kind of go back. . . . If I can't do any work then how am I going to support myself and Ruth. . . . I have to do it for my father. Directly or indirectly I have to help my father. Everything I ever considered doing, work or going to school or any of these things, has to do with my father. . . .

"RETURN TO FAMILY." The latter part of the above excerpt takes us a bit further. The "excitement in chopping wood and the gratification from this through the father's occasional expression of pleasure indicate the erotic element for the patient in such activity and the feminine identification with the mother, who also cleaned vigorously and explicitly desired the patient to be a girl, in an effort to receive attention from the father. Further, the phrase, "I can't do anything for myself," relates to the emphasis placed on self-denial in Japanese culture, and on the family as the social unit in Japan. The patient in our case spent a good part of his analysis in working through his personal feelings about this problem but, as has been said before, he ended up by returning to his family and going to work for his father. This was in line with his personal and cultural reality as embedded in a matrix of Japanese values. He was concerned in the 118th hour about his desire to return home to live and work. In this hour he related a dream in which he went back to his birthplace. This was the beginning of a series of hours during which this topic was discussed. As it relates to the material on the family, one can see the patient's search for his identity in terms of being a Nisei in the American world. He utilized the analysis to work out some of these problems and, like many successful Nisei, he did not in the end reject his heritage but rather came to terms with it.

Such a "return to the family" is a normal solution for the Nisei although there may be other equally normal solutions because of their acculturation status. It would be a necessity in Japan where a man almost literally cannot function in any sphere of life without ties to a parental family unit. For these reasons, such a return does not carry the presumption of a regressive solution to a problem such as might more readily suggest itself if the same behavior occurred in a patient from the American middle class. Nevertheless, such a return does carry with it psychological roots and consequences which are differently patterned from those in American culture.

SOMATIZATION DEFENSE. As noted in the case summary, the defensive aspects of illness and physical weakness were a part of the patient's response to his experiences in the family and at school. When the patient came for the first diagnostic consultation he had a seemingly slight paralysis of the right side of his mouth of which he was quite unaware until this was commented on by the analyst. This subject was not mentioned again until the 117th hour when the patient said:

> I always accept things out of one side of my mouth. If I would say anything my mother did not like, she would say to me that my mouth was crooked, or that I had an evil streak down my back. I thought of that the other day when you asked me where I got these ideas, and I thought about the paralysis you noticed in my face. It began sometime in high school, but I had thought about it before at the end of grade school. . . . I used to ride on the outer side of the car and there was a cold wind on the right side of my face. I noticed that my face was crooked and I used to think that it was due to an evil wind. My mother was really right. She predicted it, and here it is.

It is important that the patient began to notice his partial paralysis at about the end of grade school. From the case summary it will be remembered that this was the time when he left the rather accepting environment of elementary school and entered upon the more difficult period of high school. It is quite possible that the physical symptoms which came into consciousness at this point were related to the difficulties he was then having not only at home but also at school. Not having an adequate source of gratification in his important interpersonal situations, he turned for help and defense to the processes of his body. This is not an uncommon occurrence among many patients in America, but it has a more pronounced institutionalized context in Japanese culture than in that of the United States.

PSYCHODYNAMICS AND BIRTH ORDER. In the case summary we have seen how the patient was expected to take care of his younger brother, Tom, and thus relieve the family of this responsibility. It was also pointed out that this expectation that the older sibling will care for the younger is very much a part of Japanese culture.

In the very first hour the patient spoke of his hostility toward his elder brother and of his feeling that he was an adopted son whereas his elder brother was the true son. However, the patient treated his younger brother, Tom, in much the same way that he was treated by his older brother. For example, in the second hour he said: "I grew up with my younger brother, Tom. . . . I don't feel any antagonism toward him, but I was not quite fair with him. I used to enforce the parental rule. I would make him quit listening to the radio and start reading—admonish him about his school work." Again in the fifth hour, the patient said, "Tom is a nonentity. . . ."

The way in which the patient attempted to resolve his conflict over the parents' insistence that he take care of the younger brother during his psychotic episode is interesting in terms of the patient's position in two cultures—the Japanese and the American. In Tom's post-hospitalization period, the parents sent him to visit the patient. One attempt at resolution of his conflict occurred in a dream reported in an early phase of treatment:

I was in a male analyst's office, something like the offices of the other analysts beside you. I was taking Tom to the analyst. He went in to see him and the analyst had four patients waiting. His door was open and he was there. But he wanted two of us to come in pair by pair. . . .

In his associations to this dream the patient remarked that he had not had a letter from his parents for the two weeks that Tom had been with him, and that his parents wanted to forget and get rid of them both—that *he* really was expected to take care of Tom. He said that he had tried to help Tom, but now he wished Tom would get out of his life and out of his analysis.

In this dream one can see how the patient is caught in the conflict facing most Nisei between the Japanese obligations to the family and the desire to lead a middle-class American life—a desire which is made possible in part because of the usefulness of some Japanese values in meeting the requirements of such a life. In the dream situation here, the patient tried to get rid of Tom by turning him over to the analyst for treatment. His ambivalence and conflict in values over this solution is indicated, however, in his having the analyst see the patients in pairs so that he retains his tie to the younger brother.

CULTURAL DIFFERENCES IN MEDICAL CARE. The situation of the patient in this regard highlights some rather basic differences in the place of medical care and the role of the physician in American and Japanese cultures. Because of the small size of the American family and its geographic and social mobility, there is little possibility that someone who is seriously ill can be taken care of very adequately at home. In Japan the family system is more adequate to care for the patient at home, and less use is made of hospitals. The patient in our case, however, is caught between the two cultures, and the demands placed on him to take care of his younger brother helped to precipitate his coming to terms with the question of just how he should live his life in the United States.

ATTITUDE TOWARD WOMEN.   In the case summary we have
seen how the patient tended to reject other Nisei—especially Nisei women. He also felt that he was constantly
watched disapprovingly and suffered a good deal in any
sort of interpersonal relationship. These feelings do not
sound very different from those found in any neurosis, yet
they have rather specific references in the larger Japanese-
American study and in Japanese culture. The majority of
the Nisei men in the Japanese-American study were rather
passive and had feelings similar to those of the patient,
while the Nisei women were frequently hostile and derisive
toward Nisei men. We have previously indicated that the
Japanese view their own interpersonal relations as particularly difficult, and Japanese psychiatry has created a syn-
drome known as anthrophobia (*taijin kyofusho*) which is
manifested by feelings of inadequacy, fear of meeting people, blushing, stammering, and other signs of anxiety.

Many of the patient's problems in relation to Nisei wom-
en, and his concern over his coming marriage to a Caucasian girl, came out in the sixteenth hour. For example,
he said:

The kind of disapproval I would get from my parents and her parents—it just isn't worth it. I can understand why Nisei marry Nisei,
but I think a lot of them are not in love. The Nisei women just have
to get married and Nisei men passively accept. They don't have
any other way to do a thing. . . . There was one Nisei girl I went
with a little bit. . . . We talked about Japan and I tried to tell her
about my experiences there, but she wasn't interested. She might
have been cold towards me, but it was more than that. . . . I don't
want to get married to get devoured immediately.

From a cultural as well as a personal point of view one
of the most significant things the patient says here is that
he does not want "to get married to get devoured immediately." This certainly has reference to the patient's feelings
concerning the hostile and depreciatory treatment he received from his mother and to the more general hostility
found among Nisei women toward Nisei men. Further

than this, in the culture of Japan, a theme that is never far from the surface in literature, theatre, and art, concerns the oral aggressive character of women. Such fantasies around the behavior of women probably stem in part from the relatively unbroken tie to the mother that has been mentioned earlier.

In the next, the seventeenth hour, the patient went on to speak of the Oedipal situation and said:

Mother was very attached to the handsome young Issei minister at our church. He was the kind of man that all women liked. I hated that man and the way my mother was attached to him. And I talked about how I disliked him and everything he and my mother would do. Sometimes I even thought that she would sleep with him. . . . I really think that he was another Joe for me because I had an extreme feeling of competitiveness with him. . . . When I was a child I would go to my grandparents' house, and sometimes I would go with Tom. . . . We all took a bath together in the tub. Tom said that I was very fond of my grandmother. . . . She would put a small towel around her genitals and would be very careful so that I could never see. Before I started to grade school, mother would take a bath with Tom and me. All of us would be in the tub together. She would have a towel too, but I would try to look at her and think about her.

CHICKEN SYMBOL. In this excerpt, in addition to the Oedipal and sibling situation, one can see the tradition of Japanese mixed family bathing with its simple sensual enjoyment. In Japanese society, in contrast with the West, the flesh is not evil and is to be enjoyed. At the same time such experiences are certainly likely to stimulate the curiosities and fantasies of young children. The patient went on in a subsequent hour to report how during one of these baths with the grandmother, Tom, the younger brother, got a marble with which he had been playing in the tub caught in his rectum, thereby causing the patient great concern until it was removed. The patient's reactions to this episode are very similar to his feelings concerning the egg laid by his bantam hen.

These topics were discussed at length from the thirty-eighth to the fiftieth hour and give a key to many of the self concepts of the patient. For example, in the forty-second hour, the patient spoke of raising chickens as a means of getting close to his father. He remarked how lonely and sad he felt when he would watch the chickens being killed and dressed by his father. His own confused sexual identity was certainly bound up with the chickens as he then went on to discuss his feelings about his coming marriage and to report, in this same hour, the dream presented above in the case summary of the enemy attack on the family. In his associations, he felt that the pistol in the dream was some sort of defense and that he could not protect himself and things he loved. He went on to associate to his fear of his father and his own inadequacy in the use of his genital organ. This brought back to mind the scene of himself and his mother in the bathtub. There followed a good deal of material in which his coming marriage, his fear of sexual competition with his father, and his castration anxiety were all blended together. He was confused about Nisei girls, saying that they reminded him of his mother. Again he returned to the theme of the chickens, stating, in the forty-fifth hour, more clearly than he had done before that,

I loved the chickens and it was as though my father were hurting me the way he cut them up. Yet I knew he had to. He had to cut them up for my mother. . . . My father enjoyed dressing the chickens and he would do it very well. I wondered how and where he had learned to do it so well. He would tell Joe how to do it, but he wouldn't tell anyone else.

One can see quite clearly here the fear of competing with the father, the fear of castration by the father, a fate that seemed inevitable since he was a second son, and the realistic envy of the older brother who was taught how to do things whereas the patient was not.

COMING CAUCASIAN MARRIAGE. In the following hours the patient was able to work out some of these questions about his sexual identity and to go on to discuss many of the realistic details of his coming marriage. Part of the

working through of his problem and a type of solution were
indicated in a dream given during the fifty-sixth hour:

> I was on a vacant lot with Ruth and Dick who was a friend of
> mine. We were looking over the ground. Dick wanted to build a
> house there and we could see the foundations coming up. He was
> showing that the foundation was nearly completed and he explained
> to us that this house would cost very little. The bath had two tubs
> in it. One was a deep one, and the other was regular style installed
> with tile. And there was a quite small living room which was well
> finished. I thought that if Dick could do it, I could do it too.

The patient related this dream to his concern about housing after marriage, and went on to say that he felt more
confident than before—if a friend of his could do something,
so could he. He spoke of the two tubs, remarking that the
deep one was like those of wealthy Japanese families, and
said it seemed to have something to do with how "Jap-
anesey" he and Ruth should be after they were married.
At this point the analyst pointed out that going home would
be to do something more cheaply, and that he still had
some need to be taken care of at home because he was not
taken care of earlier.

A comment on the cultural and personal meaning of the
dream as it related to the two bath tubs might be in order.
We have seen from earlier material the patient's pleasure
in the stimulation received from taking a bath in Japanese
style with his grandmother or mother. Equally we have
seen that the patient does not wish totally to reject his
Japanese heritage, but rather to come to terms with it
so that it may be useful to him. In the above dream he
seems to have arrived at a solution symbolized by the two
styles of bath tubs—he will have both, the Japanese and the
American. We do not know what associations he might
have gone on to give to this aspect of the dream, but it does
seem to represent a solution to many of the problems he had
been discussing during his treatment.

EGO STRENGTHENING.   In the sixty-eighth hour the patient
continues through a dream his good efforts to reach a solu-

tion to his problems, a point to which he had been brought by the analytic process. The patient dreamed:

> . . . that he was on the platform loading a tender with coal and Ruth was watching him but he was afraid to go up to the cab. The engineer might not want to take such a small fireman as he was—a young Japanese, and the engine looked huge. Ruth urged him to go ahead and he did so, and the engineer smiled and shouted that he should bring a catcher's mitt with him to absorb the shock of the handle that came back with some force.

He commented after the dream that he had the feeling that he could do it. To this dream he associated the questions of whether he would be an engineer or fireman on the train and whether he would be able to manage the train or not. Ruth, in the dream, urged him to go ahead and try. Continuing his efforts toward a solution of his problems he experienced insight into the attitudes he should have towards his parents. He said:

> I am beginning to consider my parents as people, and not as someone who has almighty power. They can make mistakes as any other people. I can like them, but I don't have to feel guilty if I don't do something they ask me. . . . I was thinking about my mother's past history. Her father ignored her. After she moved to Tokyo from her village, and grandfather lost his money, she had to move to a different school. Each time she would get quite upset. She changed from the village to the city without her mother and that was a hard adjustment to make. She wasn't the favorite daughter; her younger sister was. The younger sister went to the kind of school that my mother wanted to go to. . . . My mother's oldest brother came to this country and told the grandfather to come. And he did. He wanted the family to come over and many of them did, and my mother was left in Japan. The only one who was left was my grandmother from the village and she couldn't get around to take care of the family, so my mother at 14 or 15 had to take charge and grandmother did very little. Mother took care of the younger sister and brother and had to get the passports and apply for the visas and buy the passage and so on as there was no one else to do it. Grandmother was totally helpless. She really belonged to the old school. She did not go beyond grade school, but mother did. Mother is quite hostile to my grandmother and grandfather. She feels that they could have done better with the family.

The progress the patient was making can be seen in this excerpt. He was beginning to see his parents as people, and to see that his mother had been in much the same situation as he himself had been—not being the favored child in the family and having to take a great deal of responsibility without much help or reward. Although the patient did not go on to mention it, we can see here the continuity in the kinds of problems which, often at an unconscious level, are transmitted from one generation to the next. In this case such problems were set within the cultural context of the Japanese family, but the personal feelings about such problems completely interpenetrate the cultural aspects. It is unwise to make too sharp a distinction between the cultural and the personal, but at the same time it is not possible to understand the more universal aspects of the patient's difficulties without an understanding of the structure and obligations that form part of Japanese family life.

In the next hour, the sixty-ninth, the patient continued to associate to the train dream reported in the previous hour. He felt that heretofore he had always been a passenger or an onlooker, but now someone came along and gave him a little kick and there he was as a fireman on the train. He felt he was now in the position to help operate the train even though he was not the engineer. Here again, we can see that the patient now felt able to move ahead, but only within the cultural context of still being subordinate to the father and the older brother as he is not the main person running the train but is a significant helper. This, as we know from the case summary, is the solution he effected when he went back to work with his father and older brother in the family business.

An additional point, similar to that made concerning the dream of the two bath tubs, comes from the patient's further associations to the train dream. He felt that the catcher's mitt had something to do with absorbing the shock of a long ride. He then went on to say, "It is as though I am going to wear my shoes rather than go barefooted. It is the first time I ever approached the engine of a train." This comment is probably related to many things of personal and cultural interest. Earlier, we noted that the mother spent a great deal of time cleaning and that the patient had many reactions to this compulsion of his mother. It is equally necessary to know that upon entering a Japanese house one takes off one's shoes, so that inside the house one is, in a sense, barefooted. The patient would seem to be telling us here that he is ready to give up to some extent the old Japanese home in which he was reared and to go out to make his own way as an American.

SPECIAL RELATIONS TO THE ANALYST. As in any analysis, the analyst appeared in many forms in the patient's conscious and unconscious material. A short dream in the ninety-sixth hour is of particular interest for us here. The patient reported his dream as follows: "I was going up in an elevator in a department store and it began to tip. I was afraid that it might tip over or the cables would burn." The patient's first associations were that he was always going up in elevators and this must have significance concerning his ambitions, wishes to climb, and his fears. He then went on to speak of these matters in relation to the analyst:

Most of my fear of you is irrational. Why should I be afraid of you? I am sure I think you have some kind of supernatural power. . . . When I walk in here, I feel like you know everything. That is the way I used to feel about my parents. They knew everything. They could even know when I made a mistake. . . . Sometimes I don't agree with you and I think you are all wrong, but I cannot tell you that I don't agree with you. It is impossible to do that with my father. I would lose his respect immediately. And he doesn't have much for me anyway. Parents are really very unreasonable. They never realize that we are human beings and we have the same kind of feelings that they do. . . . Everything we had to do was a command. We would never ask to do anything. I never dared ask about anything. . . . Regarding you, you are a very convenient person to start practicing being an equal with. It is convenient that you listen to me because sometimes you forget something that I have told you and that pleases me because then I know you are fallible too. . . . I am worthless, I am just nothing. . . . I can never be my father's equal. He is so omniscient and I cannot reach that level, nor yours. I feel embarrassed in your presence. There is a strong relation be-

tween this and fear of my father physically. He can use other hid-
den powers. He can crush me and he knows everything. A deity
at my mother's shrine. My dead uncle, my great grandmother, and
all the ancestors were always there looking at you. You feel the
same way every time before you go to the shrine. And you pass the
shrine several times a day. That is the way I feel when I look at
you. It is frightening. You could watch me everywhere and I am
so small that I cannot do anything.

One can see very clearly here the placing of the analyst
in the position of the parents. Equally one can see the usefulness of the analyst as a sort of catalyst for culture change
and psychological development on the part of the patient.
In this case it was probably particularly important that the
analyst was a Caucasian and a woman, as these attributes
served to aid the patient in working out many of his problems about being Japanese and about being a younger son
in the family. The analyst was not only a focus for a personal change, but also in a more general sense helped the
patient to find his place in American culture and to do this
in an emotionally as well as intellectually meaningful way.
In such a change, however, the patient still retained his
ties, as he probably always will, to the Japanese culture;
and the analyst, as do the parents in the Japanese family,
continued to occupy a more respected and powerful position in the patient's mind throughout the course of the
analysis than would be generally true for middle-class American patients. That this latter point is pertinent to the ultimate resolution of the transference problems for this patient
is well borne out in the material from the 114th hour when
the patient said that he always had to have something in
reserve, even toward the analyst. Such an attitude is very
characteristic of interpersonal relations in Japanese culture.
Around these points, the patient said:

I still have reservations with you. . . . I must have something in
reserve. . . . [The analyst asks why?] I just cannot lie down and
open my heart to you. It is too dangerous. . . . I have the feeling
that if you would meet me on the street, you wouldn't speak to me.
You would just pass me by, the way my mother always kept me in
the bedroom when the company came. She would drag me out by

the ears so the visitors could see me and make me bow politely and I would have to go back. Joe could stay out with the visitors. It was hard to keep the tears back. It is now. I am crying. Damn it, I don't like it. You make me suffer just like she did. . . . I am so angry and I cry and everyone would look the other way. [The analyst says perhaps he is afraid that the analyst won't be able to stand his tears any more than his mother could, that his mother was annoyed with him and saw him as weak. The analyst points out that all children cry, and after all there is a reason why human beings have tear ducts.] They didn't give me any sympathy. My father would run off, and Tom would sneer, and mother would leave me. I cannot trust you and it makes me feel ashamed to cry here. [The analyst points out that in addition to his feelings toward the analyst as a woman, as someone he cannot trust, that he always thinks he has to maintain his social role and to remember that the analyst is both a Caucasian and an older woman.] I know it. I would like so to trust you but I cannot. I just have to remember that it isn't proper, that I must be respectful; not trust you. At home, if the doorbell rang and it was a Caucasian, it made no matter what we were feeling or how intensive what was going on, or how angry I might be at Tom or mother at the moment, I immediately had to put those feelings aside and act as though everything was proper. . . . I was tied in every way and I tried hard to do what they wanted me to do. And I just didn't show anything in front of anyone.

The good progress of the patient, and his increasing ability to relate to the analyst and others as persons in their own right, continued to develop in the supporting atmosphere the analyst was able to communicate to him through her knowledge of the major outline of his culture as well as of its more ordinary details in his everyday life.

CONCLUSION

Perhaps the main contribution of the young Nisei case presented in this chapter was its demonstration of the close intertwining of personal and cultural factors. As we have repeatedly noted, the analytic material was rich in cultural symbolism. While it is most helpful for the therapist working cross-culturally to be well-versed in the basic parameters of the culture—its history, literature, art, and customs, such general information is less meaningful in terms of communication with patients than an empathetic understanding of

the more homely details of their background. The crucial
need is for the analyst to know how the patient feels about
the kind of house he lives in, where he sleeps, what he eats,
and all that makes up his daily life.

The present case was valuable not only in indicating the
ways that culture may determine behavior but also in demonstrating what might be called the universals of psychodynamics. These are the kinds of problems in growing up
that human beings have to meet in any culture throughout
the world. In a sense, such universals are as much cultural
in the generic meaning of the term as they are biological
or psychological. In part this arises out of the fact that
man is the only truly symbol-using animal, and that language and other behavior are learned by the small and immature child while he is being cared for by large and more
or less mature adults of both sexes in some sort of family
situation in any culture.

Japanese Postscript

Running through all five Japanese-American cases is a pervasive depression, in three reaching the point of suicidal threat or actual attempt. The depressive reaction serves as a means of expressing resentment for which the culture does not permit direct expression. Psychophysiologic reactions also serve the same purpose and abound in our material. In all cases the suppressed hostility may be traced to inadequate parentage. Both the Kibei boy and the aging Issei were sent away from their homes in early childhood. After their return they seemed incapable of establishing secure roles in their families. To them relocation came as the ultimate rejection. It precipitated young Jiro's psychotic break and supplied Aki's later developing delusional system with persecutory political content.

Mrs. Harada also had a history of parental deprivation for which she overcompensated by a double identification—with children and parents. Through her homes for children and the aged, she could masochistically enjoy giving the care she had never received and expressing a filial devotion to parents she had never known. The "maternal role" became her chief ego defense, and when threatened by her husband, her frustration was overwhelming. Since submission was required of a wife, the patient resorted to the passive aggression of suicide as a final retaliation against her husband.

The two Nisei men share problems of identification diffusion. For Ichiro the problem was more sharply focused on the father as a negative model to be avoided by eschewing all things Japanese. In the case of the other youth, neither parent exerted a positive influence since they each tended to ignore the patient in favor of their eldest son. The result was a generalized suppression of affect, experienced as apathy. A narcissistic identification object for this

449

young man was his pet hen to whom he gave the care he craved, as in Mrs. Harada's identification with the helpless.

Through psychotherapy both these Nisei patients were ultimately enabled to view their parents with greater tolerance and to fit themselves into occidental life without repudiating their oriental background.

Looking back over the cases of Japanese origin, we may note a certain cohesiveness binding them together. Distance from parent figures is conspicuous in all as well as inability openly to express resentment against them. In line with the externalization of authority and the shame-avoidance demands of Japanese tradition, hostility is consistently turned in on the self in the face-saving devices of depression and somatic illness.

PART VI

NEW WORLD SYMPHONY AND DISCORD

Preview

New world symphony and discord could easily serve as the title of the present volume rather than of merely one section, since the central problem with which the book deals concerns the dynamics of interaction between various subcultures and the dominant culture. We shall use the heading more specifically, however, to denote the acculturation process of immigrants from certain European groups who were thrown into conflict by the double standards of behavior represented by old and new worlds.

Faced with a choice as wide as a continent, we decided on a relatively narrow range so that the subtler intercomparisons and contrasts would not be submerged by the grosser variables. For our purposes, we selected two European groups equally noted for their persecutions, their ethnic cohesiveness, and their differences in cultural content. They were the Jews and Armenians. Among the Jews, we have a little boy and a young man, both from Central European ghetto background. A third Jewish case is that of a woman refugee also from central Europe, but reared in the highest social circles. The Armenians are represented by a young man who adds a new note to our symphony by attempting to repudiate his ethnic origin. The final case is that of a young English war bride who came in conflict with the tightly knit Armenian culture of her husband. The double impact of strange American and stranger Armenian ways brought this girl to the brink of psychosis.

18

A Little Jewish Boy Under Pressure of Orthodoxy

Isaac Berman and *Georgene Seward* [1]

ARRIVAL AT THE CLINIC

"Itzhak," a thin little dark-eyed boy of six was referred to the clinic because of deviant behavior at school. About two months after enrollment, he showed signs of social withdrawal: playing alone, fantasying about Superman, and crying. Soon he refused to participate in classroom activities at all and regressed to the point of soiling himself. At the same time he experienced "visions" of his mother's "passing away" and "headaches" urging him to go home immediately so that he could reach the East Coast in time for the Sabbath.

SCHOOL

The patient was attending a small, private Hebrew school from early morning until late afternoon. The atmosphere was strictly conservative, with emphasis on religious instruction. Itzhak's teacher was a short-tempered disciplinarian who tried to force the child against his will to perform all his duties, including eating up every bit of lunch. The principal was apparently even stricter, and greatly disturbed by Itzhak's disruption of the school routine. He went so far as to telephone the father during working hours to inform him that his son would not be permitted to continue

---

[1] The senior author served as psychotherapist.

at school because there was something "wrong" with his mind.

Meanwhile, the boy was being picked on and teased by his older, bigger schoolmates. His anxiety and expressed wish to be home with his mother, the first signs of his acute distress, were overlooked.

EAST COAST FAMILY

Itzhak's mother and father were reared in comparable backgrounds of Jewish orthodoxy in eastern Europe. They had in common early experiences of patriarchal family life, and later, the horrors of war, internment, and displacement. After their liberation, they met, married, and moved to the United States.

The adjustment of the young couple to their new environment was facilitated by the help of relatives on the East Coast with whom they stayed on arrival. Probably most helpful was the fact that they all lived in an orthodox section of town which preserved most aspects of their original culture and where they could speak Yiddish and practice the form of Judaism in which they had been reared. This ingrouping gave them a measure of security and a sense of belonging. Thus the transition to the New World involved little conflict with new conditions and values but, rather, provided an accepting and familiar milieu where the newcomers could hope gradually to forget the harrowing memories of their recent past.

In contrast to the young couple's easy "absorption" into the orthodox Jewish subculture were the almost insuperable obstacles in the way of their coping with the dominant culture. Their past training had failed to prepare them for suitable positions in America, and their resistance to adopting the customs and manners of the new people further obstructed their acceptance.

The birth of Itzhak, their first child, made economic matters worse. After trying his hand at a number of business ventures culminating in an unsatisfactory job which he was forced to retain in order to keep his family together, the father decided to leave the East Coast in search of more rewarding work.

EARLY DEVELOPMENT

INFANT TRAINING. As the first-born male child, Itzhak was welcomed into the family. His mother nursed him for the first few months, weaning him very gradually. She described him as a "good eater," consuming large quantities of milk. Despite these favorable beginnings, he was apparently a colicky baby, crying almost continually, and stopping only while his mother held him in her arms. The moment she put him back to bed was the signal for him to resume crying. During this period, the child developed poor sleep habits which he has retained ever since.

Toilet training was not begun until the little patient was nearly two years old. His mother's efforts in this direction, though coercive, proved ineffectual, and the child did not respond until, on her physician's advice, she relaxed her attitude.

Aside from the measles, Itzhak enjoyed a healthy infancy, and his maturation was entirely normal.

EMOTIONAL GROWTH. As a baby, Itzhak saw very little of his father, whose hard work kept him away from home a good deal of the time and made him seem like a stranger when he was there. Once, when he spent a brief vacation with his family, the patient, then nineteen months old, was afraid to play with him or even to stay alone with him. The father did nothing to alleviate his little son's fears. On the contrary, he disciplined him severely, depriving him of privileges or spanking him on occasion. He was quite proud of his ability to control the boy merely by raising his voice.

The mother, on the other hand, was constantly with the child, hovering over him and behaving in a way that she herself described as "perhaps more protective than the average." This admitted overprotectiveness, which is supported by the culture, provided her with a socially acceptable channel for satisfying some of her own security needs. This pattern of indulgence was reinforced by the other East Coast relatives who pampered Itzhak as the only child in a large family.

MOVING FROM PLACE TO PLACE

From the time Itzhak was two years old, a succession of moves kept his life in continual upheaval. The first was to a nearby state where his father was offered a better position. While the father went ahead to get settled, Itzhak remained behind with his mother, who anxiously awaited the outcome. After their reunion, the boy's renewed fear of his father gradually gave way to a measure of trust and security. The peace was short lived, however. After a few months, the father made an even more drastic change by going out West to explore for brighter job prospects. Meanwhile, Itzhak returned with his mother and a newly acquired brother to the East Coast family "for the duration." The mother, now absorbed in the new baby, was very anxious and weepy. She would leave Itzhak for a whole day at a time to the care of the other relatives. With his mother, once his exclusive companion, now dividing her attentions with a successor, and his father, whose companionship he had just begun to enjoy, gone again, it is no wonder that the child showed signs of insecurity and began to inquire anxiously and repeatedly about his absent father.

OUT WEST

PARENTS. The move to the West Coast plunged the family into a renewed struggle for existence. The father, who seemed more foreign than ever in the new environment, had difficulty in obtaining and holding suitable jobs. After three moves within the new city during the first year, they finally settled down for a year in a "mixed neighborhood" which the mother designated as "undesirable." She had to seek part-time employment as a Hebrew teacher to eke out her husband's paltry earnings. These hardships increased feelings of strain within the family. The mother reacted by tightening her discipline and then, smitten with guilt feelings, by undoing it. She shifted erratically from vague threats of punishment to actual spankings, or from "reasoning" to bribery. All these approaches were woven into a more general pattern of overprotectiveness and mutual dependency.

As for the overburdened father, he became stricter and more impatient with his boys. His efforts to train the patient according to the old tradition only reinforced the boy's ambivalence toward him.

PATIENT. As a result of these pressures, Itzhak became increasingly sensitive, timid, and dependent, possibly as a result of a defensive identification with his mother. He cried easily and made a scene every time his mother left the house, no matter how briefly. At night, instead of going to sleep, he regressively resorted to infantile demands on his mother reminiscent of his colic days, calling her repeatedly on the pretext of wanting a drink or something to eat. At other times he would talk aloud to himself, thereby waking his brother.

SUPERMAN. All day long he watched television or indulged in vivid and noisy fantasies about the TV characters. Superman played the role in his imagination of a magic father who was always strong. Incorporating his supernatural power through identification, the child no longer needed to fear either the weaker father or his own weakness. He could indulge in heroic exploits and even release the pent-up hostility he felt toward the father who had failed him in so many ways. Since Itzhak was not allowed to play with his "undesirable" age peers on the block, Superman became for him a special kind of imaginary companion.

CULTURE CONFLICT

The role played by culture conflict in this case is complex. The child's basic ethnic identification appears strong: He is proud of being a Jew. His tie to his mother, though ambivalent, is also strong. Moreover, his integration with the extended East Coast family is firmly established. He enjoyed sharing their religious observances and their holidays and longed nostalgically for them in his loneliness out West. He expressed his *Heimweh* symptomatically by the headache which told him he must get back there before Friday sundown.

The father appears as the chief source of the child's culture conflict. His frequent absences, combined with his severity and poor companionship, have frustrated the boy and prevented the usual identification. In this context, the religious rituals imposed by the father seem like a form of punishment and are resisted. Through this passive aggression, the son can retaliate, hurting and punishing his father by refusing to accept his values. This behavior, of course, sets up a vicious cycle, which leads again to the father's meting out more punishment to the child.

These dynamics are illustrated in Itzhak's reluctance to accompany his father to religious services. On one occasion, soon after the family's reunion on the West Coast, the boy had been taken to the synagogue by his father against his will. On being introduced to a friend of his father, he was seized with a crying "fit" which necessitated his immediate return home. For some time after the episode, Itzhak could not be persuaded to go and pray with his father, and he displayed fear of adult strangers. That his reluctance was due to his fear of his father, rather than rejection of his religion, seems apparent from his anxiety when threatened with exclusion from the ceremonial Friday evening dinner as a punishment for his refusal to accompany his father to the synagogue.

Itzhak's religious conflict thus symbolizes his deeper conflict with his father. It also symbolizes a broader culture conflict between East and West. In his search for security after many an uprooting, Itzhak looks for some trace of the old and familiar, but finds only the new and the strange. His former warm, tightly knit East Coast family has been replaced by a diffuse, impersonal social circle whose unpredictable practices seem to the bewildered little boy to question the eternal verities of his life. At one time he noted with fascinated horror the son of some family acquaintances casually starting the TV set on the Sabbath. Rushing to his mother, he exclaimed incredulously, "Mommy, look what they're doing!" At another time he was shocked beyond belief to meet a rabbi without a beard, which seemed to him a contradiction in terms. Under these circumstances, it is not surprising that the "why" questions so common in children of his age are largely religious in content. They seem to have taken on an air of obsessive doubting, in his attempt to reconcile the conflict between old and new, East and West, and to find some meaning and peace in his new life. For the parents, however, his persistent questions represent only an intellectual curiosity highly regarded by their ethnic group.

PSYCHOLOGICAL ASSESSMENT

TEST BATTERY.   The patient was given the following tests: Wechsler Intelligence Scale for Children (WISC), Children's Apperception Test (CAT), Despert-Fine Fables, Draw-A-Person (DAP), and other free drawing techniques. The test protocols are reproduced at the end of the chapter.

BEHAVIOR.   The boy's behavior during the examination was noteworthy. In the initial session his insecurity was betrayed by his refusal to go with the examiner and by his threats of "tearing the place apart." Once sufficient rapport was established to permit testing, there were frequent periods when the stream of aggressive fantasy prevented the child's complete cooperation in the tasks, as in the instance where he suddenly burst out, "My Daddy got cut and he started crying—he died. . . ." He showed relatively little reaction to verbal praise, yet appeared fully cognizant of what was expected of him. On occasion his involvement in the examination seemed minimal, but more often the stimuli elicited overly charged emotional reactions which were expressed in fantasy but never acted out.

WISC. The WISC (Test Summary A) elicited an extremely variable pattern, yielding a Full Scale IQ of 93, a Verbal IQ of 95, and a Performance IQ of 93. Although there is practically no discrepancy between the verbal and performance IQs, the range of subtest scores was wide. A markedly inferior weighted score was obtained on Object Assembly, and low scores were also recorded for Vocabulary, Picture Completion, and Block Designs. His best results were achieved on Coding, Picture Arrangement, and Information. One suspects that Itzhak's intelligence is above average, but the pattern seen on the subtests suggests a maladjustment which is interfering with intellectual functioning. Tests of perception, of spatial-motor skill, and of planning are most affected by the child's temporary lapses of attention. Yet his memory span for digits does not seem to suffer. His vocabulary and verbal reasoning which are important for interpersonal communication do not measure up to the level expected of a boy of his age, possibly because of his bilingualism. Coding, indicating his capacity for new learning, represents his high potential for benefiting from experience, while information and picture arrangement demonstrate how much he has already learned from his environment.

PROJECTIVE TESTS. Projective testing seemed to release an expression of the patient's rich fantasies. So stimulated was he by the human figure drawing that his verbalizations were a far greater source of material than what he drew. The CAT (Test Summary B) and the Despert-Fine Fables (Test Summary C) provided the ideal context for him, allowing free ventilation of his fantasy, while at the same time providing sufficient structure to hold him to the test stimuli.

The nature and effects of Itzhak's disturbance become much more discernible in the projective tests. One recurrent theme seen in the CAT is the fear of oral incorporation. On CAT III, the mouse wonders if the King of Beasts is "strong," and finds himself being "swallowed up." On Card X, a "mamma-dog" is spanking a "baby-dog" for eating up a rat and a cat. She in turn is ready to "eat up" the baby dog who gets away just in time. Additional information from the CAT and other tests supplies further evidence that the boy's problem revolves around orality. Unresolved dependency needs are implied in many responses. The man in the DAP (Fig. 18–1) has just gone to the market for food for his pet. Considerable shading is connected with the drawing of the food in the man's hand. In Fable 7, Itzhak talks about poisoned oranges. Eating, together with incorporation, is a persistent theme throughout the projections.

Closely connected with the child's orality is his aggression. This has already been mentioned in connection with the observations of behavior. In a sense many of the signs discussed under infantile orality were indicative of oral aggression as well. This boy does not react to his frustration passively, but in a hostile manner charged with violence, as the many wild animals in his Fables suggest. Situations are for him all-or-none. People are either "good" or "bad," and the "bad" ones are eaten up, beaten up, or severely castigated. Rarely is Itzhak the aggressive one, and then only indirectly, through identification with the punisher.

The strict moral dichotomy which Itzhak visualizes is guarded by an externalized superego in the person of Superman. Within this rigid, castelike thinking, he locates himself on the "bad" side. In drawing his family (Fig. 18–2), *he* is a conspicuous omission. Apparently he feels so insecure about his position in the family that he is led in another drawing to picture himself as falling in a parachute. He seeks mediation with his family through nonhuman efforts on his behalf, by a "friendly vulture." Such evidence leaves little doubt that the boy lacks confidence in himself and feels undeserving. In this way he is able to rationalize his feelings of frustration but not to deny them.

The recurrence of the father theme in all the projective material focuses much of Itzhak's conflict in the family setting, and is marked by feelings of ambivalence. Stories on CAT VI and VII reveal the father as the benevolent protector; in several others, e.g., II and IV, his strength and ability to save the children are questioned, while in Fables 12 and 16, death wishes for the father are entertained. The patient's ambivalence toward the father prevents strong positive identification although efforts are made in that direction, as in Fable 1, where the little bird is going to fly to the *father*. The conflict with his father is focused in his DAP (Fig. 18–1), where the man is depicted with the long beard and high hat of the orthodox rabbi. On a deeper level the symbolism of the personal details may refer to sexuality and is a further reflection of his identity problem. His distance from his father makes it doubly difficult to identify with him; both religion and masculinity are at stake. Fear of his father is further developed in his interpretation of his freehand drawings, where adult male figures are described as "ugly," "bad," and "murderers." Only through the fantasied intervention of Superman (Fig. 18–3) can the patient cope with the father figure. In Superman he has found an externalized superego that permits him to carry out limited aggressions against his father.

In general, the test results point to the existence of an emotional disturbance of sufficient severity to have interfered with the child's intellectual functioning and general adjustment. While the data do not suggest any specific disturbance of the ideational processes, the boy's preoccupation with hostile, aggressive fantasy denies him considerable opportunity for positive interaction with his environment and makes increasingly difficult any useful integration of his experiences. Basically dependent, he feels frustrated because his parents, particularly the father, are not adequately meeting his infantile needs.

DIAGNOSTIC IMPRESSION

As Itzhak presented himself to the clinic, his withdrawal symptoms, absorption in his Superman fantasy, "visions," and compelling "headaches," combined with regressive soiling, suggested a schizophrenic reaction, childhood type.

When this symptom picture was evaluated against the boy's social background, however, it appeared less malignant. His difficulties center around insecurity in his immediate family. At a time when the little boy needed support and satisfactions of his basic dependency needs, he was torn up by the roots from a warm ethnically close family group and transplanted by a succession of moves to an altogether alien climate. His father's frequent absence and forbidding presence left him without a model, ethnic or masculine, with whom to identify. His mother in her own perplexity had clung to her son in desperate mutual dependency, while at the same time she had to share her attentions with a second son.

In this unsupporting environment, even the orthodox religious rituals which had given backbone and order to Itzhak's former existence could not be counted on. In his bitter disappointment, he rejected these symbols along with the disappointing father image of which they were a part.

The new situation also failed to offer the compensation of a peer group which might have restored the feeling of belonging that he could no longer find in his family circle. But as a result of his mother's fears of contamination from "undesirable" neighbors, the child was cut off from all playmates of his own age. This left him alone with the manufactured fantasies of television, and Superman became his constant companion and guide.

The last straw came with the daily separation from the only reality left to the boy, his mother. Every day for long hours the child had to remain in the rigid school, with its cold, hard authorities and teasing classmates. This situation proved more than Itzhak could cope with, and it was at this point that he began to regress and to develop the psychotic-like symptoms that brought him to the clinic for help.

In view of the child's assets in terms of intellectual potential, sensitivity to his social environment, and ability to learn from it, as well as his capacity for affective response, the prognosis for therapy seemed excellent. So important was the mother's attitude for the outcome of the child's treatment that her cooperation in a therapy group for mothers was enlisted before proceeding with the case. Ideally, it would have been desirable for the father to have at least been counselled, but unfortunately this was not practicable.

THERAPEUTIC GOALS

Since the little patient's major problem revolved around his conflict with his father as a sexual and ethnic model, the chief aim of the brief therapy undertaken was to build a positive relationship with a man who could serve as a surrogate father figure. Through such a relationship, it was hoped that the boy's anxiety could be reduced, his negative feelings toward his family and religion reduced, and more adaptive forms of behavior developed. A secondary goal was the ultimate reinstatement of the child in a group of his age peers.

THE THERAPIST

To increase communication with the patient and his family, a therapist who understood the chief cultural values "from the inside" and yet was sufficiently different in background to be able to maintain objectivity was sought. The solution was found in a young Israeli clinical psychology trainee, who was identified with Jewish culture, well versed in the Hebrew language, but who held a more flexible religious position than that of the patient's family.

COURSE OF THERAPY

Time limitations permitted only a very brief course of treatment through play interviews. The patient was seen approximately once weekly for a period of five months, for a total of seventeen sessions. The course of therapy may be roughly divided into three stages that can be characterized as (1) establishing the relationship, (2) testing the limits, and (3) terminating.

ESTABLISHING THE RELATIONSHIP. The mother brought Itzhak to the clinic where he clung to her, a faint shy smile on his face, unwilling to leave her for the first few minutes.

On the way up to the playroom he started talking about Superman and his great strength and power. He talked rapidly, stopping only momentarily as he entered the playroom and saw with astonishment all the play things. He then went right on again with aggressive stories about Superman's "knocking people down; punishing murderers," etc., while sampling some of the toys. As though fearing his own hostility, he would quickly throw one toy down after the other, all the while weaving them into variations on the theme of Superman's aggressive prowess. Noticing the painting stand, the child moved up to it abruptly, and stood before it a long time, painting lines and circles representing Superman's special powers, e.g., his X-ray vision (cf. drawing, Fig. 18–3), by which he was able to fight off the "bad" and help the "good." Superman did not always kill bad men; if they begged for it, he would show clemency, tempered, however with the threat to turn them over to the police if they did it again.

Although Itzhak seemed to be paying little attention to the therapist, he would frequently look back to see if he were being watched and would smile slyly when choosing not to answer one of his questions. To the remark that Superman seemed very strong, the patient exclaimed, "He is even stronger than my Daddy," later adding the qualification that "Superman is not real; he is only on TV and they have tricks to make him strong."

During the first few play sessions the child's fantasies frequently included direct and aggressive references to members of his family, similar to those noted throughout testing. The father was portrayed in these stories as either weak or strong, but more often weak especially in relation to Superman. On one occasion, for example, he said, "Last night some bad men came to our home to take my Mommy away. They fought with Daddy, and they punched him in the nose and he cried. So Superman came and I punched them in the nose and they cried and ran away." When the therapist commented that he did not want anyone to take his Mommy away from him, he volunteered, "I like to stay home and play with my Mommy." His identification with Superman became evident from his interchangeable use of "Superman" and the first person singular. Throughout these sessions, the therapist played the role of a friendly and accepting listener who occasionally reflected the patient's feelings but offered no interpretations.

After the first meetings, which were dominated by Itzhak's aggressive, verbal productions mainly involving Superman, a different pattern of behavior gradually began to emerge. The patient's rate of verbalization slowed down, and he started a more realistic interaction through play activities with his therapist. On arrival at the clinic, he would now rush up to the playroom and after a flurry of excited greetings and accounts of the day's experiences would settle down to clay modeling, water-coloring, and playing with dolls and other toys. While working on the clay, he would say, "You just sit there and watch me," or while water-coloring, he would occasionally ask the therapist to help him paint his name and other words in Hebrew. The therapist took advantage of the reference to Hebrew to question him about his Hebrew studies. In this way he elicited some of the patient's negative feelings and unhappy memories at the Hebrew school. During this time, the character of the doll play changed: New, unfamiliar "people" now appeared, often attacking each other, but just as often merely visiting, or reading and playing, without involving Superman. At the end of the sixth play interview, the patient tried to open a door with a complicated lock but was unable to negotiate it alone. Succeeding after having enlisted the therapist's help, he exclaimed happily, "*We* did it!"

At the next session, he told about the family's recent move to new quarters where the landlord "was not very Jewish because he drives his car on the 'Shabess!'" Realizing the affective loading that "moving" had for the patient, the therapist suggested that they play out the moving with the dolls and miniature house in the playroom. While enthusiastically engaged in this occupation, the boy said suddenly, "Sometimes I don't want to go to the *schull* (synagogue) and my father spanks me." The therapist reflected the feeling that he did not want to be punished for not going to pray with his father.

The therapist's impression that the positive relationship with him was now on firm ground received confirmation from the child's mother who told him at this time that her son "is talking about you all the time, and anticipates coming down here." A new form of interaction made its appearance about this time that may be characterized as "testing the limits."

TESTING THE LIMITS. About halfway through the ninth interview, the patient asked to go down to the washroom, commanding the therapist, "You wait right here for me." Soon after his return he requested the therapist to play "trains" with him and follow him about. This involved running around the toy boxes, under the table, and in between the legs of the painting stand. The boy showed the therapist no mercy, forcing him to crawl and squeeze through these places to the child's undisguised delight.

Toward the end of the same session, the patient, while playing with the dolls, remarked that there were not enough soldiers to play "war," and requested that the therapist get more for the next session. The first thing he did when the time came was to check. Finding that the therapist had failed to keep his promise, he threatened, "If you don't bring them next time, I'll shoot you." He was visibly disappointed, and refused consolation in the form of a new bottle of bubble soap. Instead, he modeled a monkey in clay, naming each part as he made it. When he reached the buttocks, he could not seem to recall the English word, using instead the Yiddish, "tuchess."

His angry mood persisted throughout the session, while he blew bubbles which collided with each other and sometimes hit the therapist. During this play, Itzhak, yelling at the top of his voice, described the popping bubbles as "bad men" being killed by the police or Superman, as colliding firetrucks, or escaping murder gangs.

The following week when his new soldiers were there at last, his first words were, "You didn't forget!" That this episode was a "test" of faith in the therapist rather than an interest in the soldiers as such was indicated by the brevity of time spent in playing with them. After a very few minutes he turned to other activities.

Later in this session, while building a castle, the patient's cap, which in obedience to orthodox ritual was worn at all times, fell off. Instead of putting it back on his head, however, he slowly and slyly tucked it in his pocket, all the while eying the therapist with a guilty air. Ignoring this behavior, the therapist asked what he was building, and was informed that it was a castle "and only you and me are going to live in this castle, and no one else." Later he added, with some hesitation, "only you and I and Mommy."

In the latter phase of the therapy, the patient was reluctant to leave, and made excuses for prolonging the sessions. There always seemed to be "just one more thing."

TERMINATION OF TREATMENT. The last four sessions may be said to constitute the termination period of Itzhak's therapy. He had resumed attendance at school on a part-time basis and under the tutelage of a more permissive teacher. The boy adjusted so well to his new school regime that after a few days he would dash off into the playground on arrival without bothering to bid his mother "goodbye." During the play interviews, he spent much of the time water-coloring and finger painting "as we do at school." He proudly told the therapist of his new activities at school, of his friends there and in his new neighborhood. He also talked of the many toys he had at home and of his hope that his father would soon buy him an electric train.

When after missing one appointment because he had preferred to go to school that day, his mother brought him back to the clinic the following week, he showed little interest in the playroom and in talking with the therapist. The mother later confessed that she had "bribed" him to come that day because she was not quite convinced that he really had no more need for therapy. When asked why he had not wanted to come the previous week, he said simply, "I have more fun at school now." At this point the therapist told him he was doing so well in school now that he would not have to continue at the clinic.

THE MOTHER IN GROUP THERAPY

Under the stress of her son's "collapse," the mother displayed great anxiety and expressed her willingness to comply with anything the clinic might advise, including her attendance at a mothers' therapy group once a week. After two meetings, however, she became resistant to the group and missed several sessions. The recognition of need for psychological help, especially in group form, was foreign to her values. She "just could not see" how talking in a group, especially in a group containing a Negro, could possibly help solve her problem. Later, impressed with the improvement in her boy's behavior and his reinstatement in school, her own attitude improved and she attended more regularly and even began to participate in group discussion. She showed some important insights into her relationship, as well as that of her husband, to their son. She also began to understand the boy's need for more independent experiences than she had previously allowed him.

Despite the mother's gains in group therapy, at the end of each of the boy's sessions, she would make a point of "cornering" his therapist and questioning him closely on details of his progress as well as on the proper handling at home. Since her overtures indicated genuine concern over her son's problems rather than manipulative efforts to control the treatment, they were treated supportively, with reassurances and particular recommendations when indicated. The cultural bond between mother and therapist facilitated communication between them and proved to be a source of relief, helping her to overcome her anxiety during her initial contacts with the clinic.

PROGNOSIS

The prognosis for Itzhak at this time is very favorable. Before therapy, the harsh experiences at the hands of his father and teacher, coupled with the inconsistencies he found in his new environment, had developed in the patient an ambivalent attitude toward his ethnic ingroup which was undermining his basic self concept. The solid relationship built up through the play sessions with a trusted therapist who shared his ethnic values but was more flexible in their expression helped the little boy to stabilize his ethnic as well as his sexual identity.

The insight gained by the mother through group therapy and the brief talks with the child's therapist, together with the more relaxed attitude adopted by the father regarding his son's behavior, are hopeful signs that the positive "father-identification" may be maintained, and serve the boy as a bulwark in his later contacts with the dominant culture group.

THE LAST WORD

A check with the mother at the close of the school year regarding Itzhak's progress revealed that he had finished the term "very nicely," had gotten along well with both teacher and schoolmates, and was expecting to attend summer camp.

Test Summary

A. Wechsler Intelligence Scale for Children

Verbal Tests	*Wtd. Score*	*Performance Tests*	*Wtd. Score*
Information	12	Picture Completion	7
Comprehension	8	Picture Arrangement	12
Arithmetic	8	Block Design	7
Similarities	9	Object Assembly	5
Vocabulary	7	Coding	14
(Digit Span)	11	(Mazes)	–
Sum	55(46)*	Sum	45
Verbal I.Q.	95	Performance I.Q.	93
	Total I.Q. 93		

* Prorated.

Test Summary

B. CHILDREN'S APPERCEPTION TEST (CAT)

CARD I.

They're eating. They're birds and there's a chicken. I think a wolf's going to eat them up. First he'll eat up the chickens; then the mother and the two sons.

CARD II.

There's a bear, there's a baby bear and a great big gigantic animal who looks black and he is bigger than the father. They're fighting with the rope because they want to see who is stronger but the big creature is stronger because the father forgot to take his breakfast. He left some over. The baby bear is helping the father. The father bear gets stronger because he eats his breakfast.

CARD III.

That's a lion and a rat that's looking out of a hole to see what's going on. He wants to see if the King of the Beasts is not strong. Then the King of the Beasts swallowed him up and that's the end.

CARD IV.

Here's a mommy kangaroo. They're going to see their husband and they're bringing him lunch because he forgot it. Then the daddy doesn't know that two big bears came to swallow them up.

CARD V.

There are two animals that are sleeping in a crib. They're father and mother sleeping so they decided to go out for a walk at midnight. The father and mother saw they weren't there and said, "Let's hurry," and ran out and caught two and spanked them. They didn't do any more jokes on their father and mother.

CARD VI.

This bear is a big one and this little one opens his eye to go out of the cave. Then a wolf comes to eat up the father and then father fights with the wolf, and then when he won, he was the winner.

CARD VII.

This is a tiger that's going to eat up a monkey. But father gorilla finds out that tiger is eating up monkey and jumps down and you know who the winner was, the father. The monkey was saved and he jumped up a tree. He wasn't scared, he was only scared of the mouth.

CARD VIII.

These are a lots of monkeys, four of them. And they have a picture of sick old grandma. They don't know that the wolf swallowed her up. So they send little Red Riding Hood. Police came with father. Mother tells Red Riding Hood that it wasn't nice to tell the police.

CARD IX.

This is a rabbit and he is in his crib looking out of the open door. He doesn't know that the wolves are covering the house. Then Superman appeared to see if the wolves were dead. He landed and killed them both. And then he took them and baby rabbit was safe in time.

CARD X.

Here's a big dog that's spanking a little dog, because baby dog isn't good. Because he ate up a rat and a cat. So mother spanks him and is ready to eat him up but the baby ran away. Superman comes and tells the puppy to be good.

Test Summary

C. DESPERT-FINE FABLES

1. Little bird is going to fly to father.
2. Because he wanted to see if there were any worms. He was going to eat them up.
3. Not to eat grass but to go find a wolf. Then he'll run for help.
4. Strong.
5. The brothers and the mommys and the sisters.
6. He was going to see a wolf.
7. An orange. If it was poison, he would die.
8. I think it might be a giraffe from Africa.
9. Of wolves, and snakes, and rattlesnakes.
10. Because he looks dirty.
11. He waits with the landlady.
12. The father. And then they took another father but he was a buffalo.
13. Dreamed about Superman.
14. At end of school he'll make a bell out of it.
15. Because he saw that they left. He was in a tree looking.
16. His father died because there was an electrician man.
17. I think he won't because he doesn't want his mommy to know that he wants to tear it up.
18. Dreamed about climbing on beanstalk and there was a giant.
19. That the Suez Canal has some Americans there.
20. They will go, the boy will go (younger) and meets a bear and runs home.

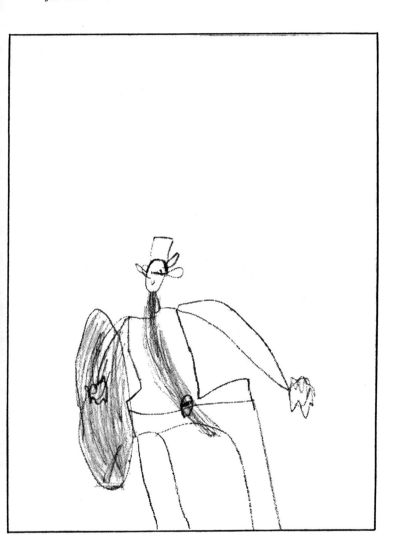

FIGURE 18–1.   Draw-A-Person Test.

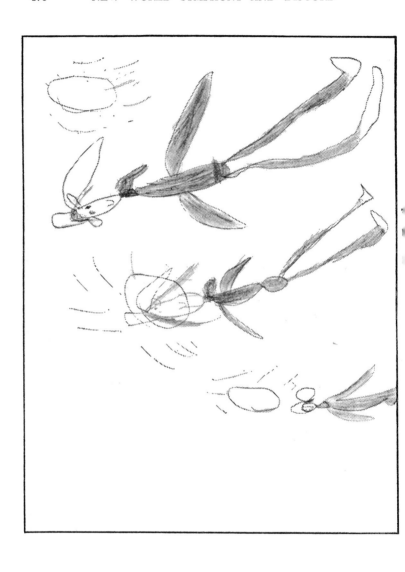

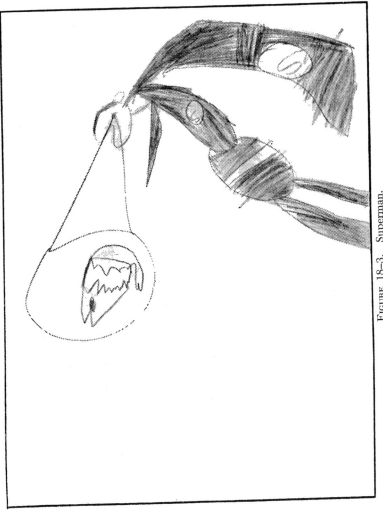

FIGURE 18–3. Superman.

19

Heritage of the Ghetto in the Second Generation

Jerome L. Singer

A VALUE TRIAD

The case of Seymour C. suggests in an unusually clear-cut way the manner in which cultural values and strivings modally characteristic of central and eastern European Jewish families are transmitted to their American-born progeny. It appears that these cultural patterns are incorporated into the character structure in a fashion that in many instances leads to a triad of salient features which may be observed in many Jewish men. These three characteristics are (1) "intellectuality," manifested by extensive resort to ideational activity frequently obsessional in nature, accompanied by considerable introspectiveness and fantasy; (2) "motor inhibition," restraint of impulse, often a deep-seated sense of physical inferiority, doubts concerning sexual effectiveness; and (3) "upward social mobility," a drive for professional attainment with vocational aspirations chiefly in fields of high status like medicine, law, pure science, and a striving for "good marks" that persists throughout life, well beyond the school years. While this general formulation may seem to partake somewhat of a cultural stereotype there seems little doubt that the characteristics described are observable in a significant number of second or third generation Jewish men raised in urban lower- or middle-middle class family settings.

Viewed as the outcome of generations of adaptation to the European urban ghettos or small town environments, this triad of characteristics in ideal proportion may be very valuable to society in making available intelligent, useful, and law-abiding participants in many of the service functions of the social matrix. The balance among the characteristics may be a delicate one, however, as a result of the specific familial pattern or a particular cultural milieu. Thus the specific family constellation which transmits the general cultural trend may be so disrupted by personal stresses between the parents as to arouse excessive anxiety in the child or to exaggerate the emphasis on one of these characteristics. Similarly the milieu in which the family finds itself may block fruitful integration of the three traits. This might be the case for a family residing in a strongly anti-Semitic neighborhood. The very fact of minority status in the nation may in itself be enough to reinforce the development of the pattern even where specific anti-Semitism has not been experienced.

The case of Seymour is an instance of intricate consequences of a neurotic family structure superimposed on the cultural pattern described above. The result is that the intellectuality, motor restraint, and professional striving are poorly integrated into the total personality and much self-defeating behavior emerges. The cultural conflict involved in Seymour's development does not stem from any obvious impact of anti-Semitism or of minority status. Rather, it would appear that the cultural values available for use by his parents as reference points for their particular personal strivings have been transmitted in a manner so enmeshed with anxiety as to distort for Seymour his own possibility of recognizing personal strengths or resources available to him as part of the American culture.

To anticipate briefly, Seymour's capacity for warmth and humor has made it possible for him to have close friends throughout his life among the boys in the street or fellow students. This facet of his personality is scarcely recognized by him and seems of little value in the face of his own competitive striving for intellectual and social status. Yet it represents a potentiality for closeness that can have productive possibilities in terms of emotional satisfactions and effectiveness in work with others. Thus, Seymour's European-Jewish focus on intellectual striving as a key to status, enhanced by his specific familial pattern, plays a disproportionate role in his perception of his own worth and of his "market value" in our society, while his knack of making good friendships which in American culture certainly opens many doors for professional attainment as well as for personal satisfaction seems to him a minor facet of his potentialities as a human being.

PRESENTING PICTURE

PHYSICAL APPEARANCE. Seymour was referred for consultation by a relative who is a psychologist residing in another state. The patient had spoken to him at a family gathering and seemed extremely eager for help since he felt that he had suffered a "breakdown." At the time of his first interview, he was dressed in a most untidy fashion, was unkempt and unshaven, and his finger nails were bitten down to raw skin. He was a young man of twenty-three, tall, extremely thin, with black hair and a sallow complexion. Seymour was rather handsome and possessed a certain dignity in his mien even in his obviously depressed state. His reasons for coming were expressed in an extremely halting manner characterized by painful blocking in speech.

> I feel I've had a kind of breakdown. It's as if my life has come to a dead stop. I can't move. I don't seem to be able to do anything and I've messed up everything I've tried to do in the past. I've been married for six months and it seems like six years. I feel overwhelmed by my wife, by school, by life in general. I've thought of suicide, of a mental hospital. I feel myself to be a terrible failure.

Seymour explained in a halting, almost painful manner that he had dropped out of law school because of inability to concentrate a few months after his first semester began. He had been too ashamed to admit this even to his wife and had kept up the pretense of attending for a month or so before revealing his situation to her. He had continued to keep his withdrawal a secret from his parents who were assisting him financially. Seymour spoke of himself in bitter terms yet with a slightly melodramatic quality as a "glorious failure," the "prodigal son doubled in spades," and as "Prufrock revisited." "I feel old, my life seems past—as if my brief glory lies behind." There was of course an ironic quality in these phrases but a savoring of them as well. One had the feeling that Seymour, although obviously depressed and unhappy, still wanted to be able to express his misery in blank verse.

SPEECH BLOCKING. Another area of difficulty included sensitivity over his blocking in speech. The long pauses and breaks in sentences (which have been eliminated from direct quotations) were a source of embarrassment to this young man in his school situations and in casual contacts with tradesmen or acquaintances. With family, intimate friends, or with the psychologist this blocking was less noticeable, and Seymour often spoke fluently and, as suggested earlier, with considerable ability for interesting and somewhat literary phrasing. In many speech situations or in classroom recitations, however, he blocked for seemingly interminable periods and in order to say something would finally blurt out vague or inept comments that often made him appear somewhat dull. The blocking in speech had been a long-standing pattern going back to early childhood but it was particularly in evidence at school from about the third grade and had become increasingly severe in the past year.

SEXUAL FEARS. Seymour did not report any physical symptoms. He had a deep sense of being "poorly put together, warped or diseased" but this feeling was not referred to any specific organic characteristic. Eventually and with great difficulty Seymour expressed fears concerning his sexual potency and capacity for sexual relations. Although this fear was not confirmed in his actual sexual behavior since he reported frequent and mutually satisfactory intercourse with his wife, Seymour felt under constant pressure to maintain a high level of frequency, to keep erections for extremely long periods, and to provide his wife with many more orgasms than himself. He kept track of frequency and became anxious about "maintaining a high average." The few instances of *ejaculatio praecox* or of temporary impotence were magnified as catastrophic proof of his ineptness with subsequent resentment of his wife whose very presence imposed a demand for performance on him despite her denial that this was her intention.

Seymour's feeling about his wife, Shirley, aged twenty-three, was extremely ambivalent and characterized by the extensive obsessional rumination which distressed him so. He realized that she was attractive, loving, intelligent, and sincere but yet felt that she had sucked away his own independence and strength. Her competence, academically and professionally (she was a scientific research assistant), remained constant evidence to him of his failures and also seemed to him a defiant competitiveness on her part. The fact that she was apparently more effective in dealing with tradesmen and in managing the household further emphasized for him her competitive striving to surpass him. He became extremely involved in each instance of even the most casual dispute between them over everyday matters or over interpretation of news events or answers to TV quiz show questions. When she proved right he became furious and withdrew into an embittered silence for hours at a time. Thus, despite much strongly positive feeling between Seymour and Shirley, a great deal of resentment had developed and he spoke often of his being trapped and "held down" by her.

FAMILY BACKGROUND AND CULTURAL ORIGINS

EUROPEAN GRANDPARENTS. Seymour's parents were both first generation Americans of eastern European Jewish descent. Mrs. C., aged fifty-three, was the eldest of three daughters of a rabbi who had come to the United States shortly before World War I from a large European town. He had assumed leadership of a small, moderately orthodox congregation in a densely populated section of the Bronx and maintained that position for the rest of his life. The congregation consisted chiefly of small businessmen, shop-keepers, and garment workers who barely managed to keep their tiny center solvent. Thus, the rabbi, although reason-ably secure in his position because of the great respect for his learning, eked out a marginal living with considerable exertion by supplementing his income through officiating at ceremonies and private tutoring for small fees.

As described by Seymour both from his own recollections and his lengthy conversations with his mother, the rabbi was a proud man, dominant in his community and in his family, extremely intellectual and pedantic. He completely cowed his wife who was a timid, somewhat pathetic woman who limited herself to caring for her children and rarely left her kitchen. Bitterly regretting his lack of a son, the grandfather sought to fill this gap by demanding an un-usual degree of Hebrew scholarship from his daughters. At the same time, since higher education was out of the question for the girls because of economic necessity, fam-ily pressure forced an orientation towards "good marriages." The intense competition already set up among the girls for the father's affection was transferred from the intellectual arena to the more practical one of material success through marriage. Seymour's mother as the eldest and least "Amer-icanized" suffered somewhat in the competition. When the two younger daughters began "keeping company" with two young men, sons of congregation leaders, who seemed likely to become professionals, the eldest daughter was under great pressure to marry first.

PARENTAL DISCREPANCIES. Seymour's father seemed un-der those circumstances as a most likely prospect. A few years older than Hannah (Seymour habitually referred to his mother by her first name at her insistence), Mr. C. was a more recent immigrant, relatively uneducated by the fam-ily standards, but extremely hard working and successful in his own business. The combination of Jacob's physical attractiveness (he was rugged in build and athletically inclined, playing soccer on a local team) and his material success proved enough to convince Hannah of his desirability despite the fact that she lacked any romantic feeling for him. She acceded to the general pressure and was thus able to marry first and have her own apartment on the "Concourse," a decided step upward socially. For Hannah her marriage was based on fondness and a sense of pressure. She resolved to make her husband develop more into the intellectual and sophisticated person she desired. Jacob's own feeling was one of enormous respect for his wife's intellectual status and family background. He felt honored and happy since he considered himself uneducated. His orientation became one of feeling that his role was to provide every material comfort for his wife and child and that, if he worked long hours at his laundry and dry-cleaning business, his reward would be an opportunity to relax quietly at home, go to sleep early, and perhaps play some soccer or handball on Sunday morning.

Neither parent found much needed satisfaction in their marriage, however, as was soon apparent. Jacob quickly grew to resent Hannah's efforts at improving his mind and social graces and withdrew more and more into "driven" physical labor. Hannah quickly became disenchanted with the possibilities of a rapid transformation of her husband into a man somewhat in the image of her scholarly father. Her frustration was aggravated by the persisting competition with her sisters. One sister had married a somewhat older man, a lawyer who had attained great success politically in the community and had become a magistrate. This sister lived in the same neighborhood and bore her first child shortly before Seymour was born so that inevitable comparisons of the children became a part of the family pattern from that time on. Hannah realized that her husband could not compete with her urbane and politically potent brother-in-law, and she began to look upon the latter as the real model for her child. Seymour thus from his earliest years heard endless tales of how Uncle Arnold would or could do this for one, or that one must behave in a certain way to impress him. Comparisons between Seymour and Arnold's son, Monroe, were constantly voiced. The family atmosphere in which Seymour found himself thus consisted of an extreme emphasis on achievement through intellect, on fierce competition for social status and prestige.

HOME PRESSURES. It does not seem sufficient to state that this atmosphere grew solely out of the specific interaction of the parents and stemmed in a "purely psychological" fashion from their specific family constellations. The peculiar emphasis of Hannah's father on intellectual achievement for his daughters and "good marriages" itself reflected a cultural pattern which emphasized male scholarliness as a supreme value. This value enhanced the feeling transmitted to the girls that the way to their father's heart or, in general, the way to real self-esteem and a sense of individual worth lay through the intellectual and social prestige of their husbands. As was often the case among first generation immigrants, the natural trend for the young mothers was to place their hopes in the sons for whom American society offered extensive educational possibilities, since their husbands in the new American culture were relatively unable to attain prestige but were limited to use of their skills and intelligence in business or shopkeeping. Hannah C. could not see her drive for status through the competitive exploitation of her son as potentially dangerous or as selfish, inasmuch as it fitted the Jewish-American cultural expectation. She wanted "only the best" for her son and "wasn't this what every mother wanted?" And "only the best" meant in America that the son must speak clearly, grammatically, be conversant with good thoughts of wise men, avoid "dirty words" or "dirty habits," and in general make the impression on others of a well-spoken "gentleman." His schoolwork would of necessity have to be excellent so that he could get into the professional hierarchy of medicine, dentistry, law, or accounting. In effect, therefore, the value pattern built into Hannah's personality in her own family constellation was further reinforced by her adult participation in a cultural milieu which sanctioned her distorted view of her maternal role and effectively prevented her awareness of the extent to which she might be crushing or inhibiting important unique potentialities in her son.

Jacob C., in a curiously negative way, further strengthened the transmission of this emphasis on intellectuality, social striving, and motor inhibition. As an adult he passively resisted the constant nagging of his wife concerning the need for self-improvement and educational growth. This resistance was accomplished chiefly by his long hours of work and regular evenings of pinochle or by falling asleep after supper. Nevertheless Mr. C. accepted the cultural values of his wife as the correct ones and did not actively resist her efforts to elevate him or Seymour; he felt incapable of following her programs but attributed this to his ineptitude. As the years went by he occasionally acceded to her educational efforts but he grew to resent her concentration on Seymour and made many bitter comments contrasting his own physical strength and mechanical skill with the boy's inexperience and awkwardness. He could not disagree with the cultural emphasis but could in frequent "snide" remarks communicate some deprecation of the "sissy" attitudes fostered by his wife in Seymour, thus momentarily enhancing his own strength and power and inadvertently reinforcing Seymour's doubts concerning his own physical capacities.

CHILDHOOD AND ADOLESCENCE

AN AMBITIOUS MOTHER. Seymour's understanding was that he was a very much wanted child and that his parents tried in vain for a child for four years before his mother conceived. He was a full-term baby in good health who suffered only the usual childhood diseases. He learned that he was bottle fed and was not a feeding problem. His recall for early toilet training or related experiences was negligible although constipation became a problem for him in early adolescence. There were no recollections of infantile sexuality although fantasy and dream material suggested the possibility that early prohibitions of self-manipulation had been severe. Seymour's earliest and most frequent memories involved a constant repetitive emphasis from his mother on his speaking properly, memorizing poetry and elocutions, and performing before intimate circles. He recalls constant closeness with his mother who spent long hours with him attempting to teach him recitations, caring for his physical needs devotedly, but attacking him in scathing terms if he seemed reluctant to continue his memory efforts. The endless references to Uncle Arnold and Cousin Monroe which were dinned into his ears served to develop in him a strong competitiveness and a need to show off but at the same time must have aroused a deep sense of futility for he recalls telling his mother at the age of eleven, "Don't count so on me—I don't think I'll be able to live up to your hopes." His mother wept when he said this, he recalls, but she continued her efforts.

Mrs. C. enrolled her son in elocution classes, a children's theatrical troupe (he appeared a few times on a radio program doing recitations), and various music courses. In adolescence she forced him to take evening classes in business practices, typing, bookkeeping, public speaking, accordion playing, and a large number of other self-improvement programs. His mother took Seymour visiting with her on many occasions and often went away over week ends or for longer vacation periods with him leaving her husband behind. Her emphasis was constantly on the boy's performing before friends and family, preparing him beforehand for each encounter in a tense briefing, and boasting afterward about his latest accomplishment.

Friends and playmates. Seymour's conscious reaction to this situation was one of acceptance. This was the way things were—Hannah meant only the best even if she did act silly about it sometimes. He tried his best in all the courses. There was relief during the afternoons when he was permitted to run free with the other neighborhood children. Actually Seymour proved very much a member of the neighborhood gang as he recalled. He made several friends who have remained close to him until the present. and he was something of a leader in various neighborhood clubs. His speech blocking which troubled him so at school was scarcely noticeable and seemed to play little part in his peer relationships. His height and accurate perceptual skill, as well as his intelligence, were assets in basketball and he was well received in this area of juvenile activity. Persisting doubt about his physical prowess, however, led him to shun the most competitive or aggressive situations. In football or rough and tumble games he seemed hesitant and used his intelligence to advantage as a referee or rules authority.

Although Seymour obviously took great pleasure in this side of his personality in childhood and adolescence he never regarded it as a vitally important value. His mother showed no interest in his relationships with friends except insofar as school competition was involved ("How come Herman got all A's and you didn't?"). She generally disapproved of the intellectual caliber of his basketball teammates but her own needs for family socialization and afternoon bridge and mah-jonng kept her from involving herself in this phase of Seymour's life between the ages of seven through fourteen.

Despite the tremendous pressure described, Seymour proved only a mediocre student at school. His grades were fair and he was never in difficulties but his enthusiasm waned quickly and he could not concentrate well. He never carried to completion any of the various evening courses he was forced to undertake. Initial interest was followed by a period of blankness and his effort more or less "withered away." By the age of fifteen, despite his continued gratification with his friends and in his basketball, Seymour felt himself a failure and his mother seemed to echo this feeling.

PSYCHOLOGICAL SEQUELAE OF PNEUMONIA. When he was fifteen Seymour developed pneumonia followed by a number of serious respiratory infections. Prolonged bed rest was prescribed so that he missed a semester and spent a spring and summer practically bedridden. During this time, Seymour developed an even greater intimacy with his mother and also withdrew into a world of heroic fantasy and philosophic rumination. Mrs. C. spent a great deal of time conversing with her son. She had made him her confidant since childhood but now long intimate conversations took place daily. This unusual closeness unquestionably aroused difficult conflicts for the boy who felt all the more that gratification and attention could come from a woman if one were helpless and passive but that a great obligation for intellectual understanding and responsibility was a concomitant of this pattern. Upsetting incestuous tendencies were also fostered. Seymour whose sexual development was just getting under way at that time was shocked by several sexual dreams in which his mother appeared as a seductive yet threatening figure (see below). His own sense of physical limitation and inhibition was heightened at this time and he also experienced considerable guilt over his inability to control masturbation. One might speculate that Seymour's emotional disturbance might have been manifested earlier and in more severe form had this period of confinement at home continued.

In the fall the family, fearing the possibility of tuberculosis, sent the boy to Denver where he lived with distant relatives and attended a private school. He remained there for two years completing his sophomore and junior years of high school. This trip to Denver proved in many ways an extremely valuable and strengthening experience, restoring to him some sense of independent worth. Here Seymour found himself capable of action and creativity. His intellectual ability and urban sophistication made him attractive to many of the young people at the private school he attended and he was much sought after by the girls. He edited the school paper, wrote a play which was performed successfully, and made decided progress in his physical health. He found himself responding with great warmth to the attentions of girls—they served as inspirations to him and he found that when "going steady" with successive girls he was more productive than he had ever been in his life. A curious pattern developed in this connection, however, for after the first burst of creative effort inspired by the current "crush," Seymour soon began to feel under tremendous pressure to maintain his high level and to continue to impress. This pressure led to withdrawal and inactivity and eventuated in terminating the relationship. Then a fresh surge of activity would begin as soon as another girl showed interest and made overtures for Seymour's attention initiating a new cycle.

PSYCHOLOGICAL RELAPSE. Seymour's "pastoral idyll" terminated with his return to New York at the end of his junior year. He responded to the change with a deep feeling of despondency which he could not shake off for months. He felt a great sense of weariness and obligation to prove his success to his mother but found himself losing interest in school work with poor grades as a result. Again he felt that he had "failed the family" and that his "glory" was past.

Seymour went on to attend a local college and lived at home although some of his friends took rooms on or near the campus. His initial career objective was medicine, a natural choice from the standpoint of his mother's values but a subject in which he had little personal interest. An early failure in pre-med courses eliminated that possibility, and Seymour was forced to alter his personal status goal to a legal career like that of Uncle Arnold.

SHIRLEY AND MARRIAGE

SHIRLEY AS INSPIRATION. Although course work proved burdensome and his record was mediocre during his first two years, Seymour found his inspiration when he met Shirley, his future wife. It was she who sought him out having been attracted by his poetic look and somewhat abstracted manner as well as by his reputation as a philosopher in the intellectual circles of the college. Apparently desirous of nurturing someone, Shirley, an attractive buxom girl slightly older than Seymour, made obvious overtures to him. He was deeply flattered since she was popular and for the remaining years at college they were inseparable although he occasionally rebelled in a passively aggressive manner to her demands on his time. Seymour worked better at his schoolwork and impressed Shirley with his productivity and the variety of his intellectual accomplishments.

Shortly after his graduation they were married in a somewhat ostentatious manner arranged for by the parents. Seymour's family was pleased with the match even though the couple married so young. Shirley's father was a dentist with a large practice and her mother a well-known music teacher. Whatever her deeper doubts and fears, Hannah C. could scarcely fly in the face of the cultural advantages of so good a match.

SHIRLEY AS THREAT. Shortly after his marriage and upon admission to a local law school, Seymour's distress became severe. The new responsibility of marriage put Seymour under more pressure to do well at school and also to prove himself sexually. Although Shirley was relatively undemanding, her own competence as a housekeeper and in her work became for him a constant source of distress in view of his competitiveness and self-doubt. Since Seymour was only mildly interested in law, the extensive reading proved burdensome even though the material was not at all beyond his intellectual powers. He began to find himself brooding endlessly about how various friends would interpret a given passage, how he might phrase his own interpretation so as to impress them most, how his instructors would feel if he made a certain point. He indulged in extensive reverie about the outcome of his career, about an adventurous life of ruggedly masculine, Hemingway-style activity. Occasionally he discussed some point in his texts and found to his dismay that Shirley sometimes offered a more adequate interpretation. This drove Seymour further within himself and he brooded bitterly over his "engulfment" by his wife. The obsessional rumination, inability to concentrate, and speech blocking became so marked that Seymour could not keep up with his assignments. Anticipating failure as imminent he voluntarily withdrew from school. To keep up a pretense of attendance for some time he went to the library every morning.

PERSONALITY DESCRIPTION

WECHSLER-BELLEVUE. Seymour's reaction to the psychological tests was one of mixed pleasure and anxiety. On the Wechsler-Bellevue (Test Summary A), he obtained a full scale I.Q. of 125, which classes him as superior. As can be seen from Test Summary A, his Verbal Scale score was nearly perfect while his Performance was only average. This finding again indicates the emphasis on cerebration and the self-devaluation and doubts in the area of manual performance. He took obvious pleasure in the verbal tests involving definitions and similarities, while on various performance items, despite his conceptual understanding of the tasks, he hesitated, began to doubt, and showed a fumbling, awkward motor response which interfered especially with his score on timed tests like Block Designs.

FIGURE DRAWINGS. Seymour's Figure Drawings (see Figs. 19–1 and 19–2) further exemplified the split between thought and action and the self-doubt in the motor area. He drew nude figures which were well executed, particularly the faces. The man (drawn first) bore a clear resemblance to Seymour, the woman to Shirley. The torsos of both figures were crudely sketched, devoid of detail except for a fulsome breast development in the female figure. The figures lacked hands or feet and the male figure lacked a penis although Seymour had drawn a tentative line in the pelvic region and then had discontinued working on that part of the torso. The over-all effect again was one of motor impotence, of the need for a dependent relationship on a strong female figure. His failure to draw hands may possibly reflect a denial and fear of aggressiveness.

RORSCHACH ANALYSIS.   The Rorschach record was a rich and complex one (see Test Summary B). Although the response total of 39 was not unusual, each percept was elaborated in detail and involved considerable integration of separate blot elements. It was apparent that Seymour viewed the examination as an intellectual challenge and his elaborate efforts at integration whether of Whole or Large Details suggested the driving need for impressing others with his conceptual skills. At the same time he showed some flexibility and the actual balance of his location scores was within normal limits according to Klopfer's scoring.

Structurally, Seymour's Rorschach protocol was characterized by a marked emphasis on introversive experience. There were no less than nineteen responses primarily determined by movement (M) (plus five additionals), with a relatively equal balance between Human, Animal, and Abstract content for these percepts. Seymour's Experience-type $(M:$ Sum C ratio) of 6:10.5 is misleading if taken literally since six of the eight color-determined responses were symbolic pure C and further exemplified his need to impress and his intellectual approach to affective experience. There were in actuality very few reactions to the color or shading of the blots other than in this symbolic fashion. Thus, on Card VIII where he offers the response "Passage of Centuries, each color represents a different epoch in the growth from the medieval darkness to modern times."

Without proceeding to a detailed analysis of the Rorschach profile it may suffice to point out the support found in the test performance for the general indication of the triad of motor inhibition, intellectuality, and social striving. The richly introversive pattern of movement responses suggests considerable introspectiveness, awareness of problems, and the capacity for creative imagination and conceptual thought. At the same time the large number of Animal Movements (FM) is evidence of drive and sensitivity to primitive needs, while the abstract movements exemplify the extensive and painful experience of inner conflicts and tensions. All this internalized fantasy activity characterizes the obsessional, ruminative, self-doubting aspects of Seymour's personality which block overt activity.

Failure to use either the gray-black continuum as "color" or even to give clear-cut bright color responses, except for the intellectualized C-symbolism percepts mentioned above, further suggests that Seymour will be unlikely to act out aggressive or conflictual material or to express overtly emotion of a diffuse or egocentric kind. He is obviously capable of strong emotional experience but his intellectual approach prevents overt manifestation and is more likely to take the form of self-dramatization, of attempts to see his failures and despair as part of the "cosmic sweep of the centuries," in his phrase. The ambition and need to impress are further manifest in his "whole compulsion" and in his elaborations of simple responses. So great is this pressure that bizarre constructions emerge, as on Card III where the central red "bow-tie" area is seen as the "breaking hearts of the natives, symbolic of the deeper meaning of the ceremonial of ripping apart the animal."

The content of the Rorschach blots lends further support to the pattern of striving and competitiveness but adds another element, a deep-seated rage and aggressiveness that probably cannot find expression in direct action but only in the type of introverted, self-defeating behavior which characterizes Seymour's life style. Thus response after response involves a fierce competitive struggle with destructive implications. Seymour's first response is "Two birds fighting over their prey, noble birds like those seen on Assyrian kings' tombs . . . in the center being torn to pieces a foetal rat or vermin." Later this blot area was seen as a vagina. On Card V he sees "Two stallions rushing together in battle. Neither side victorious. A pyrrhic victory, both getting their lumps," while on Card X the upper central figures are "scorpions, angry, a simulated aggressiveness, each trying to climb a stalk and saying, 'I'm going first.'"

TAT STORIES.   Seymour's TAT stories (Test Summary C)
reflect a similar pattern of competitiveness, excessive striving, and sense of failure.   Card I evokes a long story of a
boy who wants to be a "great violinist," "striving for perfection," whose efforts do not "come up to expectations."
Thus, "He will come short of being one of the greats and
this will haunt him, leave him unsatisfied and he will count
himself a failure." Another story involves father and son
in a competitive alliance based on misinformation which
the father gives the son against a third party. The son lives
to suffer the consequences of his father's misleading him.

DREAMS AND FANTASY BEHAVIOR

Seymour reported with some reluctance that, as suggested
by the Rorschach, he has an extensive fantasy life. It consists chiefly of recurrent heroic achievement fantasies such
as one in which he sees himself as a soldier of fortune, two-
fisted but clever, serving in the employ of nations like In-
donesia, Burma, or India in developing their resources and
fighting bandits. In all of these he is unmarried and definitely a rover but a native woman, attractive and sensual,
is always available to him. This pattern of fantasy recurs
constantly in similar forms, sometimes with the patient as a
successful but itinerant public health physician for the U.N.
or a free-lance writer obtaining material from his travels.
These fantasies occurred to him generally early in the day
while he was shaving or riding the subway to his classes,
and he would find himself absorbed in them to the point
of occasionally missing a subway stop. Although he was
quite aware of the unreality of his day dreams, he enjoyed
them and felt that they bore an essential core of truth, that
he indeed was capable of leading the life of the hero if
only. . . . Here, however, Seymour could go no further.
He felt engulfed by his marriage, yet obviously the inhibition of action had existed long before he had met Shirley.

The patient also experienced a less voluntary type of fantasy in the form of painful obsessional thoughts generally

occurring during periods of stress. They appeared as fragmented ideas with a morbid quality. One recurrent obsession dealt with an image of his penis as withered by disease. Another involved a picture of eating canine feces. Seymour's associations to the first of these fantasies led him eventually to recall a frequent prohibition against childhood masturbation by his mother who stressed that touching his penis would lead to its infection and that death would follow. Thus for Seymour the penis became a symbol of a delicate organ yet one of great importance since harm to the penis meant death. Undoubtedly this type of experience may have enhanced the conflict over motor activity and given rise to a sense of danger in the uncontrolled use of one's hands. The second fantasy led to an association to the Passover ritual, the eating of bitter herbs as a symbol of the suffering of the ancient Hebrews in bondage. In effect Seymour seemed to feel that he had sold his individuality into bondage in order to stay in his mother's good graces and that his fate was to swallow his anger and suffer inwardly.

Two night dreams supplement the picture. One of these recurred during Seymour's adolescence at the time of his serious illness when he spent so much time with his mother. It was a frankly sexual dream involving her; she was the aggressor encouraging intercourse with Seymour. In the dream the woman's vagina actually consisted of a penis with a suction-like opening. The other was experienced about the time of the patient's initial consultation and consisted of a depiction of his wedding except that the ceremony at the altar involved a ritual circumcision. In effect both dreams suggest a deep confusion of wife and mother, a view of women as needed, but with loss of manhood as the price exacted for maintenance of the dependent relationship. It is as if the arousal of incestuous and dependent wishes which Seymour's mother undoubtedly fostered in him by her seductive confidences were experienced by him as attainable only at the cost of denial of genuine assertion and vigor.

CONCLUSION

It would appear difficult indeed from the data available to differentiate the cultural from the idiosyncratic elements in this case. Viewed along several dimensions one can see the extent to which Seymour's personality and his distress are the products of cultural and religious traditions in a transitional phase and the specific pattern of relationship between his parents. Historically the urban background of central European Jews, involving their isolation in ghettos as well as their tradition of talmudic scholarship, must be kept in mind in evaluating the goal setting of Seymour's mother and her peculiar interpretation of her maternal role. The transitional phase of the family, moving from a patriarchal European-Jewish structure to the changed relationship of father and mother in America, must also be kept in mind. This change was further complicated by the specific family background of Seymour's mother, coming as she did from a family that stressed sibling rivalry and masculine achievement.

The particular nature of Mrs. C.'s relationship to her husband further emphasized the likelihood that the mother would place great emphasis on her only son as in many ways a more desirable "husband" in the image of her father. Whatever natural or "maturational" tendencies toward an Oedipal development already existed in Seymour were thus greatly enhanced by his mother's seductiveness and setting him off against his father who, himself, became defensively antagonistic to the boy.

The emphasis on verbal and intellectual performance, on motor control and social striving, undoubtedly coupled with natural intellectual endowment, led Seymour to develop great skills in symbol manipulation and in the time-free dimension of planning and imagination. Yet the suppression of much of his individual assertiveness and boyish "high spirits" must have enraged him, making him feel weak and incapable of motor responses. His actual capacities for affective warmth or physical skill became partly dissociated from his conscious value system and emerged only in ruminative fantasies of adventurous achievement. Thus, the constellation of factors operative in Seymour's early development served in effect to offer him a rich world of imagination and thought, a striving for achievement and prowess, but at the cost of his ability to move toward a realistic goal or to feel capable of acting.

In a sense, therefore, the long shadow of centuries of Jewish ghetto life was still cast upon Seymour. The imprint of the intellectual vigor and motor restriction that characterized the European Jew were evident in this young man combined in so disjunctive a way as to cripple him and threaten to crush a human being with much to offer to society and himself.

FOLLOW-UP

Following referral by the writer Seymour entered into intensive psychoanalysis and seems to have made progress at least in terms of improved social functioning. He has been able to find a job and has gradually taken up his education, preferring to go on in more academic phases of political science and sociology.

Test Summary

A. WECHSLER-BELLEVUE INTELLIGENCE SCALE, FORM I

Verbal Scale	Wtd. Score	Performance Scale	Wtd. Score
Information	14	Picture Arrangement	14
Comprehension	16	Picture Completion	14
Digit Span	13	Block Design	10
Arithmetic	16	Object Assembly	10
Similarities	16	Digit Symbol	10
Vocabulary	15		
Sum	90(75)*	Sum	58
Verbal I.Q.	133	Performance I.Q.	110

Full Scale I.Q. 125

* Prorated.

Test Summary

B. RORSCHACH PROTOCOL

(Response only; inquiry excluded)

CARD I. 19″

1. Two flying animals tearing apart something between them. Two birds fighting over their prey, noble birds like those seen on Assyrian Kings' tombs. Mythological or Oriental.

W   FM   A, Myth   O

2. The prey in the middle singularly reminds me of a vagina.

D   F   Sex

3. Now on the outside these flecks remind me of feathers flying off, perhaps from the birds' fight.

dd   MF   A, obj

4. The thing in the middle now looks like a sort of weasel—a miserable little animal.

D   F   A

I feel I am looking down on this scene from a bird's eye view. I feel a preference for the noble bird rather than to the prey—it looks like a foetal rat or vomit, I mean vermin, being torn to pieces.

CARD II. 9″

1. Looks like a scotty; puppy dogs anyway. They're not kissing. They're not fighting over it. They seem to be sharing food or chocolate.

W   FM, Fc   A   P

2. As I look closer, the thing in center I said they were sharing—I get the impression of a vagina.

d   F   Sex

3. The red part—almost like a spark of happiness—as if the dogs were enjoying each other. Or else to make it more fanciful, the symbol of love to be.

D   C,symb.   Symbolic

4. The red lines between them could be an idea, an idealization, a dream, a pink or red dream—that they're identical. This is a study in sameness.

5. The food in their mouths keeps them from really joining. Their progress is halted by the food in their mouths.

d   F   Food

CARD III. 6"

1. African Ubangis ripping apart the ribs from a dead animal.

W   M   H   P

2. The thing in the center down there—a sea horse or sea vegetable.

D   F   A, Pl

3. A subplot—their hearts in the center. How each one's heart is sort of breaking as they're ripping the animal to pieces. Of course they're not angry at each other for this is a ceremonial.

D   Fm, Fc   Hd, Symb.

4. Or this part looks like a nose plug used in swimming.

D   F   Obj   O

If we take the center there's a deeper meaning. Friends share a common problem. They're doing something symbolic showing each other that there are similar occurrences. The breaking hearts of the natives, in effect, the deeper meaning of the ceremonial of ripping the animal apart.

CARD IV. 20"

1. A man with very long feet; he's jumping up in the air or is being lifted off his feet. His arms look like swans but they're arms and they're broken.

W   M, FM   H   O

2. Behind a screen, feet of two girls shooting upward as he is, hiding in fear.

D   M   Hd   O

3. As you go to the top there's a walnut at the head.

d   F   Food

He seems glancing over the top of the screen and he's angry. He hasn't quite looked over the screen yet and the girls behind don't have any anxiety yet. This thing is full of foreboding.

CARD V. 10″

1. Two stallions rushing together in battle. A pyrrhic victory, both getting their lumps.

W   FM   A

2. Dark in front—symbolic of the force of battle—as if armies entangled dark clouds.

W   MF, CF   Battle

3. On top fops like satires in the Court of Louis XIV. Very dignified, pompous, superficial.

d   M   Hd

They're in opposition to the carnage below which they're observing.

4. An ominous bird hovering over battle. Defeat or doom.

W   FM, FC   A

CARD VI. 7″

1. Initially again a picture of a vagina.

D   Fc   Sex

2. Fountain, the water coming out and it spins around.

W   FM   Obj

3. Two snakes or salamanders looking at each other on top.

d   FM   Ad

CARD VII. 10″

1. Two rocking chairs. Nobody sitting in either. As if hooked in back. Don't need anybody pushing. Seem capable of rocking themselves.

W   F, FM   Obj

2. Two statues like bookends with pretty young girls on style of Jean Simmons. On pedestals—marble quality.

W   F, Fc   H, obj

CARD VIII. 3"

1. Pretty historic. The color reminds me of travel to the West. Recalls a time. The Grand Canyon, Painted Desert, Petrified Forest. Geological portions of the earth.

W   C   Na, Geo

2. The cosmic sweep of centuries here. Sort of an invention. The different colors correspond to the passage of time or different geological layers.

W   C,symb.   Abstract

3. The two beavers on either side are like two balancing stages. The process personified. They're coming up from darkness to modern times.

D   FM   A   P

The green—fresh farm land, young but then the decay of modern times but a ray of hope. The gray area pointing to the future. The beavers symbolize work, diligence, application, responsibility. Moving up from the pink-dark ages to green. Egypt and Greece, the cradles of civilization. A stream of life. The life force.

CARD IX. 15"

1. A carnival effect or Mardi Gras.

W   C,symb.   Abstract

2. The green areas remind me of men dressed up in as old beings. Almost like the Magi on horseback with beards. Oldish, possibly negroid but happy, gay.

D   M   H

3. Plums or peaches.

D   FC   Food

4. Pregnant stomachs. Only the stomachs of the women seem alive.

dr   M   Hd

CARD X. 11"

1. An aquarium. Idea of the different genus and species. All are exhibited in parts.

W   F   A

2. Crabs.

D   F   A   P

3. Scorpions. Angry, a simulated aggressiveness, each trying to climb a stalk and saying, "I'm going first."

D   FM-M   A

4. Cliffs again. Travelogue idea. The color.

D   CF   Nature

5. Bugs. Caterpillars crawling on their bellies.

D   FM   A

6. Broken branch near edge of a cliff. Not in danger of falling but to show that there once were fertile areas here.

D   F,m   Pl

7. Running stream, rivulet flowing down into canyon.

D   Fm, CF   Na

8. Yellow splashes are symbols of the burning sun drying out the land.

D   C,symb.   Abstract

There are all kinds of wasted animals.

RORSCHACH PROFILE

R= 39	W%= 35
M= 6	D%= 45
FM= 8	d= 15
M= 5	DdS= 5
F= 11	
Fc= 1	RT (Achrom.)= 12.1″
FC= 1	RT (Chrom.)= 8.8″
CF= 1	

$$C= \quad 6 \qquad \frac{F}{R}=28\% \qquad W{:}M=14{:}6$$

$$\frac{A+Ad}{R}=26\%$$

$$P=4$$

M: Sum C $=$ 10:6.5
(FM+M):(Fc+C+C′)$=$13:1.0
Responses to Cards VIII, IX, X$=$35%

Test Summary

C. THEMATIC APPERCEPTION TEST

CARD 1.

Young boy, sensitive and intelligent-looking, who has been taking violin lessons for a rather long time, is thinking about music and violin-playing. He wants to be very good, if not great, and has been striving after perfection. He wants to be a great violinist. He now, though not dejectedly, meditates upon what he thinks has been his failure to achieve the perfection he seeks. The time preceding this picture he spent practicing. There is one sheet of music on the table, so he has been striving to master it completely. After many repetitions his playing has not come up to expectation and he has laid the violin and bow carefully and lovingly on the table. As for the future, I don't know. I imagine he will continue to practice and probably have a concert career and achieve some notoriety. But he will come short of being one of the greats and this will haunt him and leave him unsatisfied and he will count himself a failure.

CARD 3BM.

A young teen-age girl is crying against a couch. I say girl because of the shape of her buttocks and general shape of her torso. But I am not fully convinced. I find it difficult to imagine what's happened but I assume she's met some failure; possibly loss of a boyfriend, scolding by father. She seems to be wishing to be dead. She hates life. As for prognosis—it would be good. I would guess that the sun is shining outside. I would also guess that she will forget about this present boy-friend and shortly find another which will make her happy. If that is not her trouble and it is her father, arguments will blow over and she will be reinstated in his good graces shortly.

CARD 6BM.

It is a son. No—adopted or a friend. He has come to tell her something about her son—or father. The son has uncertain look on face—I mean the man. He's uncertain. A tragedy—father killed. Or son has run away or been divorced or hurt—but there are extenuating circumstances. She's taking it stoically. She seems too old to be the gentleman's mother.

Mother looks lonely for either her husband or son. She will miss either one and her life will sort of come to an end unhappily. She will mope her concluding days away and the gentleman will go away and follow his own life. He will have earned something from this mixup that's been going on and even with a feeling of satisfaction—it'll not happen to him.

CARD 7BM.

It is a picture of a father and son chat. The father does not seem to be scolding the son. Rather the father seems to be cajoling the son into hatred or anger against a third party. The son seems like college sophomore home on vacation. The preceding events would be the homecoming of the son from college. Something has occurred in the house or neighborhood that he has not heard about. The father then has quickly taken him aside and by not telling the son the entire truth, has deliberately engendered a false picture in his mind. The son now dislikes the person the father wants him to dislike. Future: an alliance has been formed between father and son against the third party. The son will go back to school with the misunderstanding implanted there by the father. The father is happy. The son will live a long time in misunderstanding. The father may have been jealous of a third party.

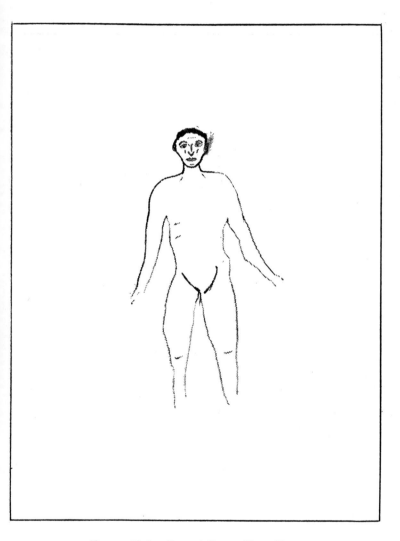

FIGURE 19–1.   Draw-A-Person Test: Man.

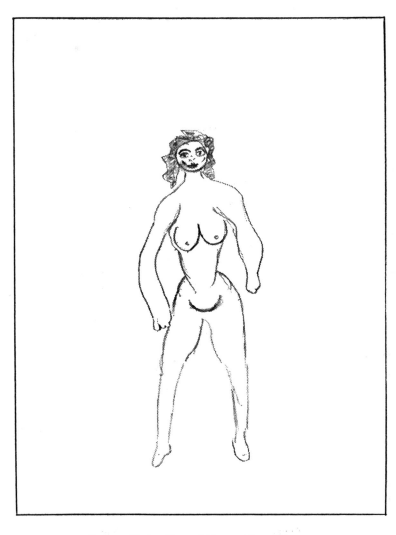

Figure 19-2. Draw-A-Person Test: Woman.

20

A Displaced European Molds Herself into an American

Charlotte Buhler

PRESENTING PICTURE

APPEARANCE. Ilona T., a tall, well-preserved woman of forty-nine, made a striking impression with her proud carriage and black, well-cut clothes. She introduced herself as a Hungarian who had left Europe when Hitler marched into Vienna. She belonged to a wealthy, as well as highly cultured, Jewish family that had provided her with social advantages and professional training in sculpturing. Her mother and sister had gone to Paris to stay with relatives while she had come to the United States by herself, where, soon after her arrival, she married an American business-man.

The patient stated that she had not wanted to consult a psychologist, but came only because she had heard of the writer in Vienna and had been interested to meet her. As for going into therapy, she did not think well of it. Moreover, she and her husband could hardly afford it so that under the circumstances she would feel guilty about spending the money on herself when she should be able to manage her own affairs without help from outside.

DEPRESSION. Ilona was referred by her physician in conjunction with a severe depressive reaction which had climaxed in an acute breakdown. She had been suffering from

509

sleeplessness, headaches, and crying spells. She claimed that she had lost interest in life to the point where she found the ordinary household duties more of a burden than she could carry. The statement of these complaints was followed by a recital of self-reproaches to the effect that it was ridiculous that she could not do what everybody else was doing and that she was probably too perfectionistic about everything. She had been accustomed to doing things extremely well and had been admired for her efficiency and orderliness. All day long she reproached herself for being so demanding and dissatisfied but, try as she would, she found that she was simply not up to overcoming these moods of distress and coming to terms with life.

PREDISPOSING PICTURE

HUSBAND'S DRINKING. She herself attributed her present condition to her husband's recall to the home office of his firm because of excessive drinking. The couple had been living during the past five years in Calcutta, India, where she had had an unusual opportunity to develop her artistic interests in addition to enjoying family and social life. Her husband, a representative for a large establishment of antique dealers, had specialized as a buyer of oriental art and could have stayed indefinitely if it had not been for his drinking. Since he was too valuable to be dropped, his firm had recalled him to the home office so that they might give him an assignment under their more immediate supervision.

Questioning Ilona elicited the information that her husband's drinking was not of recent origin but had worsened as his position demanded greater independence. The alcoholism had affected her the most at the beginning of their marriage. She had met and married him only a few months after her arrival from Europe. During their short engagement he had not indulged in alcohol. When he started immediately after marriage, she was appalled. Since heavy drinking was rare in her cultural background, she had never encountered it before. It frightened and revolted her. She did not feel that her marriage was a failure, however, in view of the many compensatory features involved. Her husband had provided the escape she needed from her insecurity as a displaced person. He had also proved to be a good father to their two little girls.

INTERVIEW WITH HUSBAND. An interview with the husband was suggested by Ilona herself. She felt that the therapist should be acquainted with him and get his point of view. Burt M. was a youthful looking man of forty-seven. He gave the impression of bewilderment and helplessness with regard to his wife's condition, and volunteered the opinion that his drinking must have contributed to her depression. He said he deplored it and was determined to get control of it—a decision which he actually did carry through after his business transfer. Burt stated how much he loved and admired his wife. In fact, he was inclined to put her on a pedestal. To him they were a well-mated couple who could be very happy once his wife was convinced that he had stopped drinking. He also expressed regret at the loss of his position in India, but hoped to get equally good opportunities after he had overcome his habit.

INITIAL IMPRESSION

After the initial interview, the impression made by the patient may be summarized as follows: Here is a woman steeped in social and professional success, beautiful but quite cold and neurotically driven by personal ambition, who in the middle of a successful career and an interesting social life was uprooted by political upheaval. Suddenly she lost the security to which her high social position had always entitled her in the past and found herself a member of an outcast group, in a strange land among strangers. She attempted to meet the crisis by throwing herself into a hasty marriage with a man alien to her in cultural background, language, and religion. By her precipitate behavior, she hoped to acquire the protective coloration of the new group. This precarious adjustment was maintained for over a decade until the new uprooting occasioned by her husband's instability culminated in her breakdown.

EARLY YEARS

MONEY AND MANNERS.   Ilona T., born and raised in Budapest, was the elder of two daughters of a highly respected Jewish banker. Her father died during her elementary school years and she grew up in a household reigned over by a continually ailing mother and a strict governess. Financially they were secure, but the family capital was not large enough to allow them the lavish life that the father's career might have provided for them. The mother's retiring personality added to the limitations of the family's life after the father died. A frustrated society woman, she was constantly preoccupied with her obesity and other health problems.

The girls were for the most part left to the governess who required them to conform to her antiquated and rigid ideas about good manners. Every day of the week they had to walk through the park near their home at the side of their "dragon," as the girls called her between themselves. During these walks, they had to keep themselves in perfect posture and to converse in French. Furthermore, their play time and other recreational activities were regimented. They attended a private girls' school reserved for the children of the upper classes, which reinforced the stilted behavior learned at home.

The only fun the girls knew was in their play. They played very well together and obviously got some release for themselves in their doll house. From an early age Ilona also enjoyed drawing, painting, and work with plastic material in which she excelled. In all this the girls were left to themselves as long as they conformed in their daily duties.

UNCLE PAUL.   The complete boredom of this life was only occasionally interrupted by visitors, some of whom were entertaining, like Uncle Paul who took the children on sprees to a *konditorei* where they could gorge themselves on hot chocolate decorated with whipped cream and with *Dobos* or *Sachertorte*. Uncle Paul, a bachelor brother of the father, also brought some worldliness into their lives by sometimes telling the growing girls daring jokes or somewhat unsavory stories, with the admonition, "Don't tell your mother." He would also take them to museums and to the opera, always providing interesting comments and mental stimulation.

Apart from this uncle's regular visits, there was very little social life in Ilona's childhood home. She had no intimate friends since she met no children outside of school. Stilted parties, occasional visits of cousins, the addition of dancing lessons later on, were the extent to which Ilona and her sister were permitted to socialize.

Boys. The dancing lessons at sixteen were the patient's first opportunity to meet boys. There was no dating, no meeting without adult chaperons. Once when a young man wrote her a love letter, the mother was outraged and forbade further contact with this boy. Ilona, seventeen at the time, was still completely conforming and subdued. But at eighteen she allowed herself for the first time to be talked into an amorous relationship that might have become an affair had she not cut it off in panic.

VIENNA

Art and love. Her one outlet was art. She was gifted in drawing and at her request was allowed to visit an art school when she was fourteen. Later she switched from drawing and painting to sculpturing and, at twenty-three, she suddenly picked up enough courage to announce that she was going to Vienna to visit the art school there. She had been advised to do this by one of her teachers who was also able to persuade her mother of the need of developing the girl's talent.

Ilona's art school years in Vienna with subsequent employment in a china-manufacturing company at last brought her some degree of personal emancipation. She made friends with people who lived extremely unconventional lives and she threw herself into this bohemianism in an attempt to overcome her training and her inhibitions. She had one affair without love and then fell in love with a man who kept her on the string for two years with empty promises. Parting from him at twenty-eight left her disillusioned and somewhat embittered. She summed up her feelings with the words, "This had to happen, when I finally had broken down with my silly principles."

After this she had one or two affairs with men who appealed to her physically, but whom she did not care to marry. "What did I wait for?" she asked somewhat desperately. "Perhaps for that perfect match that never seemed to offer itself. I wasted my life at that time; I whiled it away."

With respect to her art, she said, "I used it for self-expression, but I had no goal, nothing that I was working toward."

THE NEW WORLD

ESCAPE INTO MARRIAGE. When in Ilona's thirty-fifth year the Nazis marched into Vienna, she was forced to flee, and made her way to Washington together with another artist, with no other plans than to continue her career there. This, however, proved to be more difficult than she expected. Although she had good introductions, she was not offered the type of job she had been hoping for and felt lost and lonely in the big city in the company of people whose ideas and interests were completely foreign to her.

When a few months after her arrival, she met Burt, an American businessman, who instantly fell in love with her strange beauty and her fascinating personality, she accepted his marriage offer with the same desperate courage with which ten years earlier she had suddenly decided to leave her parental home and to go to Vienna to study.

The new life that opened before her contained more disappointment than fulfillment. Her husband was a complete stranger from a world about which she knew nothing and cared less the more she found out about it.

Burt was from an American family out West. His father was a minister in one of the Protestant sects and a rather unctuous and talkative old man. Burt himself was an excellent businessman and the typical "jolly good fellow"; when not drunk he was charming, witty, and very good company.

CLASH OF VALUES. With her background of high culture and social stability she was lost in the mobile, breezy ways of her American-Western husband. Moreover, she longed for the intimate closely knit circle of relatives and friends so characteristic of the European-Jewish life in which she had grown up and so utterly unfamiliar to her gentile husband with his casual acquaintances. She felt that she could never bridge the cultural gap between them no matter how much Burt might admire culture and look up to her for help in attaining it. Since under the circumstances she was too preoccupied adequately to respond to him, she decided that her only salvation was to devote her life to her children.

Burt's career took the family first to the West—away from the few friends Ilona had made on the East Coast. They were then sent to India where at least the external arrangements made things easier and where art and continental friends created for her again some semblance of the cultural climate in which she felt at home. It was no wonder that she reacted strongly against their recall to the United States where she was forcibly reminded of the basic inadequacy in their relationship once the external props of their lives were removed.

RORSCHACH STUDY

The Rorschach (Basic Rorschach Score = +4) reveals a complex psychoneurotic picture with anxiety reactions predominating. (See Test Summary for complete protocol.)

In the interest of social conformity, indicated by her high
$FC:CF$ ratio and the generous use of "populars," the patient
holds in check her impulsive tendencies (FM). She tries
to cope with the resulting tension (m) by intellectualizing
(note "X-rays") and by sublimating her hostility in the
many "dancing" percepts throughout the protocol. One of
her chief defenses is to seek refuge from her present problems in the world of art which takes her back to her past.
The Rorschach content gives eloquent testimony to this in
such responses as the cut glass, stylized figure, and gar-
goyles "like decorations on a cathedral" (Card I), and the
"angel heads on clouds . . . like on Italian paintings" (Card
VII). Related to this defense is her attempt to create distance from the reality around her through masks and costumes. Potentially inimical people appear not in flesh and
blood, but in the less threatening form of caricatures (Card
III), clowns, and stuffed figures (Card VI). They may be
derogated to the subhuman level of chimpanzees (Card
III) or elevated to the superhuman as angels (Card VII).

On Card IV, her first response of "a cow, her head bent
down," etc., is followed by, "a big boot, riding boot . . .
reminds me of my father's riding boots; black." This chain
of associations suggests the fearfully submissive attitude of
a European Jewish girl toward her patriarchal father. Further evidence of submissiveness appears in the "profile of a
woman; she looks down" (Card IX). The response, "angel
heads on clouds," etc., on Card VII suggests a glorified concept of woman—mother (?).

Of psychodynamic significance in connection with Ilona's
insecurity are her repeated projections of holding onto something, such as the "two bears who cling to something" (Card
VIII), "two lambs balancing something on their noses"
(Card VIII), "two dogs in a circus act holding something
in their mouth" (Card II), and "two bears which cling to
something, perhaps a snowed-in tree" (Card III). The last
response makes one wonder whether the patient is trying
to derive security from something cold and unyielding, perhaps the new country and people. The preoccupation with

physical contact revealed in such responses as "two elephants; they touch each other with their trunks" (Card I),
and "two clowns' heads touching each other with their
backs" (Card VI) may have homosexual overtones as well
as the more manifest need for security.

Throughout the Rorschach the large number of human
movement responses (M) and the many examples of superior form-level attest to the patient's high intellectual ability, which, however, is often blocked by her emotional disturbance. Her creative talents are an undoubted source of
strength, and a good prognostic indicator for a favorable
outcome of intensive psychotherapy.

PSYCHOTHERAPY: OVER-ALL COURSE

Since long-term intensive therapy was out of the question, briefer treatment was planned for Ilona, with the aim
of helping her to channel her resources into socially constructive directions. The patient would be guided to a better understanding of her needs and the defenses that hindered their adequate expression. Her immediate "culture
conflict" would be viewed as a rationalization for earlier interpersonal conflicts. In the light of a revised self concept
acquired through the therapy, it was hoped that Ilona might
be able to see the significance of her entire life's course and
to build new goals for her future.

The patient had a total of 113 interviews which stretched
over a period of two years, with several months' interruption at the end of the first year when her husband entered
treatment. After that she returned for four months of weekly
interviews. During the first year she averaged two visits
per week.

FIRST PHASE: CONFUSION

In Ilona's therapy, three phases can be clearly distinguished. The first period was characterized by a confused view of her problem, according to which her various
difficulties were seen as distinct and unrelated. She com-

pared her present inability to cope with her marital, maternal, and professional roles with an idealization of her former efficiency. What she failed to perceive at this stage of her treatment was her underlying core problem of relating adequately to other people.

FEELINGS ABOUT SELF.   Some quotations from a very early session give the flavor of her confused feelings about herself:

I was always extremely efficient, used to enjoy working. Now, when I see all this disorder in the house, I cannot decide to just bring some part in order—I think of the rest that I cannot manage on one day, and do nothing. From early in the morning on, I think about all that we did wrongly the day before and I lose courage. I cannot even tell the children what to do anymore—have lost all confidence in myself . . .

Occasionally, however, she shows some glimmerings of insight:

But I had really always doubts in myself. I was really never happy in my life, just pretended to be. I was always a worrier—had inferiority feelings and worried about doing things well—small things; in big things, in big decisions, I let myself suddenly drift into them; I allow people to talk me into things . . .
Therapist: How was it with your marriage?
Patient: Exactly like that, he talked me into it. I let myself be convinced. It all happened fast; I did not want to think about it. . . .

FEELINGS ABOUT HUSBAND.   During this first period her attitude toward her husband was brought out by her therapist in the following exchanges:

Patient: I must admit that I never loved him. He was very attractive to me; he seemed a decent sort—but how can one live in a marriage with a man with whom one never can talk as one feels it? I must always "treat" him, think carefully what to say and what not.
Therapist: Was it a mistake to marry him?
Patient: I can never get close to him—have never talked with him about anything important, not even about the children.
Therapist: Did you ever try?
Patient: Yes, he does not want to. He says, "You decide, you know best."
Therapist: Since he was physically so attractive, was then the sexual relationship gratifying?

Patient: Sex? Oh, no, not particularly. I had only once in my life an orgasm with a man with whom I had a short affair. He did not even count.

Therapist: Is that perhaps why you could react?—because he did not count?

Patient: Oh no, I don't think so—what do you mean? I thought in a marriage all that is important for the physical relationship is that the man is physically attractive, agreeable, neat—and all that Burt is . . .

Therapist: Yet you could not really react too well.

Patient: No. I always thought sex would have nothing to do with our lack of understanding and with my horror of his drinking—but all this repression of my feelings has not helped.

RESISTANCE. By the seventh interview she begins spontaneously to work into the dynamics of her own development. She starts out by saying how she dislikes this analyzing:

It disgusts me but I admit I don't really understand anything. I am frustrated, tense, even our dog senses my tension and eats better when somebody else feeds him. The smallest things upset me, but how can I ever be different.

RELATIONSHIP WITH PARENTS.

Patient: I wonder how my *mother* could stand her life, being so ill and having no happiness at all.

Therapist: You mean she accepted things?

Patient: It seemed as if she did, she was complaining a lot about her health. Otherwise she did not express dissatisfaction, but was always friendly.

Therapist: Did you ever talk with her about things?

Patient: Never. Once when I was older she told me that at four or five, during a promenade in the park, our governess had said, "All the people look at you," referring to mother. I said, "Perhaps they look at *me!*" We were both very good looking.

Therapist: Do you think you competed with her in looks?

Patient: Compete? I don't know, maybe. Mother had very beautiful sisters—always wanted to be told how beautiful she was. I remember, as a child I never was allowed to wear what I liked. Always we had to wear these ugly uniform dresses.

Therapist: Did you feel your mother did not want you to look pretty?

Patient: Do you think so? I always thought it was just the way children in our class of families were being dressed in those times, but maybe there is something in what you say.

Therapist: Did you feel your mother loved you?

Patient: Mother always reproached me that *I* was cold, that I never wanted to hug her, that I criticized everything. I always felt my mother preferred my sister; she was easy and sweet. She still is—takes care of mother and has no life of her own.

Therapist: What about your father?

Patient: I hardly remember him. He had never time for us children—was quite detached. He never talked with us children about anything. I remember only one nice scene with him, how he took us on a walk on Christmas eve, before we got our presents which mother laid out under the tree while we were gone. That was a happy excitement. I also can see him at the dinner table. He asked often why I did not say something; I was a very quiet child—quite timid.

Therapist: But your father *did* show some interest then? Do you feel he loved you?

Patient: Oh, I am sure our parents loved us in their own way. . . .

SECOND PHASE: THE KEY PROBLEM

In what might be called a *second phase* of this therapy process, Ilona began to see that her marriage was perhaps "the key to everything" (twentieth interview) and that the problem of this marriage had a double origin in her personality and in the cultural heterogeneity between herself and her husband.

OVERCONFORMITY. She began to see the significance of her mother's domination in her development. She said:

My mother—I must think of her so often recently. I suppose to a great extent her physical ailments were psychological in origin. Mother would of course be indignant if one told her that. But I can see it must have been her way of escaping life because she could not cope with it.

I can see now if psychotherapy does not change things for me it would be my own fault. For years I did everything under protest. I always had tried to force myself—I am cramped up. Was it just fortuitous that all my friends married around 21 and only I did not? I was the prettiest of the whole circle. Even my father asked: "Why do our girls not marry?" Of course, he did not realize that we never had any casual social life; Mother always chaperoned us when any young man came to call. But why did I not rebel for so many years; why did I always conform with these outmoded ideas? I just made excuses for myself; in reality I was afraid. . . . I always say I cannot talk with my husband, but did I ever talk with anybody seriously? I realize I have no goals at all—my children were the only sense of my life.

PERSPECTIVES.   In her twenty-ninth interview, Ilona made a kind of survey of her life in terms of phases.   She said:

First when I came out at 18, I conformed, and continued to conform until at least 24, showing no initiative of my own; then from 24 to 35 I rebelled. I went off by myself and worked on my art, but as far as my personal life is concerned, I was squandering it. Then at 35 I drifted into this marriage, but then I set myself the goal to make it a go—to have these children and a home—and now at 49 I must recognize that it was all a failure, except for the children. I lost the professional independence that I had gained in my twenties and I did not make my marriage a success. I am ashamed of how blind I was, and how false my decisions. I realize I am confused—have never thought anything through at all. . . . I really like to talk to you, but I need your interesting comments and questions. Sometimes I feel considerably better now.

IDENTIFICATION WITH MOTHER.

Patient: When I visited Mother in Paris a few years ago, we talked about home. She could not understand how little I remembered of our childhood. She was quite angry.
Therapist: What do you think about her now?
Patient: I feel Mother had inferiority feelings as a child, because she was not as pretty as her sisters. Later she admired me because I was pretty, but still she was a little jealous, too. But you know, for a long time I did not know that I was pretty, until I heard people say it. I thought my sister was prettier.
Therapist: Seems the same as your mother did, doesn't it?
Patient: Yes, it does.   And also in other ways Mother was also influenced by others as I am.
Therapist: How about your marriage and hers?
Patient: Yes, there are certain similarities—we both married without love; we married men with whom one could not talk at all—to whom one never could get close, although for different reasons. Father was a distant neurotic, while my husband is a distant American.

DISTANCE FROM HUSBAND.

Therapist: Do you still feel you cannot talk with him?
Patient: Well, I suppose my husband and I must have something

in common, something intangible. In many ways I am very fond of
him. But I cannot talk with him—we have a different language. He
has a good sense of humor, yet in my whole marriage I could not
once really laugh at his jokes. About books, about movies, I just
could never make him understand what I think. I play a farce identifying with his Republicans. I threw myself into all this stuff—I
wanted so badly to assimilate this.

In a later statement along the same line, she showed fuller
insight.

Sometimes I realize now, and I am ashamed to admit, that I married this American for vanity's sake. I wanted to prove to myself
how I could conquer him and master this whole situation here.
Therapist: You wanted to belong, again by way of conforming. Is
it so different from what you did at home with your own parents?
Patient: Maybe not—maybe I *do* repeat my pattern as you showed
me I did, but then, for what can a European such as I live here? I
have no civic interests, you know; all this is completely foreign to
me—all that interests him.
Therapist: But your mutual art interests?
Patient: His art interest—oh, my goodness, he looks at art as a com-
mercial product—he cannot just look and feel it.
Therapist: I wonder whether this is quite fair?
Patient: Maybe not—maybe it is not. But I feel things. To him
there must be either a business or a political value; art is nothing in
itself.
Therapist: How about his feelings for you and the children?
Patient: Sure he loves us, but then we decorate his home.

CULTURAL DIFFERENCES AS A SCAPEGOAT.   As her therapy
proceeded, Ilona began to remember more of her childhood,
particularly it came back to her that she had liked her father
very much. It was with sentiment that she thought of him
and she remembered his interest in history and family trees
and his absent-mindedness. With little help she clarified
for herself how the lack of closeness with her father, his
early death, and the entirely female environment in which
she grew up had prevented her from developing any heterosexual relationship and had prevented her from getting
close to men, American or European alike. Perhaps her
husband's "foreignness" was a good excuse for her not to
have to come close.

She soon discovered that his looking up to her and putting her on a pedestal made her into a kind of mother image to him, which he seemed to need and she seemed to encourage, "just as my mother did with my father. I am always the sensible one with my husband—that is a mistake."

At this point, Ilona persuaded Burt to go into psychotherapy in order to combat his own neurotic needs. She hoped that the therapy would aid in keeping his alcoholism under control. She talked at length about his alcoholic episodes and how they affected their marriage, and she ventilated a great deal of resentment and hostility in connection with it.

Six months after she had started psychotherapy, Ilona declared that she wanted to save and to improve her marriage.

INTERRUPTION AND SETBACK. For financial reasons Ilona had interrupted her therapy when her husband began his treatment. But this interruption caused a setback in her condition. When she returned to psychotherapy, it was with a skeptical attitude and a negative transference. During this period she went back on most of what she had recognized and admitted to herself and made many oppositional statements, such as that she had always had a goal, but never could reach it; that she had never found what she wanted; that she could not see the use of therapy; that she could not change so late in life; and that she had an inferiority complex like her mother and was completely identified with her.

Her hostility against the therapist during this period was apparent in one of the very few dreams that she reported. She dreamed that the therapist put a piece of cloth soaked in chloroform round her neck. She tore it away, screaming, "I do intentionally again everything badly. I do not want to learn anything new." She refused to accept the interpretation that perhaps she did not want her husband to improve and gain an understanding equal to her own, so that she would no longer have an excuse for not coming close to him. Her conscious attitude, however, was belied by her less guarded statements:

I have to admire Burt—how hard he tries. Yet it can never, never become the right human relationship; it cannot be—*I do not even want it.*[1] This immense basic difference between Burt and me—we only live side by side. I must admit he went more honestly than I into this relationship. I am simply not up to things.

AGAIN THE CULTURAL SCAPEGOAT. At this time, she also doubted her effectiveness as a mother, and expressed regret at having given up her art work. She summed up her feeling of failure by saying:

It all did not succeed in this wrong cultural climate. What I could have accomplished is lost. I have no goal anymore, no plan—I don't want to.

In the same vein, she remarked:

My husband has always this optimism, but I feel hopeless—I am neither American nor European now; I hang in the middle somewhere . . . He used my European culture for his background. . . .

In all this, Ilona unwittingly validated the therapist's interpretation that she was seeking an excuse for avoiding intimacy in personal relationships. Culture provides a most convenient scapegoat.

RELEASE FROM EARLY EMOTIONAL RESTRAINTS. During this period her resentment of her mother, who forced upon her a superficial conventionality at the expense of her deepest needs, and her guilt feelings regarding this resentment were worked through.

THIRD PHASE: TOWARD A CONSTRUCTIVE SOLUTION

A *third phase* in Ilona's therapy was represented by her attempt to work toward a constructive solution of her life problems. Unfortunately, this phase was prematurely dis-

---

[1] Italics supplied.

rupted because the family had to move East suddenly for Burt to take over a special assignment that had come up unexpectedly. Even though there remained many unresolved problems, the development of this phase went far enough for her to reach a better relationship with her husband in spite of their cultural disparity.

SEARCH FOR LIFE GOALS.   Ilona now looked more honestly for what she and her husband had in common and could share, rather than for their differences. She also tried to find for herself a more positive orientation in life, a philosophy of some sort which would serve as a guide for the future.

On a number of occasions she deplored her lack of religious training:

Nobody had any conviction about anything—no faith of any sort. . . . How do I get a conviction about something? I feel there must be something. . . .

Yesterday I was in a European circle; I felt I do no more belong to it. . . . But the world of my husband? He just needs people for his business.

Therapist: There are cultured Americans, you know. You might meet someone in one of your classes.

Patient: Maybe . . .

She also showed the beginning of a renewed interest in her artistic career:

It is so strange how little a career of my own meant to me then. I like to sculpture, like to meet artists, like this free life. . . . I know I should still be able to do it. Yesterday my husband said if I would do again some sculpturing at home, it would be his greatest happiness. Does he mean that? Our relationship is still so empty, so superficial, but if I were now with the right sort of people, I could pull myself out of this dissatisfaction of my life. . . .

By the time of her move back East, Ilona was making rapid progress. She had signed up for a class in sculpturing, and even decided to learn to drive—this "most American occupation" that she had always been strongly set against. She thinks she may have learned things from her husband, not only he from her. Her increased insight is revealed by her significant statement to the therapist: "You will be glad to learn that I suddenly see again in proper proportion how much you have helped me."

OVERVIEW

Ilona has presented a picture of unquestioned culture conflict which on the surface, at least, appeared to be the central, causative factor in her emotional disturbance. As pointed out, she had grown up in Europe in the intimate atmosphere of a closely knit circle of relatives, friends, and fellow artists who shared a common language, cultural symbolism, and personal interests.

All this had changed after the political upheaval that resulted in the dispersal of her group, along with others, and in her flight to America. Here she found herself among cheerful but casual people whom she did not understand. The privacy and privilege of the ingroup she had enjoyed in Europe had no counterpart in her new environment. Now for the first time, the patient was faced with the need to build new relationships in the absence of external group supports. Lacking sufficient ego strength to cope with this major readjustment problem, she resorted to her old familiar defense of overconformity. Through a hasty marriage, she plunged headlong into the new culture, hoping thereby to become completely immersed in it. Instead, she was overwhelmed and left feeling more isolated and alone than ever. In her frustration, she blamed the ensuing difficulties on the disparities between her original and her adopted culture. The very real culture conflict was unwittingly exploited as a scapegoat for her deeper-lying difficulty in relating adequately to others that originated in her earliest childhood experiences with her parents.

It was only through treatment with a psychotherapist who could empathize with the patient sufficiently to mobilize her remarkable ego assets that she gradually oriented herself toward finding a new identity in a new world.

Test Summary

RORSCHACH PROTOCOL

Response	*Inquiry*

CARD I. 11″

1. Two elephants. They touch each other with their trunks.

Just their shapes and the way they stand.

2. Stylized female figure, standing.

I see her from the back, her hands are raised.

3. V A glass held in a stand.

The stand holds it up at the sides, it is decorated. The glass is transparent.

4. V Gargoyle-like faces.

Like decorations on a cathedral.

CARD II. 20″

1. Two dogs, in a circus act, holding something in their mouth. Cannot get away from the dogs.

They run, there is rhythm in their movement, they hold their snouts up, and the snouts are turned.

2. V Well, a spot of blood is all I can see besides.

Just a blood spot.

CARD III. 15″

1. Caricature of two men who take off their hats and bow to each other.

Evening clothes.

2. V Two chimpanzees, no, better, two men, their arms up in a dance.
The red is only disturbing, does not mean anything.

Negroid heads, fuzzy hair.

3. Bones, chest bones.

Just shape.

CARD IV. 13″

1. A cow, her head bent down, body does not fit well; the eye fits.

2. A bat, hanging by his wings.

There is the body, the tail.

3. A big boot, riding boot.

Reminds me of my father's riding boots, black.

Response   *Inquiry*

CARD V. 16″

1. Feet of an animal with big wings, whole animal there standing.

2. A dancer, she is dressed in a costume, with wings.

   She wears a mask.

3. A hunting trophy, animal fur rug, hairy.

   Hangs on a wall.

4. Bones of an animal.

   Perhaps with hooves.

CARD VI. 23″

1. A figure, again with arms outstretched, standing.

   East-Indian, perhaps stuffed.

2. V Two clowns' heads touching each other with with their backs; more like masks, laughing expression.

3. Two more profiles.

   Open mouth, nose, they look into the distance.

CARD VII. 13″

1. Angel heads on clouds, with their hair standing up. The wings are below. With blown cheeks, they blow into the wind.

   Like on Italian paintings.

2. V Two lambs; they balance something on their noses.

   They look wooly.

3. > A dog sniffing on something.

   A Scotch-terrier, shape.

CARD VIII. 7″

1. Two bears who cling to something, perhaps a snowed-in tree.

   Furry bears, not this color, snowy tree, whitish, ice on them.

2. V Skeleton, X-ray perhaps.

   Chestbones.

3. > This way, they look like some walking animal.

4. ∧ Like Napoleon hat, sitting on a uniform.

   On a stand, like in a museum.

Response	*Inquiry*

CARD IX. 22″

1. Caricatures of animals, they are turned back; little animals, sit on something green.

   More like gnomes perhaps.

2. ∨ A blossoming tree, full of pink flowers, fluffy.

3. Profile of a woman, she looks down.

   Her hair is tied up in a knot, see the texture of the hair.

CARD X. 12″

1. This is like undersea nature, many colored animals.

   They are alive.

2. Here are green worms.

   They are crawling.

3. There are bugs, they have caught something.

   Not this color.

4. Sea horses.

   Just the shape of them.

5. A sea animal with many tentacles.

   In motion.

6. Bones in X-ray.

7. Birds with blue heads, their beaks touch each other.

   They sit on a gray branch.

21

An English Bride in an Armenian-American Family

A. William Hire

SEPARATION ANXIETY

Dorothy was an English "war bride" who had married an American GI of Armenian descent. At the end of World War II she came to the United States, settling into her husband's family in an Armenian section of New York. Apart from letters from her mother, the only contacts with her former home land had been occasional visits with other English "war brides." From the beginning Dorothy had difficulty adapting to the new family, new neighborhood, and to her role as mother and housewife, but of late, at the age of twenty-six, she had become burdened with symptoms that frightened her and her husband to the point of seeking psychiatric aid.

STRANGE SENSATIONS. When first seen at the Clinic Dorothy recounted recent episodes of unusual sensory experiences involving perceptions specific to parts of her body as well as to her environment. She had attacks of "nervousness" and was seized with the fear that she was "going crazy."

Her distress had begun two weeks following the birth of her third child, and increased throughout the three months prior to her coming to the clinic. Strange sensations of numbness and tingling in her arms suddenly alarmed her as she sat talking one evening with her sister-in-law about the new baby. Her husband who was also in the living room was watching television and not engaging in the conversation. Dorothy left the room without comment in an effort to regain her composure. The sensations lasted for a few minutes and then she rejoined her sister-in-law and husband. Her arms seemed weak and a vague fear continued throughout the evening. That night she slept poorly. The next day she went to a doctor who gave her a sedative which "did me no good." After a few days the disturbing feelings subsided. Her previously poor appetite, however, now became even worse. She lost weight, became irritable, and neglected the children and her housekeping. Her husband told the interviewer at the clinic that he had taken her to innumerable doctors since the onset of these symptoms and that nothing had been found wrong with her except that she was "extremely nervous."

Two weeks after her first attack she was bathing the baby one day when suddenly she saw only his hands and arms waving in the air. Frightened, she screamed and ran out of the bathroom. The panic passed after a few moments but a vague uneasiness associated with a fear of going crazy lingered. Shortly afterwards she was undressing, preparing to retire, when her husband entered the bedroom. He was talking but she could hear his voice only faintly, "as if he were away at some great distance." This was followed by feelings of anxiety and the thought that "something was going to happen" to her.

Episodes continued in which she became acutely aware of either her whole body or of her hands, arms, or legs, feeling as though these parts of her body did "not belong to me" or that her whole body felt strange, as though it "were not me." This might occur suddenly while at home with the children or while walking along the street. Once when putting on her coat to go out she became "very conscious of my right arm" as she was putting it into the sleeve and became so anxious that she had to take off the coat and stay in the house.

Complaints also involved her eyes. She concluded for a period of time that it was "my eyes and not myself" which were causing her difficulties. She commented on these difficulties by saying that her eyes were "so small and yet they see so much." She was at times seized with "fear" as she saw the children together. Once, as she looked into a pot while cooking, the pot appeared to extend to a great depth and she experienced the same "fear." The eyes of other people made her feel uncomfortable, especially those in her neighborhood where she felt she was being "looked at through Armenian eyes."

During her attacks she often tried to maintain her equilibrium and sustain herself by concentrating on an object and then continuing to think about it. For example, she directed her complete attention to the refrigerator and repeated: "This is a refrigerator; this is a refrigerator." She likewise held her attention on objects such as chairs, mirror, thimble, and sewing machine. After fifteen or twenty minutes, attacks ordinarily would pass, but when they were over she would become disturbed at the thought of having to resort to such unusual devices and continued to worry lest it mean that she was going crazy.

STRANGE CUSTOMS. Dorothy had met her future husband while he was stationed in England during World War II. After a courtship of two years, they were married ten days before he was to return to the United States. She followed six months later and they established a home within a tenement house owned by his mother and in which she also lived. Another daughter-in-law shared the house as well.

Dorothy was not welcomed by her mother-in-law. Instead, she was greeted with the remark: "I don't see why my son had to marry you when there are so many nice Armenian girls in the neighborhood." Many difficulties followed as the mother-in-law criticized Dorothy's housekeeping for its many discrepancies from Armenian customs. When the mother-in-law's friends came to visit they would call Dorothy in and discuss her in Armenian. They examined her clothing, took off her shoes for comparison with domestic products, and would not let her leave the room, even though she was completely excluded from conversations. A source of continued irritation for Dorothy, and one which she verbalized many times during therapy, was the inclination of the people of the neighborhood to speak in the Armenian language even though they knew English. She excluded her husband from this criticism except for one lapse which was outstanding in her memory when he spoke to some friends in Armenian in her presence.

"ARMENIAN" BABIES. Two months after Dorothy arrived from England she became pregnant. Her husband was quite pleased but she thought it was too soon after coming to a new country. She had hoped she would have time to become accustomed to her new home before having the responsibility of a child. After a few months when she had begun to busy herself with knitting and sewing for the expected baby her misgivings disappeared. She had no difficulties with pregnancy or delivery. The new arrival, a boy, resembled his father and was "dark-skinned like an Armenian." Dorothy cried and felt she did not know how to care for him. She wished that her mother were there as "she would know what to do." Her husband rushed about but "did not know either." She became accustomed to her baby, but there were disagreements between her and both her husband and mother-in-law regarding the child. There was bickering about naming the child as well as about his baptism.

As Dorothy got used to her little son, she began to think that she would like more children. A second child was planned three years later and she and her husband looked forward to a baby girl. Pregnancy proceeded without complications until the eighth month when Dorothy was hospitalized for bleeding and kidney infection and swelling of her legs and face. Three weeks after she was hospitalized labor was induced and she delivered another boy. The first thing she asked when coming out of the anesthesia was whether the baby had dark skin like an Armenian.

In less than a year she was pregnant again but this time without having planned it. Her doctor had advised her to wait a few years before having another child. However, no serious difficulties arose during the pregnancy or delivery except for the loss of several teeth due to nutritional deficiencies. This time she was acutely disappointed that the baby was not a girl, but was consoled by his light skin and resemblance to her.

APPEAL FOR HELP. It was shortly after the birth of this boy that the symptoms began to develop which eventually brought her to the clinic. She came for a few interviews and then interrupted treatment for five months while she took the children to England for a visit. Her husband urged this in lieu of psychiatric treatment on the ground that her problems were related to homesickness. Very little benefit was derived from this venture and, within a few weeks after her return to America, she made urgent calls for clinic appointments.

LIFE IN ENGLAND

Dorothy was the fourth in a family of seven children. She went to school for nine years until she was fourteen, the usual procedure for people of her laboring class. She was trained for six months in dressmaking after which she entered factory work. A portion of her earnings went to her mother as her contribution to family finances.

ANGRY FATHER. Her father earned a small but steady wage. He was a strong, robust man who did not object to hard labor. He was very strict with his children, especially his daughters, but he himself suffered from a lack of self-control before his family. He drank quite heavily and frequently came home in an argumentative mood, during which he would threaten to strike the children. On these occasions he was also prone to provoke verbal battles with his wife over the care of the home and the family budget. Many times his wrath took the form of overt physical expressions in which he slapped her. Dorothy was perpetually fearful of what would happen to her mother when the father arrived home intoxicated.

Her father demanded to know the details of his daughters' behavior, where and with whom they went, and what they did. Dorothy, in contrast to her sisters, obeyed all his rules very scrupulously.

AMBIVALENT TIE WITH MOTHER. From early childhood until the time she left for America Dorothy spent more time with her mother than did any of her siblings. In retrospect she says: "I never really appreciated my mother until I left her." She then recalled sentimentally how hard the mother had worked, sewing and knitting clothes, going out to work when funds were low, and trying her best to hold the family together in the face of the animosity among the children.

Once when Dorothy arrived home with her week's pay she threw it across the room at her mother, calling her a "money grubber." She said that to this day she did not know what possessed her to do this. "It just came out of me," she stated. Both she and her mother cried about this. Dorothy spoke of how she wept even now when she thought of it, especially if her mother had recently asked for money in one of her letters.

One evening during the heavy bombing raids of the war her mother became feverish and felt ill. When the sirens sounded Dorothy was caring for her and became very frightened and felt unable to decide whether to stay with her mother or go to the shelter for her own safety. She finally went to the shelter but could not sleep as she was thinking about her mother who remained in the house with the father. The next day the mother was taken to the hospital with pneumonia. Dorothy felt very guilty, believing that her mother would have been all right if she had stayed with her.

SISTERS. Dorothy had three elder sisters, one younger one, and two younger brothers. The eldest sister was Dorothy's favorite sibling. They slept together because they were congenial. Through her marriage this sister was enabled to live on a higher standard than anyone else in the family. She talked with Dorothy about contraception and spoke highly of Dorothy's suitor before they were married.

The other sisters were fun loving and always sought a gay time. They went out with "fast men," never came in on time, drank, and did other things for which the father was always admonishing them. Each had a premarital pregnancy or illegitimate child. The eldest of the three was the first to become pregnant. Their father had flown at her throat a few months previously for coming home late. When she became pregnant he threw her out of the house to live with some relatives elsewhere. This upset Dorothy very much and she went to visit her every day.

Dorothy's next older sister was always getting into difficulties over her many love affairs. It was this sister, two years her senior, who introduced Dorothy to her future husband in an informal gathering of soldiers in a theater lobby. The young Armenian took an immediate interest in Dorothy but she was repelled rather than attracted to him. She did not like him for the first six months of the two-year courtship. The relationship was sustained by the sister's urging double dates, and finally threatening to "cross-date."

Dorothy's younger sister was quite vivacious and had many friends. Dorothy was envious of the fact that she was able to assert herself. In describing her Dorothy said: "She never took back talk from anyone." She was, however, quite promiscuous in her relationships with men, became pregnant at the age of fifteen, and was married at sixteen.

THE BROTHERS. The youngest siblings, the brothers, were constantly fighting with each other. The older teased other members of the family. He used to taunt Dorothy by calling her "fat face" because she was chubby as she was growing up. The younger had a violent temper and would go after the older with a kitchen knife in a mad fit of fury when provoked beyond his tolerance. Their fights and arguments did not diminish with increasing age and Dorothy was frightened by them. She used to stand by the knife drawer when she perceived the beginnings of a bout so that the younger could not get a knife. It also embarrassed her to have anyone visit the home for fear the brothers might start one of their frequent tussles with each other.

SEXUAL DEVELOPMENT.   What Dorothy learned about sex was gleaned from playmates and from references or remarks by her sisters. Her earliest memory with sexual significance was of seeing her youngest brother bathed when he was an infant. Her father bathed her and the younger brothers together until she was eleven years old, at which time she rebelled. She always dreaded these occasions and found them "humiliating."

She was introduced to the menstrual function by seeing an older sister walk through the bedroom with used menstrual pads in her hand. When the sister noticed Dorothy's interest she said: "Don't look at that; your time will come soon enough." The girls in the factory told her that if she did not get a period by the time she was twenty-one she would go crazy. This made her anxious for her menses to begin.

Her first period occurred during the latter part of her fourteenth year while she was at work in the factory. She saw blood stains when she went to the bathroom and became so nervous that she had to leave work. She hid her stained underwear under her mattress at home where her mother found it a few days later, and, contrary to the girl's fearful anticipation, she explained the function to her without scolding.

Some months following the onset of the menses Dorothy's brother-in-law who lived in the house made advances to her while lying next to her in the air raid shelter. She was afraid to make a scene or to protest. She consequently said nothing but was tense all night and frequently got up to urinate. Finally, toward daybreak she fell asleep. When she awakened she was frightened as to what had happened while she slept. Next month she missed her menstrual period. She was afraid to tell anyone but finally confided in the sister whose husband had made advances to her, that she had missed her period. She suggested to Dorothy that she see a doctor who reassured her that she was not pregnant and told her it was not unusual to miss periods at the beginning of menses.

A love affair that Dorothy considered "serious," before meeting her future husband, occurred when she was fifteen. For six months she went out with a fellow a few years older than herself who worked in the same factory. She would wait on street corners on her way to work just to see him. Usually, she would just watch him pass but sometimes she would muster enough courage to pretend an accidental meeting and walk the remainder of the way to work with him. She described the relationship as being one which was very discreet. He later married and she "stopped thinking about him."

COURTSHIP. The mixed feelings with which she met her future husband focused on her dislike of his appearance, especially his dark skin. He was stationed about ten minutes' walk from where she lived and she was soon seeing him almost daily. They went walking, to movies, and out dancing. This she enjoyed very much. They did not indulge in any kind of sexual play or intimacy but when they were double dating with her sister they had to wait on the way home from the movies and dances while the sister and her escort lingered in darkened doorways during the blackout. She did not invite him to the house for a year after she met him because she was embarrassed about the family situation and was afraid her brothers would get into a fight while he was there.

It was during the first year of her courtship that she remembered her father's berating her sisters for their behavior. Referring to the premarital and illegitimate pregnancies of the other sisters he said the only good one was the eldest one, adding: "There's Dorothy, but she's still young. We'll see what happens to her." Dorothy cried after this because she felt it was unfair that her good behavior should be doubted.

During the second year of their acquaintance, her suitor came to the house frequently, and her parents became very fond of him, considering him a gentleman. Dorothy was much impressed by her mother's approval, saying, "Mother could tell about those things."

An incident which affected her father very much in the young Armenian's favor occurred one night when bad transit connections made them late getting home. Although they were not very late, Dorothy was quite upset and her suitor insisted upon explaining to her father, who accepted the explanation and was quite courteous and reassuring to her suitor.

During the two years of courtship her suitor never spoke to her of love and marriage. She wondered if he was just spending time with her and planned to go back to the United States without her. Finally, after obtaining her parents' consent, he declared his intention of marrying her.

In-laws. Dorothy and her husband were married ten days before he was to return to the United States. Before the ceremony he explained to her that they would be living in an Armenian community with his mother.

Six months later Dorothy followed him to New York where she and her husband took an apartment in his mother's house. She was very lonesome and cried frequently during the first few months. In addition to her mother-in-law's critical attitude she was troubled by her husband's absence nearly every evening on his job as postal clerk. She joined a club for English war brides but lost enthusiasm for it when she found that her husband would not attend the social occasions with her even when he did not have the excuse of having to work. He protested that he was not interested and went away to gamble with his friends instead. Dorothy got the impression that her mother-in-law was suspicious of her leaving the house even though it was with another English girl and her American husband. Allusions were made to English girls as "fast" when friends of her husband's family were visiting the house. One remark by her sister-in-law made Dorothy wonder if they thought she

had been a street-walker when her husband met her. Her
mother-in-law's friends constantly stressed to Dorothy that
her husband was "a wonderful man." This she took to mean
that they thought that she was "no good."

DEATH OF MOTHER-IN-LAW. During the latter period of
her first pregnancy and after the child was born, Dorothy
stopped going to the club. Two of her friends whom she
had met there continued to visit her, but for the most part
she felt more lonely than ever. Two years after the birth
of the first son the mother-in-law suffered a stroke and became a partial invalid, requiring a great deal of care. It
was necessary for Dorothy to check on her frequently. On
two occasions she arrived just in time to extinguish fires
caused by the mother-in-law's carelessness.

After the mother-in-law's death soon after the birth of
Dorothy's second child, the house was sold, and Dorothy
and her husband moved to an apartment within the same
neighborhood. Her husband resisted any idea of leaving
the neighborhood, saying that he did not want to be away
from his friends. Although Dorothy was pleased to be out
from under her husband's parental roof at long last, she was
not able to find new neighbors with whom she felt friendly.
She visited the landlady frequently and enjoyed their conversations except when the landlady's friends came in and
spoke in Armenian. Then she felt "left out" and that she
"did not belong."

DECOMPENSATION. With the arrival of the third child
Dorothy soon lost her grip on managing the household. Her
husband would tell her to "snap out of it," that the doctors
had found nothing wrong with her, that she was just "weak-
minded." He told her that if she would realize that she
was a married woman with three children everything would
be all right. Later on, as a gesture which he meant to be
sympathetic rather than critical, he told her that she was
not capable of shouldering family responsibilities, that the
whole situation was just too much for her. "Instead of getting married," he would say to her, "you should have stayed
home and worked in the factory where you were happy."

These complaints were also repeated to the therapist when her husband visited the clinic for a conference in which he talked privately about his wife's condition. He appeared cooperative and voiced eagerness to help in any way that he could but had very little understanding of the difficulties she experienced and could not give any elaboration of her symptoms beyond her own quotes. He expressed sympathy in that he thought that the adjustment to his mother had been difficult for her, but at the same time observed that his wife, unlike Armenian girls, had always done her housework "with an effort" and could not seem to perform her tasks "without wearing herself out." He also reiterated his opinion that she should never have married at all, that she was "really happy doing stitching in the factory."

ATTEMPT TO ESCAPE. The trip to England was arranged as a last resort. The visit itself seems to have had both pleasant and unpleasant aspects. Although she enjoyed some good times with her sisters, the children proved difficult to manage and she found their nostalgia infectious. In her eagerness to return to her husband she cut the trip short by a month. On her return, her husband was delighted at first to find her apparently much improved. It was not long, however, before he was faced with the same old complaints, which discouraged him to the point of resisting her return to the clinic on the ground that it had not helped her. After a few weeks he relented in exasperation and she took up regular appointments once a week for a period of approximately a year.

SPECIAL EXAMINATIONS

NEUROLOGICAL CHECK. Dorothy's complaints about peculiar sensations necessitated a checkup of her central nervous system functioning. Neurological examinations and electro-encephalography yielded negative results and reduced to an absolute minimum any probability that she was suffering effects of organic brain disturbance.

BENDER GESTALT TEST. The Bender Visual-Motor Gestalt Test was administered as one of the psychological tests.

The designs were all reproduced without difficulty and the results were consistent with the negative findings of the neurological examinations and E.E.G.

RORSCHACH AND TAT. The Rorschach and Thematic Apperception Tests were each administered twice. They were originally given early in the clinic contact and again when termination of treatment was under consideration. During the testing, it was difficult to obtain elaborations from her since she was extremely hesitant about describing what she saw. In spite of much reassurance it was not possible to allay her anxiety. On the TAT she would ask permission to surrender the picture with obvious eagerness to get rid of it. She also seemed relieved when she had completed the testing and was able to leave the office.

APPRAISAL OF RORSCHACH AND TAT

Generally the test results revealed Dorothy as an extremely guarded, restricted, apprehensive person, uneasy about expressing herself. This was not surprising in view of her stated fear that she was going crazy and her probable assumption of the special meaning of the testing in relation to this. The uneasiness, however, had implications beyond the threat of the test situation. In fact, the test situation was capable of provoking anxiety to such a degree only because she was struggling so desperately not to become aware of what was going on within herself.

The tests showed a lack of tolerance for disturbing fantasy characteristic of people who repress and deny thoughts and feelings as a means of coping with them. These defenses were endangered by the impact of the projective testing. Specific indications from the Rorschach material of her struggle to maintain repressions were found in the particular manner in which she failed to utilize the human movement determinant with a consequent shift to animal content. Even within this category we noted her inability to "recall" the names of animals and her difficulty in verbalizing responses. These tendencies reduced the quantity of responses on both the Rorschach and TAT and prompted the refrain of "I don't know" which occurred throughout both. The precariousness with which she was holding off a breakthrough of repressions was indicated by her need for support from the examiner during both procedures before she could give expression to "imagination."

The nature of the disturbing fantasies which she sought to ward off was inferred from the responses to the TAT. As may be noted in Test Summary B, the content was marked by deep hostilities, intense guilt, and masochistic fantasies. Thus, the basic orientation was presumed to be a sado-masochistic one. She was preoccupied with conflictual elements of sexuality with the result that relationships between men and women were perceived as leading to fear and unhappiness. Fundamentally she saw relationships as triangular so frequently and so intensely that her current mode of relating was apparently close to the original prototype of her parental relationships in the Oedipal situation.

No evidence of a relationship with the mother figure could be found in the TAT material. A punitive, deserting mother who aroused feelings of rivalry was portrayed, with attendant feelings of fear and guilt (see, especially, Cards 2, 7GF, and 18GF in Test Summary B). The roles of husband and father were fused. This comes out strikingly in Cards 3GF, 6GF, and 13MF. Men were perceived as aggressive and destructive toward women in sexual relationships. Fear was the most outstanding feature of her attitude but, beneath the surface, there were indications of strong feelings of hostility with consequent guilt. In dealing with men a placating attitude rather than one of open conflict was dictated by a sense of inadequacy in the women.

The dangers and insecurities thus seen to be inherent in relating to people resulted in emotional isolation. This is further elaborated in the Rorschach (Test Summary A) through the patient's manner of responding, with its particular content on the colored cards. Feelings of coldness, anxiety, and of personal inadequacy appear even in the face of fundamentally appealing affect (note, especially, "ice" and "polar bears" on Card VIII). Hostile feelings were seen to lead to fears of punishment through rejection rather than to a turning of destructive impulses against the ego.

Although severely burdened, the ego had not relinquished reality contact when confronted with the very strong pressures from the threat of erupting repressions. Reality testing was impaired by marked uncertainties and fear of failure as indicated by the patient's repeated pleas for support from the examiner lest she misjudge or fail to know reality.

RORSCHACH AND TAT AGAIN. The second administration of the Rorschach and TAT showed little change in the direction of increased strength and confidence on Dorothy's part. Certain features of the Rorschach indicated even greater inhibition: There were instances of outright rejection of cards. At the same time there was less hesitation in some of the elaborations, presumably reflecting a more adequate rejection of unacceptable impulses without discernible progress in working through to an understanding of them.

Repetition of the TAT showed changes in the direction of more explicitness with respect to story details, revealing deeper-lying material previously warded off by repression. The counter-struggle had been reduced. This is shown, for example, in her changed response to picture 13MF, in which on the second administration the patient saw the attacking man as the girl's father rather than as the formerly unspecified man.

13MF. This looks as if the man here is fairly old. Probably the father may have hurt the girl, the way she's laying there like. (Why?) The way he stands here. (Happened?) Gee! I don't really know—unless he killed her. (Why?) Well, the way she's just laying here—or maybe he just hurt her. (Before?) If it was her father probably she did something wrong also. (For instance?) Probably she was a bad girl. (How?) Yeh—well, I mean she didn't obey him, but he looks kinda sorry if he did hurt her. (Outcome?) Well, if he did hurt her, beat her, I think she'll forgive him if he's her father—I think everything will work out ok.

In other stories there were also changes with respect to the straightforwardness with which the original theme was elaborated. There was now a somewhat more hopeful tone in which the ego showed less helplessness and inhibition.

18GF. To me it looks like a mother and daughter and the girl probably came in late. She went with a boy the mother dislikes. She looks kinda angry. The mother looks as though she's trying to tell her not to go with him. (Thinking and feeling?) I think she'll listen to her mother anyway. The mother seems to know whether she's going with the right person. She'll understand her mother. (Outcome?) She'll understand her mother. She'll find another boyfriend, you know.

8GF. I don't know. She looks kinda contented. Maybe she's waiting for her husband to come home from work or maybe she's just thinking. (What?) Probably about the future—if she has children. (Thinking?) If she's not satisfied in the house she's in she might be thinking of a nice home. (Outcome?) She looks nice in the picture. Things will come good for her. She'll have all she wants.

THE TREATMENT PROCESS

RELATIONSHIP TO THERAPIST. The treatment sessions were characterized by desperate pleas for reassurance with little capacity on her part to pursue thoughts and associations which would lead to uncovering the conflicts and impulses underlying her symptoms. For a very long period it was difficult to establish even an adequate description of her feelings and symptomatology.

Why this should be true became clearer when her desperate struggle to prevent the emergence of frightening fantasies was understood. She related well to the therapist in the sense that she was quite willing to unburden herself and seemed to cling tenaciously to her trust in his ability to help her. Her strong denial defenses kept negative feelings from overt expression, and the pressures of her preoccupations determined the themes discernible through most of the material and the treatment sessions. She was highly suggestible and would accept any attempt to rephrase her thoughts for her.

When the pressures of her anxiety receded she was ready to discontinue treatment by mutual consent with the therapist. Consequently, she never arrived at any impressive de-

gree of insight nor did she face her feelings about the
therapist, which rose very close to the surface as her fears
abated. She remained rational and highly critical of her
unusual thoughts and sensations throughout treatment but
was quite tense and at times rather depressed. On a few
occasions she wept during interviews.

INABILITY TO "SWALLOW" HUSBAND'S COLDNESS. Dorothy
dated the onset of her difficulties from the time of her first
pregnancy during a visit of an army friend of her husband
whom she had known in England as a "fast" sort of fellow.
In planning his entertainment, her husband told her that
he was going to "show the friend the town" and that they
would sleep somewhere else. Inwardly, Dorothy became
very angry, wishing to throw something at him, to hurt him.
Outwardly, she showed no sign of her feelings except to request that they return home to sleep. They left saying they
would sleep elsewhere. The husband, however, did return
very late while his friend rented a room. The next morning Dorothy could not swallow her food. From that time
on she could only take small bits of food even though she
felt hunger. This inability to swallow periodically bothered her thereafter and occurred as one of the many complaints reported from time to time throughout treatment.

Many of her mixed feelings about her husband involved
her frustration with his inability to demonstrate any kind
of protective or sympathetic attitude. She complained that
he was talkative with his friends but when with her he
would only watch television. She said that only once did
she venture to tell him of her symptoms. When he dismissed her problem by telling her she "sounded silly," she
never mentioned them to him again because he "wouldn't
understand." Actually, they did continue to talk of her
symptoms since she would report from time to time his telling her to "snap out of it" and that the trouble was "all in
her."

Her feelings of isolation from her husband and loss of
identity came out episodically in her fear that something
was going to happen to her, that her body did not belong

to her—"it was light or something." She reported first having had this feeling when she learned that she was pregnant for the third time. On a later occasion the symptom
recurred while she was washing dishes, and it stayed with
her as she went into the living room to join her husband.
Without comment, she reported having sat down but *not
near him*. In reply to the therapist's question as to what
she thought might help her at such times, she made the
significant remark, "Someone to hold me."

While speaking in one of the interviews about her "scary
feelings" she told how at these times she tried to think of
her name as "Dottie," as she had been called in England.
Then she began to think: "What am I doing *here?*", and
the "scary feelings" arose. At other times she thought of
what would have happened if she had not been born—she
"wouldn't be here if my mother hadn't had me." She added
that these were not actually "thoughts" but "just a kind of
feeling."

MOTHER-IN-LAW TROUBLE. One of the focal themes to
which Dorothy frequently returned during therapy was
the difficult time she had had when she first arrived in the
United States. Late in the series of interviews when she
had become somewhat more free in discussing details of
her experiences she spoke of how her mother-in-law's dirtiness offended her. She would get her hair in the food while
cooking and would soil her clothes and floors until the whole
house "smelled." Some rooms in the house were rented to
people outside the family. The mother-in-law wanted Dorothy to clean these rooms but she was so repelled by the
filth that she could not bear to enter them.

Another source of irritation was her mother-in-law's over-
concern about childbearing: "When we first got there and
didn't have a baby right away she would say, 'You're just
fooling around.' . . . What did she expect? I got pregnant in two months!" After the first child was conceived
the mother-in-law would call her friends in and they would
laugh and talk in Armenian finally calling for Dorothy to
"come in and let us feel your belly." If Dorothy resisted

the mother-in-law would threaten to tell her husband. The husband defended Dorothy when this happened. Within this context, Dorothy related her frequent preoccupation with how things were "before we were married and had kids and worries."

CONFLICT OVER HER "ARMENIAN" CHILDREN. Her attacks of anxiety were specifically associated with her marriage and care of her children as well as with the broader facts of environmental change. This relationship became more focal and clear-cut as therapy progressed. Dreams which she reported were also of interest in this connection. Soon after her return from the trip to England she dreamed that she was on a boat with her children and the boat was being rocked violently. Finally, it capsized and she saw the face of her eldest son looking at her through a porthole as the ship went down. All the children were lost and she awakened feeling "very nervous."

Some days later she saw a neighbor's child with the measles. That night she dreamed of seeing this little Armenian boy sitting on a stove upon which there was also a frying pan. The pan caught fire and the boy jumped off. She added that the stove was like the one in her kitchen and that the boy was dark and the same size as her oldest son but "they don't look like each other at all." The following afternoon she was sleeping with her youngest son and dreamed that she was all alone "with nobody around her." She awoke with the "fear" and tingling sensations all over.

When treatment had progressed far enough for her hostile feelings concerning the children to emerge into consciousness she dreamed one night that she was in bed and an Armenian girl of her acquaintance was telling her she ought to be up taking care of the children. Dorothy "flew at her throat" and awakened with feelings of fright. In discussing the dream the therapist remarked that the slur on her motherhood seemed to infuriate her. Her subsequent thoughts were that she stayed in bed too long and that her husband had to get up with the kids. He berated her for this. The Armenian girl in the dream was someone she had

met soon after coming to the United States. The girl had
made Dorothy angry at that time by saying that England
"starts all our wars."

In connection with her conflict over her children, it is
significant that she tried to avoid discussing the death of
her sister's illegitimate child. It was clear that Dorothy
thought the sister had murdered it. Dorothy had heard the
"strange cry" of the child before it was found dead in its
crib. The doctor said it had smothered to death but Dorothy strongly suspected that there had been more than
neglect.

FEAR OF LOSING CONTROL. The following is a representative interview at the point in treatment where she had begun
to sense a relationship between her impulses and her symptoms. The recounting is based on notes from an interview
which took place during her treatment about four months
before termination. Where possible the coloring and structure are preserved.

Dorothy smiled as she entered the office. The therapist
asked how things were. She responded:

> Not bad, doctor; not good, but not bad. I'm still getting the feel-
> ing, but it's better. I noticed something this week that's also hap-
> pened before. I will be taking some milk from the ice box and I
> say to myself—"You're taking milk from the ice box"—like I'm con-
> centrating on it. I do it when I have the feeling I'm going crazy—
> to make sure I know what I'm doing—because I'm afraid I won't
> know, I guess.

The therapist attempted to restate her problem for her
in terms of "losing control" but it did not appear to have
meaning to her. He then asked if there were any special
day when this was likely to occur. She replied that it was
more likely to happen on week ends when her husband was
working and she was at home with the children. She added
that it was not the children that made her feel bad, it was
that her husband was not home. She then spoke of the
loneliness of Sundays because it was such a quiet day and
followed this by nostalgic remarks about late rising and
Sunday movies in England.

Returning to thoughts on the children she said,

They are really good kids but sometimes I lose my temper at them. I let it build up and then I could kill them. I'm afraid I'll really hurt them sometimes when I get mad. The big one should know better. But I don't hit them much. I think it's because I'm afraid I'll really hurt them that I don't hit them half enough sometimes. The woman downstairs is hitting and hitting, but I don't do that. Once I hit Frankie (the oldest) and his nose bled and I thought I'd really done it then, and I was frightened.

Sometimes when they go to bed Frankie will tell Eddie (the next younger) not to go to sleep and they'll fool an hour and a half before they go to sleep and I'll be getting madder and madder. I'll say: "Frankie, if you don't want to go sleep at least let Eddie." They keep it right up till I go in and hit them. Then they go right to sleep. My husband tells me I should hit them right off but I don't.

Her thoughts then turned to the two older boys' liking for nursery school and the fact that the youngest would be going. She wondered what she would do then, saying that he was all she had now unless she got pregnant again.

There was some talk about her working when the children are all off to school, about having sent some money to England for Christmas, and about the pleasant look on the faces of her children when they recently got their Christmas toys. Her husband was home on Christmas day and all had gone well even if he had worked at night. She had been reminded of her own former loneliness and of a new neighbor, a French girl who was struggling with nostalgia as she had once done. This interview was followed by a series in which she continued to speak of her fear of hitting the kids.

The next trend in her therapy sessions was away from discussion of aggression on her part, but was concerned with the danger of the children's getting hurt in accidents. She had had an anxiety attack after seeing a movie in which a hypnotist had caused someone to commit murder. Her fear specifically of hurting the youngest child was brought out through continued reference on her part to anxiety attacks while caring for him. The therapist finally was able to help her to focus the import of what she was saying in terms of the feelings involved, and to help her gain insight into the fact that to feel angry does not necessarily lead to killing. Some of her associations during this effort involved memories of her father striking her sisters and her childish fantasy that he would kill them. It was during that phase of treatment that she dreamed of the Armenian girl telling her to get out of bed and care for her children.

RELIEF. Following this there was a period of lessening frequency of her attacks along with improvement in morale. She began to find excuses for breaking appointments. The therapist considered the alternatives of continuing treatment to a point of better insight or of letting her accept the symptom relief as an adequate accomplishment. When he broached the possibility of her stopping she seemed to feel that she was able to get along without further treatment. It was agreed that she would come in occasionally over the following months to consider any problems that might arise. She arranged to work part time as a stitcher in a factory. The additional money was of course welcomed by the husband and they began thinking of buying a house in some other community which made her feel better too.

REORIENTATION. A visit from her three years later revealed that she had had some recurrence of symptoms but she did not regard them as severe and they no longer frightened her. The children were all in school and she was working a full shift in the factory. She emphasized how fortunate she felt in having a good husband, one who was not mean to her or the children. She remarked on how frequently her friends told her this, and in the same context she spoke of how they also told her that the United States was now her home. She added that she regarded herself as fortunate in having come to this country to live in comparison to "what people have in England."

INTERPRETATION

CONFLICTING CULTURAL DEMANDS. An overview of the problems of this English war bride in her attempt to adjust to her Armenian husband's way of life leaves no doubt as to the important role played by the radical cultural change in producing the stressful context in which her loss of personal identity developed. Her marriage required that she give up all her former ties and relationships apart from the contact she still maintained with her mother through letters. In addition to experiencing the loneliness of being in a foreign country with a husband who, in terms of her background, did not give freely of his companionship, she was restricted to a totally unfamiliar and uncongenial subculture within the adopted country. She was called upon to fit into a community which held itself aloof from the new culture and clung tenaciously to the old.

A full understanding of Dorothy's difficulties requires an analysis of the specific ways in which the culture affected her behavior. Why she was so unadaptable and reacted with symptom development are the questions which must be dealt with.

DISCREPANT MARITAL EXPECTATIONS. First, the disparity between the types of family life in which the patient and her husband grew up resulted in the creation of certain expectations with respect to roles in marriage which neither was able to fulfill for the other. He expected her as a wife to have a high degree of self-reliance and tolerance for a life of relative apartness from the broader world of her new home land. These expectations were reflected in his reactions to her symptoms, especially when we consider the context of his assertions that her difficulties would be solved if she would accept her role as wife and mother. He seemed to see nothing amiss in the situation except for her inability to work according to his image of Armenian girls, without complaint or excessive use of energy. Apparently he expected her to assume the matriarchal role with which he was familiar.

The matriarchal image presented to the young wife in the aging and repulsive person of her mother-in-law dismally failed to meet her need for support and help with reality testing, which her own mother had customarily supplied.

Instead, she spoke a language Dorothy could not understand, offered "advice" which in its import was a condemna-
tion and rejection, and expressed an outspoken frankness
toward sexuality and pregnancy which were at variance
with Dorothy's inhibited attitudes.

UNRESOLVED CONFLICT WITH MOTHER. Dorothy had previously learned neither to see nor speak of pregnancy, to
rely on her mother for help in the more trivial aspects of
sexuality as well as in the more important evaluation of
men with respect to their potential sexual danger. Even
in the matter of marital choice itself, her mother's judgment
of her prospective husband was crucial. Presumably the
patient's hope of being saved from more dangerous sexual
men was reflected in this. Her future husband did not
arouse her anxiety by making sexual demands during courtship, and he supported her in the role of good girl in the
eyes of both her parents. An incident in which she interpreted her husband as identified with the ways of sexual
men stood out in her memory and coincided with the development of her first symptom.

Outside the sexual area as well as within it Dorothy had
depended on her mother's judgment, as when she sought
her advice about a contemplated change of job. In all instances reported, Dorothy never gave the slightest indication of having questioned her mother's wisdom. Nevertheless, beneath this outward deference and dependency, strong
undertones of rivalry and hostility were revealed by projective techniques. Her marriage, by forcing a radical separation, unconsciously was an attempt to resolve her conflict
concerning her mother. The attempt failed, however, because the conflict had not really been worked through to
the point where new attachments could be formed that were
not re-enactments of the old. The girl continued to seek
replacement of the mother figure. The new landlady, for
instance, was a definite improvement on the mother-in-law,
but she, too, lapsed into the distant inadequacies of a foreign person.

MEANING OF SYMPTOMS.   It was significant that Dorothy's major symptom development took place while she was confronted with disappointments both in marital expectations and in the discovery of an adequate mother substitute.   It was no accident that her most alarming disturbance occurred just after she had given birth to her third child, a child representing a psychologically illicit pregnancy inasmuch as it had been forbidden by her doctor, and which was conceived, at least in her fantasy, because of her excessive passion, also forbidden according to her standards.   The symptoms represented a re-enactment of the real or fantasied murder by her sister of her own literally illegitimate child.   The patient's improvement in therapy was the result of her becoming able to deal with her murderous impulses toward her children, especially the "illegitimate" one.

The understanding of her symptoms assumed a unified pattern when interpreted as representing different aspects of the fundamental need to escape from the threatening features of her marriage.   The symptom which occurred in connection with bathing the baby seemed to represent a "disappearing child," one which vanished before eyes that "saw too much" and therefore aroused hostility and the consequent anxiety.

The children were all "foreign" and of the "dark people" among whom she lived unhappily.   Her concern over darkness seemed to involve a contrast with or difference from herself.   A comprehensive meaning of this preoccupation did not emerge but the association to sexuality is suggested by her explicit perceptual interest in the darkness of Card III of the Rorschach.   She was originally repelled by the dark complexion of her prospective husband but accepted him when he proved not to be sexually threatening to her. A related association that dark people are dirty was suggested by her inability to enter the rooms of boarders in her mother-in-law's house and the disgust aroused by her mother-in-law's personal dirtiness.

The fearful aspects of sexuality were connected in her mind with fears of destruction and of the dangers of pregnancy itself, which her mother implied but refused to discuss with her during adolescence. The destructive fears involved also the fantasied sadism of the male as portrayed in her image of an assaultative father who explicitly sexualized his relationship to her by bathing her.

Dorothy's difficulties arose because of certain inabilities stemming from a weakness in ego functioning which hampered her expression of impulses of any degree of intensity. She could not speak aggressively to her husband even though she felt like throwing something at him. She could not protest the advances of her brother-in-law but merely alternated between complete passivity and withdrawal from the scene. She once threw money at her mother and upon another occasion interceded with her over the drunken father, but immediately cried in both instances. She felt very deeply the hurts at the hands of her mother-in-law, but her complaints to the therapist were such that, at times, it was almost as though Dorothy felt the trouble were in herself.

Many of her symptoms involved strange bodily sensations which occurred on occasions when strong feeling was aroused. They seemed to represent a depersonalization that served to deaden the underlying feeling. She felt she was "not herself" in a way that went beyond the symbolization of her reality situation of "detachment" from her former life in England. It should be noted, however, that not every girl undergoing a similar cultural change would have developed Dorothy's psychopathology. In her case, the unresolved conflict with her mother, leaving in its wake an inadequately integrated ego, predisposed her to breakdown. The particular circumstances of her marriage, adding the dimension of culture conflict to her already confused identity, exposed her fragile ego to more stress than it could tolerate. Decompensation of her hysterical defenses ensued, and collapse into psychosis was narrowly averted by psychotherapy.

Test Summary

A. RORSCHACH PROTOCOL [1]

Response	Inquiry

CARD I. (Examiner suggests patient hold card) 9″

1. I don't know . . . it looks like a butterfly. I imagine (laughs), I mean . . . you can stop and think for a while? I think that's what I'd . . . (asked to smoke)

(Location, W) The wings, a piece jutting out there. (Dd22) I don't understand the names . . . (of different parts) (Alive?) Oh no . . .

CARD II. (Looks puzzled) 25″

1. Can you just guess or something? . . . I can't make this one out . . . (encouraged) . . . I'd say it looks like a couple of animals . . . It is hard to puzzle out . . .

(Location D1) The ears (Dd31). The way it's bent, I do figure it's the whole animal. (Kind of animal?) No, I don't know . . . Maybe a rabbit of some kind, the ear . . .

CARD III. 35″

Is it really that they represent something or do I tell you what I think it looks like? . . . I can't make out this one . . . I don't know—wouldn't be like a shadow of somebody would it?

(Location, D9) Way it's pointed like. (Points out edges of shoe.) I really don't know. (Much questioning elicits: "looks like a person") (Else about shadow?) (No response.) (If as D2, D3? Meaning red color?) That's what I mean; it's really the darkness of it.

CARD IV. 15″

1. This one reminds me of the skin of an animal, I mean the fur . . .

(Location, W) It looks like fur when opened up. (Fur?) It looks like it, the way it's painted, the sharpness of it . . .

CARD V. 12″

1. That reminds me of a bat (laughs). I've only seen bats in pictures, but . . .

(Location, W) I've seen them in pictures; it reminds me so much of that, and the wings. (Wings?) I mean to me it looks more raggedy (points out edges). . . .

---

[1] The numbering of Rorschach locations follows S. J. Beck, *Rorschach's test, I. Basic processes* (2d ed.; New York: Grune & Stratton, Inc., 1949).

Response	*Inquiry*

CARD VI. 90″ (Hints at side turn with sort of side tip. Examiner says ok to turn.) ∨ ∧

1. I don't know . . . > ∧ < I don't know about this one. To me they all resemble an animal. (Reassured) To me it wouldn't be a big animal. I am imagining it in half (blot) and then . . . (embarrassed, apologetic).	(Location, W) When you see it as if you would bend the card. (i.e., sides together) It reminds me of an insect with this (D8) as being the head part (notes "eyes"). . . .

CARD VII. 80″ > ∧ > <

1. Looking at it like this, it reminds me of an elephant . . . Are these actual pictures or . . . just what we think they are? (Reassured)	(Location, D1) There is the trunk (D5); the rest is the head. I don't know about the rest of it.

CARD VIII. 45″ < ∧

1. I know. That reminds me of the ice.	(Location, D8) It is a mountain, like in a picture. (Ice?) The way they put color in too; it isn't blue, but it's like . . .
2. With polar bears or something.	(Location, D1) Head, feet. (Alive?) No . . .

CARD IX. 55″ < ∨ ∧ <

1. This one looks hard (smiles) . . .> ∧ < ∧ > ∧ > I don't know. The top reminds me, but the bottom I don't know. (Top?) (Can't think of name of animal, "not reindeer"), but horns or something. Haven't you got to guess what the picture is like?	Mainly, (D7) horns. (Unable to recall what animal)

CARD X. 22″

1. This here resembles a flower but I don't know about this here . . .	(Location, D9 & D11) I don't know the name of it . . . but it has color to it (D9) and it's long . . . You probably know what I mean—and prettiness to it too, and this looks like the stalk (D11) to me.

TESTING THE LIMITS

Liked best: VIII (Why?) When I first saw it I could imagine everything, bears . . .

Liked least: III (Why?) I don't know . . . although others are all dark too . . . don't really know, just the way it caught my eye, I guess.

Test Summary

B. THEMATIC APPERCEPTION TEST

CARD 1. 15″

Well . . . I don't know. How would you start? . . . There's a little boy. I don't know. To me it looks as if he loves the violin . . . Have you got to end it now, like? (What do you think will happen?) Well, I think he'll eventually play it. (In picture, why isn't playing?) Well, I don't know, probably the violin might be broke or something . . . what else? (i.e., should she tell about?)

CARD 2. 10″

I don't know. Would that be a farm? . . . To me it looks like a love picture or something . . . I don't really know what to say. (Story?) The girl here looks very miserable. That would be the pattern we'd be going by. She doesn't look very happy . . . (Unhappy because?) Probably in love . . . (Others fit in?) I don't know. In a way, I think that would be her mother . . . unless you could say man was . . . (Part mother playing?) She seems to be in the way. (Whose?) Girl's way. (Will happen?) What do you mean, to all of them like or . . . Probably, the mother will go away; although, this girl looks as if she's ready to go . . . but in a way she looks so determined here—the mother.

CARD 3GF. 15″

The girl looks in a bad way, I mean crying and everything . . . I think she could be sick . . . Should you have two things like that? The woman . . . her lover or someone left her. She came out and found him gone . . . Another thing, she could be sick and trying to get to the phone or something. Is that all? (Happens?) If she is sick, to me it looks as if she's just drop down; or if it's her lover or somebody she'll probably have a good cry and they'll come back tomorrow (laughs) maybe . . . (The patient apologized saying she did not "know how to express it." Reassured by examiner.)

CARD 5. 37″

I don't know. It would probably be a woman calling her family in for supper or something . . . That's all . . . (Sort of woman?) I don't know. She looks like a nice woman, I think.

CARD 6GF. 22″

The girl looks kinda worried in the picture. I don't know whether that could have been her husband, or what; but she looks as if she doesn't want him near her, or something . . . I don't know. (Happens?) . . . (long, long pause) . . . I don't know. The way she's looking, it looks as though she's scared he's going to do harm to her or something. I don't know what else to . . .

CARD 7GF. 17″

The mother looks as if she's reading to the little girl . . . The girl don't seem interested . . . (long, long pause) . . . (Why might not be interested?) . . . (long, long pause) . . . Well, I don't know . . . The way I'm looking at the woman, it doesn't look like her mother. Probably her parents went out or something.

CARD 3BM. 32″

She couldn't have shot herself would she? That's what it looks like . . . (Led up to it?) It could be her husband died; or she had family trouble, or something.

CARD 10. 10″

It just looks like a love picture, is it, or . . . (More about people?) The way they look here, they look so much in love with one another. (Happen?) The way they are, I think it's already happened; probably they will get married, if they aren't married already.

CARD 18GF. 25″

I don't know . . . She looks as if she's going to hurt the girl there—strangle her or something—probably because she (girl) did wrong. (Did wrong?) . . . It might be with a fellow . . . (Who is hurting girl?) I would say it was the mother . . . (Happen?) . . . I don't think she'll hurt her. I don't know.

CARD 13MF. 22″

It looks as if he might have killed her . . . (long, long pause) . . . Maybe she wasn't good to him or something. Probably he will give himself up to the police. That's the way he looks . . .

CARD 12F. 26″

That couldn't have been the girl when she got older or something, could it? I don't know. I just think of that. It probably is her when she got older. (What is she like when older?) She looks like she was the devil . . . a witch, or something.

CARD 8GF. 27″

I don't know . . . The girl looks kind of happy, but yet she looks lonely . . . I don't know what to think of this . . . (Happen?) I don't know. She looks as if she will be angry. I don't know.

22

Upward Social Mobility in a New American

Howard E. Mitchell

PROLOGUE

Picture a somewhat tall, slender, dark-complexioned handsome boy tensely ruminating over the problems of adolescence as he lies in bed in a drab, meagerly furnished second-floor rear apartment shared only by him and his father. Deftly someone raps on the door. It opens and in walks the boy's uncle. Albert has learned years before that "when the men talk, I keep quiet." Consequently, he pretended to be asleep as his uncle and father talked in low tones. As he cringed beneath the warm sheets he suddenly became cold when he heard his uncle say, "They found her dead about two hours ago. It happened sometime during the earlier part of the night—she strangled herself." He was referring to Albert's mother.

As Albert's account of the early trauma in his life unfolded, much of his emotional difficulty could be understood. Yet, understanding of another nature was necessary in order to help this young man effectively. This encompassed a knowledge and understanding of certain features of his cultural heritage and its conditioning influence upon him. It took the writer scurrying to learn about the essential features of the Armenian-American subculture with its cohesive structure, intense nationalism, lasting hatreds, gay festive occasions, central role of the church, and paternalistic family constellation. All these factors contributed to his discomfort.

THE SHAPE OF THINGS TO COME

MEMORIES OF MOTHER.   Seventeen years later when we made our first contact with Albert, he related how he feigned being asleep in these words, "I never told anyone about this incident—sort of kept it to myself." In fact, Albert had so firmly repressed this incident surrounding knowledge of his mother's death that when reminded of it in a later therapy session he looked surprised. Other things about his mother were consciously vague at this time. "Isn't it funny," he remarked in his third treatment hour, "I cannot remember having a single conversation with my mother." Primarily, his early memories of his mother were of seeing her wave to him from a distance through the barred windows of a New England State Hospital where she was interned until her death. His mother was hospitalized after the birth of his one younger brother, Edward, when he was three-and-a-half years of age, and remained there for seven years. As therapy progressed, he recalled that she had blue eyes, was light complexioned, but "her hair was dark, just like mine." He also recalled that when about five or six years old his mother came home on a trial visit from the hospital. On this occasion she was supposed to give him a bath and began washing his back with cleaning fluid when one of her sisters came into the room and stopped her.

His two earliest memories produced early in treatment also touch upon the portrait he paints of his mother and his relationship with her. The first dealt with a cane which both his mother and father had bought him for his third birthday. By mistake, he left his prized cane on the train in which the family was traveling. He clearly recollected having had a temper tantrum when the train departed with his cane. The second memory was of an event occurring around four years of age, when his younger brother was born. He stated rather precisely, "My brother was born and they took me into the next room. One week later my mother had a breakdown and was committed to a mental institution."

Loss of home: "They kept shifting me around." Following the mother's hospitalization Albert was sent to live with an aunt in a small nearby New England village. He remained with this aunt for one year during his initial kindergarten experience. By prior agreement he was sent to live with his mother's sister in another New England state for the next two years. In this setting he negotiated grades one and two. Then, for another two years he was sent to live with his mother's cousin back in his native state, about forty miles from his home. "This relative had several children of her own and couldn't really take care of me, so I lived with my father from the eighth grade through high school," Albert said. It came as no surprise when he added, "They kept shifting me around—guess I was a burden."

During the crucial adolescent period following his mother's death he determined to become self-sufficient. He obtained odd jobs, sold newspapers, and served as delivery boy for a neighborhood grocery. The larger share of his earnings he gave to his father, but some of it he concealed because he had to look out for himself.

Meanwhile, his one younger brother, Edward, went to live with his father's younger brother, Mr. T., who resided in a large city four hundred miles distant. In talking about his academic achievement during elementary and junior high school Albert referred to his brother. He indicated that while he himself had never been a good student because he was continually shifted from one school to another, "Edward made all A's—he went to one school."

Hostility toward father: "I won't be like him." Albert remembers little about his father's family. His father had been a farm laborer reared in rural Armenia before coming to the United States during World War I. Settling in New England he usually kept employed as an unskilled factory laborer. Then a few years prior to Albert's mother's death his father achieved an appreciable degree of vocational status. His two brothers enticed him into a business partnership with them. "They put up the money and he put up the labor," Albert stated. After the mother's breakdown, his father became despondent, gambled away his savings and newly acquired earnings, drank excessively, and engaged in numerous affairs with women.

Albert's father eventually sold his share of the business to his older brother, "a scheming selfish individual," as the patient describes him. He added that this particular uncle took unfair advantage of his father, giving him, "little aid when my father needed it most." He spoke of how his father passively accepted the dictates of his older brother and how foreign this seemed in view of the fact that all his uncles "really ruled their households," according to the paternalistic orientation of the closely knit Armenian-American subculture.

Early in treatment the patient remarked that, in spite of his father's difficulties and the low estate he assumed, he always felt inferior in his presence. This was in contrast to his feelings of superiority to other people. Usually, no matter how many advantages in life the other person had, Albert could reassure himself with the thought, "I know that what I've got I worked for. . . . Nothing was given to me." The reaction formation against his deep-seated feelings of insecurity and isolation had begun to take on a distinctive character.

Albert felt that his father kept his distance from both his brother and himself, contributing little to their care. His associations to his initial "therapeutic" dream [1] points up his unconscious feelings toward his father's neglect. This dream dealt with the patient's taking a bundle of dirty clothes to a cleaning establishment. When he asked the proprietor the amount of his bill, the latter indicated three hundred dollars. Albert was both amazed and irritated at this and pro-

---

[1] We are not concerned with the obvious transference implications of this initial dream at this time.

ceeded to take his clothing to another store. Behind the counter he recognized a department head at his place of employment. This individual, by contrast, was friendly and charged him a reasonable price. Then he was sorry he had left part of his clothes at the first establishment. It was at this point that he awoke.

Spontaneous associations yielded nothing. When asked to associate to "dirty clothes," however, he recollected an early memory. Albert was reminded of an incident when he was ten or eleven years old.

> I was living with my father then. My mother was in the hospital. My father always used to check pedantically to see that my fly was buttoned, shoes tied, but never really looked at the condition of my clothing. On this particular morning I put on a shirt which had a dirty streak in front but covered it up with a sweater. When I got to school the teacher—I still remember her name, Miss Bonner—made me take off the sweater. When she saw the dirty shirt she made me stand in front of the whole class. I looked like a fool. I hated her after that.

Discussion of the implications of this dream led to his feeling of hostility and embarrassment over his father's indifferent attitude toward him. He sensed that among his Armenian relatives and associates "the father was a source of strength"—a powerful ego ideal from whom advice and counsel might be sought. In his case, his father was dependent on the son rather than being able to provide paternal support.

Albert continued to live with his father until he had completed high school at age seventeen. He immediately enlisted in the navy, never again living with his father. His final decision to leave was precipitated by his father's request for a loan from the patient ostensibly to pay his godfather but actually to gamble away. Albert explained that when this happened he had to get away from his father and "everything he represented." We shall see that this included concealing his ethnic identity when in the service.

SIBLING RIVALRY: "HE HAD IT BETTER." Albert's brother Edward, who was legally adopted by his uncle, Mr. T., after his mother's death, "had it better." While Albert was shifted from relative to relative, unable to establish roots firmly in any family setting and gain the resulting satisfactions and security, Edward developed adequately, acquiring marked determination and a feeling of independence. Edward completed high school with honors and successfully matriculated at an outstanding Eastern university before induction into the service. When discharged from the army he taught high school before resuming his educational program; currently, he is a graduate assistant in the humanities at his alma mater while completing his doctoral dissertation.

The seeds of sibling rivalry were perhaps sown early in Albert—in the conflicts and misunderstanding engendered by being removed from his room when his brother was born and his mother's removal from him following the child's birth. He had strong feelings that his brother's birth caused his mother's mental illness. Nevertheless, in treatment most of Albert's resentment of Edward was caused by the fact that he had been able to gain autonomy from his father and foster parents. This was first expressed in terms of Edward's lack of gratitude for everything that had been done for him. Special reference was made to Edward's marriage in 1952 which has its cultural implications. Edward, though threatened with subcultural excommunication, married a non-Armenian girl. Besides Edward was culturally disrespectful to the strong Armenian paternalistic family orientation by having his aunt and uncle who had adopted him introduced as his parents. Albert admitted envy of Edward's ability "to get away with such a move and still be accepted by everyone in the family."

THE PRICE OF A NEW HOME: "BE A GOOD ARMENIAN." During his service experience Albert resolved that he would never return to live with his father. His uncle, Mr. T., had for several years been trying to persuade him to join them "after he saw how I was treated." His household consisted of Mrs. T., Edward, and their son Frank.

Upon discharge he went to live with the T.'s. His aunt immediately began to dominate him. The price of his new home was clear—"Albert, you must be a good Armenian." He was expected to be devoutly religious, only date daughters of their Armenian friends, revel whenever she cooked shish-kabob, and become an active member of the Armenian Revolutionary Federation. This organization had been established after World War I with the aim of eventually liberating Armenians and avenging their ancestors who were slaughtered or starved by the Turks in 1915 in their effort to stop their aiding the Russian Army.

In one sense his aunt's pressuring played into his own neurotically driven independence strivings. She kept after him to better himself and not be like his father "who will never be anything but the poor farmer he was in Europe." He should amount to something since his father had not. At her insistence he went away for three years and completed a business school course, majoring in accounting.

It was on his return to the T.'s that Edward had married his non-Armenian wife, and his aunt began with renewed and increased force to structure his life so he would not also "betray" them. He quit one job to accept another with "less pressure." As his ego defenses crumbled his symptoms became intolerable and he sought treatment. The price asked for his new home had become more than he was able to pay.

THE EMERGING PERSONALITY

THE PRESENTING PROBLEM: "I CAN'T SLEEP." Seven years following discharge, Albert appeared at the Veterans Administration, Mental Hygiene Clinic, requesting treatment. Although neat and tidy in appearance he was pale, of asthenic build, and gave the impression of a lack of stamina. His principal complaint was, "I can't sleep." After finally getting to sleep, he experienced nightmares from which he would awaken in a tremulous state, with his stomach extremely tense. Then he would get out of bed and frequently walk the floor in a near panic until dawn. Once daylight appeared he became less tense. Knowing the early trauma he had experienced "in the night" it was easy to speculate about the meaning behind this behavior. He also complained of becoming so irritated that he feared "blowing my stack."

ONSET OF ILLNESS IN THE SERVICE: "THINGS WENT BLACK." Interestingly, Albert's initial debilitating symptoms during his naval service took the form of epileptoid seizures. He traced his acute symptoms back to 1943. During the return trip from the Mediterranean Theater of Operations he sustained an infection in his right leg. On reaching a New England port he was put ashore and hospitalized for thirty days until his leg healed. On release from the hospital he found that he had been replaced by another radio-man on his old destroyer. He was sent to a smaller craft—a destroyer escort for its initial "shake-down" cruise. "Here my symptoms really began."

One day when his ship pulled alongside a destroyer tender in a Southern harbor, Albert noticed that he wasn't feeling well and went below to rest on his bunk. "I had an upset feeling—I was feeling low, then things went black and the next thing I knew I was being examined by the ship's physician." His shipmates told him he had had "a fit," during which his toes and fingers became rigid. This was the first such attack he had ever experienced.

Three months later a second episode occurred. Albert and several shipmates were returning from liberty in a Southern port. They were all engaging in some "horseplay" when Albert tripped and several personal effects fell to the ground. As he groped around in the dark for his possessions, he seemed to lose consciousness. The next thing he remembered was awakening in the base hospital. His companions told him that he suddenly became raging and wild and it took several of them to subdue him. The physician who examined him wanted to keep him hospitalized, but at the patient's request he was "sent back with the gang."

Back aboard ship his work in communications began to suffer. Treatment later revealed that a focal source of irritation to Albert at this time was a new communications officer with whom he had to work intimately. Differences between them reached a climax when the officer, on learning that Albert was foreign born, stated, "no wonder you have so much trouble; all you foreigners are made of poor stuff." The hostility he felt towards this authoritarian figure was internalized, and he became increasingly agitated, depressed, and ineffective until he was finally transferred to the neuro-psychiatric ward of a base hospital in May, 1945. Following three weeks' stay in a locked ward, he was assigned to shore duty in New England. "I was perfectly happy then, because I could get home every night."

A subsequent physical examination suggested cardiac difficulties, and he was transferred to another naval hospital for further study. This examination failed to indicate heart disease "and so they put me in the psychiatric ward for a couple of weeks." He was granted a medical discharge three months later with a diagnosis of "Psychoneurosis, anxiety state, moderate–severe."

The salient emotional component in the onset of his illness in the service appears to be separation anxiety. Witness the disturbing effect of not being assigned back to his original ship after his first hospitalization, his wanting to "go back to the gang" in preference to staying at the hospital, and his happiness when based near his old New England haunts and able to get home every evening. It seems as if he was unable to tolerate again being "shifted around."

THE DYNAMIC PICTURE. Any attempt to formulate Albert's dynamics in capsular fashion points up the prominence of hostility, guilt, depression, and independence strivings in a setting of personal and cultural dislocation. The traumatic events of his early childhood served to augment his deep-seated feelings of isolation and anticipated rejection from those about him. He seems to be threatened continually by a loss of self identity and to have the unconscious desire to assert himself, to ally himself with powerful figures and success. On the other hand, such an alliance further threatened him by putting him in danger of being totally "swallowed up" by these powerful individuals. In Albert's philosophy, all aspects of one's environment must be approached cautiously. Only as a last resort does one make an emotional investment with its risk of rejection or ridicule. He evolved a safer method: Keep one's distance, compulsively size up the entire situation and in a calculating, intellectual manner decide on a course of action. This course of action was characteristically directed toward the accomplishment of tasks that would bring success, achievement, power, and hence, security. This psychodynamic formulation of the patient was greatly aided by the psychodiagnostic study presented below.

PSYCHODIAGNOSTIC STUDY

On applying for treatment in December, 1952, the patient was studied by members of the neuropsychiatric team. We shall concentrate here on the psychological test findings since physical and neurological examinations, including an electro-encephalogram, were negative. He was administered the Bender Gestalt, Rorschach, and M-M Sentence Completion tests. Albert was a cooperative subject despite his concern over his slowness. Other than expressions of tension during the session, no irrelevant or incoherent behavior or statements were noted.

BENDER VISUAL MOTOR GESTALT.   His performance on the Bender Gestalt was generally poor (Fig. 22–1). It reflected considerable constriction, rigidity, and the need for stabilizing external cues without which his performance became somewhat disorganized. The principal diagnostic contribution of the Bender Gestalt was that it further ruled out the possibility of organic brain damage or epilepsy as suggested by his history of blackouts.

THE RORSCHACH.   Albert's productivity on the Rorschach (Test Summary A) was below average, and the profile reflects the constriction of affective expression already inferred from his Bender Gestalt performance. He possesses a strong need to achieve and master the total situation. On the other hand, there is an inability to analyze a situation into its discrete parts for fear of revealing his inadequacies.

It is interesting that his one rejection was Card IX, on which it is difficult to achieve a *W* unless color is used.

Not only the profile but the content of his Rorschach responses demonstrate the extent to which Albert denies affective expression and is threatened by his environment (see Test Summary A). He perceived a human head on Card I, remarking, "it's cut off, not smiling, not frowning, no expression to it . . . ." Also on Card 1 he saw, "a voodoo mask of a witch doctor used for evil purposes, not for good." Another striking feature of his Rorschach protocol is that all shading and color responses are additions elicited during the inquiry, showing a potential for being sensitive and responsive to his environment.

In summary, the Rorschach showed poor integration of emotional response, denial of affect and personal involvement, as well as efforts to withdraw from emotion-producing situations. This appeared against a backdrop of tension and anxiety indicating the ineffectiveness of these defenses. Occasional depressive signs and low productivity in an individual of superior intelligence, combined with strong success strivings, round out the picture.

M-M Sentence Completion Test.[2] Albert's responses to this test are presented on the classified score sheet (see Test Summary B). The numbers refer to the random sequence of items as they appear when the test is administered. In spite of his need to use repression and give conventional responses, this test revealed material of significance in understanding and treating the patient.

The seeds of environmental thwarting are prominent in his sentence completions, as, for example, the suggestion of insufficient paternal support and maternal warmth. This inference was drawn largely from the responses to the

---

[2] This particular version of the Sentence Completion test was especially designed for use in the VA Mental Hygiene Clinic, Philadelphia, by Drs. Julian Meltzoff and Howard E. Mitchell. It is referred to as the "M-M Sentence Completion Test."

The score sheet form is similar to that developed by Dr. Bertram Forer of the VA Mental Hygiene Clinic, Los Angeles.

"father" and "mother" items. There is an underlying theme of dependency denial in interpersonal relationships and a feeling that: *"A man who would* go places has to work for it." A basically dependent orientation is suggested, however, by his response to the item: *"If he were king he would* relax for the rest of his life." His dependency also is evident in his portrayal of women as "nice" in so far as they cater to his needs and have characteristics similar to his own. Another aspect of this prominent theme is his disturbance and agitation by aggressive stimuli. In the light of the Rorschach and Bender Gestalt findings of emotional constriction, we may even go beyond this and infer that the expression of any strong feelings regardless of their nature is threatening to Albert.

Hostile attitudes toward the "father figure" appear nearer the surface than those toward the "mother." In recognition of the patriarchism of the Armenian subculture, added significance should be attached to some of the authority items. For example, resentment is clearly expressed in the item: *"His father always used to* do nothing to help him." At the same time, the patient submissively seeks the guidance of authority. Repeatedly during treatment he cited examples charged with envy of Armenian peers who had an easy time because their fathers saw to it that their eldest sons learned "the business and they merely had to take over."

As regards Albert's motivation for psychotherapy, there were positive expressions revealed in the following items: *"Talking about his troubles made him feel* better"; *"After he left the interview he felt* better"; *"Because of his illness* he wants to be cured."

On the other hand, consistent with his difficulty in expressing feeling and allowing himself to make an emotional investment, were the responses to the items: *"Doctors usually* ask a lot of questions"; *"What he really thought would help him* was to go to school." His defensive use of intellectualizing is apparent.

DREAMS MIRRORING THE CONFLICT. Albert's dreams were productive and meaningful throughout treatment. Out of a total of sixty-five sessions, he related approximately thirty-five dreams, 70 per cent occurring within the first half of treatment. Apparently during the early stages of the therapeutic relationship, dreams were the principal medium for the expression of his feelings. The great majority of these dreams had the dominant theme of the patient's serving as passive pawn of some threatening, aggressive person or circumstance. Albert interpreted these dreams as showing how frightened he was of being "taken advantage of." Nevertheless, in the majority of these threatening dreams, there was hope of being helped or saved by a benevolent individual. As already noted, this feature was conspicuous in his initial dream, and seemed to have a bearing on his relationship with his father. It was also the major theme of his second dream in which he finds himself in a night club with a friend when a tall actor turns on him and chases him from the place. He is saved in the nick of time by his friend who rushes them away in his Cadillac.

As we shall see in our discussion of Albert's treatment process, his dreams also mirror the various stages of the transference relationship.

THE THERAPEUTIC COURSE

A RELATIONSHIP DEVELOPS.   The patient's therapy extended from January, 1953 until May, 1956. Until the terminal phase of treatment, he was scheduled for weekly interviews. He had previously had brief continuous therapy with two psychological interns under the writer's supervision. When treatment was temporarily disrupted by the second therapist's leaving the clinic, he was assigned to the writer, a permanent staff member, in an attempt to correct an impression of his "being shifted around" again.

Both the previous therapists felt that Albert might best be helped in the context of the patient-therapist relationship. One wrote in his transfer summary, "this patient has to feel that he is accepted and appreciated by the therapist, and under such conditions he will no doubt find it easier to ventilate his hostility."

When first seen in treatment in January, 1954, Albert's circumstances and complaints were much the same as he had presented when he came for help the year before. He was still bothered by insomnia. On the other hand, he was beginning to ventilate his hostility toward his father and the aunt with whom he lived. Positive gain was made out of the transfer by interpreting it as an anxiety-producing repetition of his father's passing him around from relative to relative.

Transference dreams were much in evidence at this time. In the second interview with the writer he told of being terrified by a dream in which he was in a glass house in a foreign country which was invaded by Japanese. The invaders kept probing around until he sought the help of friends who rescued him. In the previous hour the therapist had explored rather specifically his relationship with his father.

Gradually these dreams with obvious transference implications began to disappear. He was more positive in his approach to treatment and appeared ready to explore his hostility problem, his inability to accept and gratify his dependency strivings and his inability to tolerate his vulnerability to the rejection that he perceived in all human relationships.

WORKING THROUGH HOSTILITY. After a year of treatment Albert had achieved sufficient ego strength from both the therapeutic relationship and his job to make significant gains in working through his hostility. Besides the therapist's attempt to provide a stable, supporting father figure, his immediate superior on a new job not only was kindly and sympathetic to him but appreciated Albert's potential for vocational advancement.

The hostility he felt toward his father was triggered and ventilated in a rather dramatic session. Albert had been home alone while his aunt and uncle were on vacation. He complained about his sleepless nights and fatigue on awakening. The content of the hour led to the therapist's pointing out the relationship between his insomnia and hostility. The interpretation was made that he had difficulty in dropping his guard and falling asleep for fear of being attacked. Furthermore, it was pointed out that his fear of aggression was a projection of his own hostility. This suggestion reminded him of a motion picture, *The Living Swamp,* which stimulated him to dream about being chased by a bear. He then associated this experience to his last big argument with his father before leaving home to live with his aunt and uncle. He stated that his father's main concern was not whether he was leaving, but how much of his savings he was going to give to him. He recalled running from the house at the height of the argument and when he returned his father had locked him out.

The other major focus of his hostility was his aunt, Mrs. T. Once Albert had ventilated his hostility toward his father, he began to recognize his unconscious identification with him. They had much in common. Both of them had been exploited by a hostile, rejecting world. As this took place Albert expressed increasing resentment toward his aunt's ridicule of both his father and himself. He began to defend his father's actions in arguments with his aunt. Then as a next step he expressed resentment of her domination. It was in this area of content that the interplay of culture and personality was most pronounced.

The aunt's domination largely appeared in a cultural context. She demanded that he like Armenian food, girls, religion, and political ideals. At the same time that she told him to be strong, virile, and masculine like his Armenian forefathers "who were slaughtered by the Turks," she unwittingly destroyed such a concept by the effeminately dominated atmosphere that she created.

Initial acceptance of his hostility toward his aunt's domination followed by exploration of the cultural basis of her beliefs and attitudes began to bring about changes in the way Albert viewed those around him. This followed an explosive incident in which he demanded his rights and to his surprise found that his aunt not only did not withdraw her supply of affection but granted his demands.

PERCEPTUAL CHANGE AND GROWTH.   The idea that a person's self image largely determines how he thinks others view him was interpreted to Albert. In addition to the changes we have attributed to certain therapeutic efforts, no small measure of the change in Albert's self concept resulted from his rapid vocational advancement at this time.

Soon after he began treatment he again accepted a position of greater responsibility with a large manufacturing concern. He compulsively and rigidly worked long hours in this new position. He had no interest in seeking heterosexual relationships after work or going out with his buddies—he was always too tired or having to try and get a little sleep "because of a monthly inventory beginning the next day." In perspective, this devotion to duty, to the neglect of social life, was interpreted as laudable, but also as a defense against putting himself in a position where intense emotional investments are made.

About this time his firm made a sweeping reorganization of its personnel. While still perceived as a little boy at home by his aunt, his manly contribution was recognized on the job. He advanced rapidly until in late 1955 he was made head of his department at a salary more than double his beginning wage of five thousand dollars. With the help of guidance and support he achieved a new sense of security and adequacy as he advanced vocationally. Changes consistent with the above came about in his self concept. It was at this point that he fought for his autonomy with his aunt "because for the first time I'll be what I really want to be."

SEX AND MARRIAGE.   Throughout treatment the patient made abortive heterosexual contacts. As mentioned above, he was generally too tired or too busy. On occasion he would double date with one of his Armenian friends, taking the girl to dinner, dancing, or to the motion pictures. Significantly, no matter how much Albert claimed to have enjoyed the evening, he made no effort to follow up with any of these girls. Equally significant is the fact that he met one girl who was an exception to this practice. He dated her frequently for six months until her mother wrote him stating she was mentally ill and becoming more upset by their relationship. They advised termination of the affair, which he did not challenge. Exploration revealed that this was the first woman who confided in him and gave him the feeling of being wanted. While he had been somewhat aloof and suspicious of this young woman all along, he did make a somewhat positive response to her.

His next affair began in the summer of 1955 with a young non-Armenian girl of twenty named Helen. Albert, in the process of working through his hostility toward his aunt, dated Helen "for spite." She became the battleground for his aunt and himself. He took her to an Armenian family wedding "just to see how my aunt and other members of the family will act." Helen's going to this Armenian affair was the issue already referred to over which he demanded his rights and won.

As his use of Helen in his interpersonal struggles was made clear to him he reacted with guilt. Then Albert sought to shelter her in every way from his aunt, his family, and his subculture. As self-respect continued to grow, a genuine respect for Helen as an attractive personality developed. In March, 1956, Albert announced that he was ready to make a lasting emotional investment: he and Helen had become engaged. They were married in June, 1956 in an Armenian church with his aunt and both families in attendance. When contacted for a follow-up interview in August 1956, the patient reported they were making a satisfactory marital adjustment and his upward mobility was continuing but on a new basis. Now he could sleep.

Test Summary

A.   Rorschach Protocol

Response	Inquiry

CARD I. 6"

1. Bat.

   W   FM,FC[1]   A   P

1. Location: Whole. Black, spread out, tail, 2 wings and 2 feelers. In flight.

Response

2. Face, top of head cut off, 2 horns, big ears.

W   F—   Hd

3. Halloween mask.

W   F   Mask

4. Voodoo mask—like natives might wear in Africa.

W   F   Mask

CARD II. 21″

1. Squashed insect

W   F—,FC¹,C   A

CARD III.

1. Two people in front of a pot with hands in pot. Cooking some- ‧thing . . . red stuff is vapor. Have hoofs like a horse. Looks like natives. They are female.

W̶   M+,K   H   P

2. Branches of a tree.

W   F   Na

CARD IV. 6″

1. Skin of an animal flattened out —eyes, tail.

W   F+   A,obj

CARD V. 3″

1. Bird flying in air, a black bird—

Inquiry

2. Location: Whole. Not smiling, not frowning, no expression, a human face. Out of proportion.

3. Location: Whole. Of a demon. Used for disguise.

4. Location: Whole. Reminds me of something in a novel. A witch doctor might wear it. (Why a witch doctor?) Looks like used for evil purposes not for good.

1. Location: Whole. Back squashed. Secretion from insect blurting out. Also because it's black. Somebody stepped on it. Secretion is the red because insect doesn't have blood. Looking at its insides—intestines.

1. Location: W̶, all except upper red details. Females. (What about blots give impression of females?) Their breasts and the way they are dancing around like women do.

2. Location: Upper red details. Leaves growing in one clump at the end of it. Don't know what kind of tree.

1. Location: Whole. Its appearance, outside of skin because you can see its eyes.
Add. 1. Location: Whole. Shape of a bat

W   F   A

1. Location: Whole. Might be an

Response   *Inquiry*

a vulture. Bird which would   eagle. Big bird that preys on small
swoop down on a rabbit or small   animals.
animal.

W   FM+,FC¹   A   P

CARD VI. 3″

1. Cat with whiskers. A Siamese   1. Location: Whole. Nostrils, whisk-
cat or a leopard. Member of the   ers, no eyes. Comic cat. Fur looks
cat family.   like a heavy or big cat. Tiger or
                                   something like that.

W   F   A   P

2. X-ray of an animal. Some parts   2. Location: Entire center detail.
are darker, no eyes, nostrils and   Backbone, 2 holes for nostrils big
tail.   for small nose. White spot on back
                                    of neck.

D   Fk   A,obj

CARD VII. 14″

1. Two profiles of monkeys looking   1. Location: W×, all except bottom
at each other. No, 2 Indians be-   center D. Looking at each other
cause they have feathers in their   frowning. Ready to fight, waiting
heads.   for somebody to start.

W×   M+   Hd

CARD VIII. 8″

1. Two rats on each side—hanging   1. Location: Side animal details and
on a tree.   center tree D. Seems sort of like
                                     rodent. Forelegs, head and has fur.
D   dr FM+,Fc   A   P   (Fur?) Fuzzy all over. Definitely
                                     see eye. Christmas tree hanging on
                                     to—green and comes to a point.

2. Tree growing out of stone.   2. Location: W×, all except side A
                                     details. Trunk goes all the way into
W×   F   Na   stone. Blends into stone which is
                                     orange and pink. But it's just the
                                     general contour.

CARD IX.

Doesn't look like anything—just an
ink blot.

CARD X. 17″

1. Crabs, four of them, 2 blue and   1. Location: Center top, outer blue
two brown, grabbing hold of   and center pink details. Legs stick-

Response

pink rock. Two blue ones holding onto yellow rock. Brown ones hanging onto stick.

dr   FM+, FC—   A,Na

2. Two yellow dogs looking up.

D   F+   A

Inquiry

ing out. Hanging onto green seed weeds.

2. Location: Inner yellow detail. Poodles, French. Heads, nose, sitting with front legs up.

RORSCHACH PROFILE

W	12	M	2	H	1	F%	50
D	2	FM	4	Hd	2	A%	43
d	0	K	1	A	7	P	5
Dd	2	F	9	Aobj	2	S	0
App:	W ((D))	DdSFc	(1)	Na	2	Orig	0
Seq.	Orderly	C¹	(3)	Mask	2	SUM C:	0
		FC	(1)			M:C	2:0
		C	0			W:M	12:2
						Rejection:	IX

Test Summary

B. M-M SENTENCE COMPLETION SCORE FORM

I. INTERPERSONAL RELATIONS

A. *Father*

48. *Whenever he was with his father he felt* OK.
53. *Because of his father* he went away.
70. *Many fathers* don't care about their children.
93. *His father always used to* do nothing to help him.

B. *Mother*

7. *Because of his mother* he left.
18. *Many mothers* are good.
56. *His mother always used to* help him.
90. *Whenever he was with his mother he felt* good.

C. *Family*

6. *He depends on his family for* nothing.
10. *His family treats him as* he should be treated.
42. *He feels that his family* is good.

59. *When away from his family* he was alright.
72. *If his family would only* stop nagging him.
82. *When there's a quarrel in the family* he doesn't feel well.

D. *Males*

23. *Most men act as though* they were men.
52. *He felt the other fellows* are OK sometimes.
73. *The men who work in his department* are weak.
89. *Lots of fellows* are satisfied to be left behind.
91. *A man who would* go places has to work for it.

E. *Females*

5. *Some women* are good.
9. *Most women should* be seen.
38. *The women in his life* are pretty nice to him.
64. *In the company of women he feels* very good if she is nice.
83. *A man wants a woman* who can have the same likes and dislikes as his.
98. *Women usually think he* is attractive.

F. *Authoritative Figures*

14. *His superior officers* are good to him.
37. *Most people in positions of authority* should be trusted.
44. *The men over him* are very nice.
69. *A fellow can work best when his supervisor* is nice to him.
81. *Taking orders* does not please him as giving orders.
85. *When he saw his boss coming he* smiled.

II. Social Situations and Relationships

30. *When he is with a group of people* he likes to be seen.
45. *At social gatherings he* likes to be seen.
60. *His neighbor* didn't have much to say.
80. *When with others he tends to* want to be heard.

III. Dominant Drives

1. *Sometimes he wishes* he were not here.
11. *Most of all he wants* security.
17. *If he were King he would* relax for the rest of his life.
19. *He would be happy if* he were able to be happy.
22. *He daydreams about* nothing.
77. *More than anything else he needs* money.
99. *The main thing in his life* make a success of himself.

IV. Reactions to:

A. *Aggression*

97. *When he is criticized* he doesn't like it very much.
35. *When they tried to get his goat* he got angry.

43. *When he was bawled out he* didn't feel good.
 3. *When the other fellow challenged him to a fight* he fought.
21. *If the bully hit him he would* hit him back.
84. *When he was knocked down he* got up.

B. *Rejection*

66. *When she refused him he* didn't care too much.
47. *When she walked out on him he* didn't care.
57. *When they didn't invite him* he felt bad.
75. *When they passed him by without speaking he* laughed.
28. *When they turned him down for the job he* looked for another.
68. *When they left him flat he* got new friends.

C. *Failure*

31. *Seeing that he could not make the grade he* tried harder.
54. *When he failed he* studied and passed.
71. *When he realized that he was going to fail he* studied and passed.
88. *When he saw that he was not getting ahead he* quit and got a new job.
92. *Whenever he does below average work, he* tries harder the next time.
96. *His lack of success caused him to* try harder.

D. *Responsibility*

25. *When others have to rely upon him he* tries to help.
40. *When he was completely on his own he* did very well.
58. *When he has to make a decision he* did it without asking.
62. *When asked to take over the job he* did it well.
67. *When given new responsibilities he* did them very well.
78. *Having responsibility makes him* feel superior.

E. *Sexual Stimuli*

27. *When it comes to sexual relations he prefers* women.
33. *His greatest sexual difficulty is* not being married.
49. *His sexual desires* are OK.
61. *His first sexual experience* was very dumb.
76. *Following the sexual act he usually feels* satisfied.
86. *Sexual intercourse* is good if not abused.

F. *Wife and Marriage*

13. *When he thinks of marriage he* thinks some more.
15. *Compared with other women, his wife* is OK.
29. *A wife usually* is good to his husband.
36. *His marriage* is a failure.

51. *The main thing in marriage is* getting along together.
63. *In many marriages* people are not suited to each other.

V. Attitudes Towards Illness and Treatment

  8. *Before entering the doctor's office he usually feels* funny.
16. *Doctors usually* ask a lot of questions.
24. *Ever since he became sick* his work has been failing.
32. *Talking about his troubles makes him feel* better.
41. *The doctor who is treating him* is OK.
46. *Because of his illness* he wants to be cured.
55. *After he left the interview he felt* better.
65. *What he really thought would help him* was to go to school.

VI. Causes of Anxiety, Fear, Hostility, Guilt, Frustration, etc.

  2. *He felt held back by* nothing.
12. *He got sore when* he is needled.
20. *Nothing is so upsetting as* not getting when credit is due.
26. *The thing that gripes him most is* nagging.
34. *He is afraid of* most anything anybody else would be.
39. *He is ashamed of* nothing.
74. *It makes him nervous when* people say he is nervous.
87. *He often worries about* his health.
100. *Anybody would become angry if* he were knocked down.
79. *He felt to blame when* things didn't go right.

VII. Self Concept

  4. *His personality* was good.
50. *He thinks of himself as* a nice guy.
94. *Compared to most men he* is pretty good.
95. *His standards are* better than average.

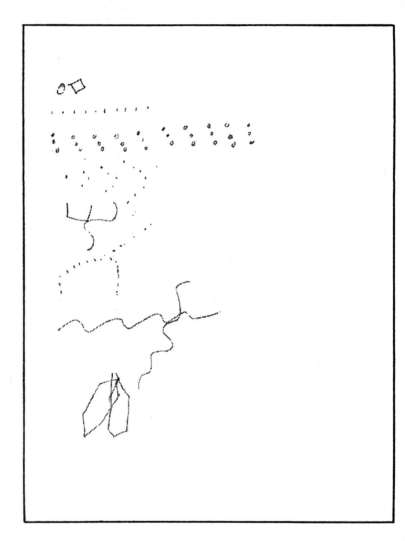

FIGURE 22–1. Bender Gestalt Test.

New World Postscript

Despite disparities of age, sex, and social background, the cases in this section have many problems in common. The Jewish child and man, Itzhak and Seymour, share a Central European ghetto heritage with its rigid orthodoxy, tradition of talmudic scholarship, and emphasis on emotional control. In both, the presenting problem involves academic difficulties associated with social withdrawal. Intense mutual overdependence between mother and son, with the father a relatively remote authority figure, have complicated the picture by making masculine identification difficult. Psychotherapeutic intervention enabled both individuals to establish sounder identities that did not stifle their affective needs.

The upper-class European Jewish woman, Ilona, although coming from a background in which Jewishness played only a minor role, shares with Itzhak and Seymour a rigidly conventional upbringing within a closely knit social circle. When the anti-Semitic forces of National Socialism forced Ilona to flee Europe, she sought to restore her feeling of ingroup belongingness. By marrying a "typical" American, the very antithesis of her original culture, she tried to embrace the new and become a part of it. Far from representing a disidentification with her past, this was actually a desperate effort at restitution, at least of her former *feelings*. The repeated movings, however, made it impossible for her, as it was for Itzhak, to get her roots down anywhere.

As in the comparative male cases, Ilona had been guided by the values of intellectuality and control to the detriment of her emotional needs. Because of their congruence with middle-class American ideals, these values facilitated social articulation on the surface, but failed, as in Seymour's case, to meet her deeper frustrations. Deficient early parental relationships made it difficult for both these people to get close to their spouses later. In Ilona's case, her husband's "foreignness" provided a convenient rationalization for her inability to build a close relationship with him.

An interesting comparison is possible with Dorothy, an English girl who came to the United States after the war and also married a member of an outgroup, this time, an Armenian. Not a political refugee, Dorothy fled her home in an unconscious effort to escape the ambivalent tie with her mother and fear of her sadistic father. The cultural discrepancies she encountered were too much for her weak ego to integrate. Under the strain, her repressive and denial defenses failed and depersonalization feelings, with dissociative reactions, took their place, signaling a fragmentation of her precarious identity. In this case, the culture conflict paradoxically plays both a crucial and, at the same time, a fortuitous role. With the girl's basically fragile ego, other stresses might have been equally effective in precipitating a break. Culture conflict *just happened* to be the triggering mechanism.

Albert, the Armenian young man, adds further interesting comparisons. Although, like the Jews, he is a member of a cohesive ingroup, his neglect by an improvident father, in contrast to his brother's adoption by a respectable uncle, developed in him strong ambivalence, with active repudiation of everything Armenian that his father represented. Unlike Ilona, Albert's "passing" and zeal to become assimilated was negatively motivated. In both cases, the inadequacy of the intellectualizing defense was indicated by their mounting anxiety, but timely psychotherapy helped them to face their underlying conflicts.

In all these cases can be traced difficulties in relationships with parents which created identification problems. Cultural factors, of course, were necessarily involved even at this depth because of the parents' cultural affiliations which were transmitted more or less explicitly through the direct contacts of child training. Culture affected the individuals on a surface level as well. Finding themselves minorities attempting to adjust to a dominant culture, their difficulties could be readily rationalized in terms of cultural differences. Thus they could escape personal responsibility for their problems as well as indirectly blame them on the parents who in their opinion had failed them.

Epilogue

As noted at the outset (Chapter 1), the various types of culture conflict are not unique to any single subculture but may occur in all. In these case studies we have found problems of identification failure in an English girl as well as in a Negro-Indian woman; acting out behavior in a Hopi as in a Puerto Rican; intellectualizing in a Mexican-American as in a Jew, and so on. Moreover, the shame-guilt ratio in superego control has been found to vary within as well as between the groups studied. Patterns of social articulation, similarly, are not limited to certain subcultures: Congruence, for example, while characterizing the Nisei authority attitudes also characterizes Jewish upward social mobility, while resistance is typical of certain other aspects of the Nisei and Jewish subcultures.

The point in all this is that the human raw material does not differ with culture or subculture, but that different cultures tend to select, out of the total range of personality potential, certain aspects for special reinforcement. These aspects then become the modal points around which individual members cluster, and give rise to group differences. This does not mean that a separate treatment process is necessary for each subcultural group. Nor is it necessary that the therapist match his patient in skin color, eye shape, or any other ethnic feature. What is essential, however, is that the clinician add to his equipment sophistication and information as to the variety of values found in the cultural backgrounds of his patients.

Index of Names

Page citations in italics refer to bibliographic listings

Index of Subjects